PAIN IN OBSTETRICS AND GYNAECOLOGY

RCOG Press

Since 1973 the Royal College of Obstetricians and Gynaecologists has regularly convened Study Groups to address important growth areas within obstetrics and gynaecology. An international group of eminent scientists and clinicians from various disciplines is invited to present the results of recent research and to take part in in-depth discussions. The resulting volume, containing the papers presented and also edited transcripts of the discussions, is published within a few months of the meeting and provides a summary of the subject that is both authoritative and up to date.

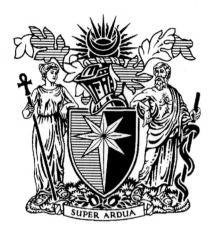

Previous Study Group publications available

Antenatal Diagnosis of Fetal Abnormalities
Edited by J.O. Drife and D. Donnai

Prostaglandins and the Uterus
Edited by J.O. Drife and A.A. Calder

Infertility
Edited by A.A. Templeton and J.O. Drife

Intrapartum Fetal Surveillance
Edited by J.A.D. Spencer and R.H.T. Ward

Early Fetal Growth and Development
Edited by R.H.T. Ward, S.K. Smith and D. Donnai

Ethics in Obstetrics and Gynaecology
Edited by S. Bewley and R.H.T. Ward

The Biology of Gynaecological Cancer
Edited by R. Leake, M. Gore and R.H.T. Ward

Multiple Pregnancy
Edited by R.H.T. Ward and M. Whittle

The Prevention of Pelvic Infection
Edited by A.A. Templeton

Screening for Down Syndrome in the First Trimester
Edited by J.G. Grudzinskas and R.H.T. Ward

Problems in Early Pregnancy: Advances in Diagnosis and Management
Edited by J.G. Grudzinskas and P.M.S. O'Brien

Gene Identification, Manipulation and Treatment
Edited by S.K. Smith, E.J. Thomas and P.M.S. O'Brien

Evidence-based Fertility Treatment
Edited by A.A. Templeton, I.D. Cooke and P.M.S. O'Brien

Fetal Programming: Influences on Development and Disease in Later Life
Edited by P.M.S. O'Brien, T. Wheeler and D.J.P. Barker

Hormones and Cancer
Edited by P.M.S. O'Brien and A.B. MacLean

The Placenta: Basic Science and Clinical Practice
Edited by J.C.P. Kingdom, E.R.M. Jauniaux and P.M.S. O'Brien

Disorders of the Menstrual Cycle
Edited by P.M.S. O'Brien, I.T. Cameron and A.B. MacLean

Infection and Pregnancy
Edited by A.B. MacLean, L. Regan and D. Carrington

Pain in Obstetrics and Gynaecology

Edited by

Allan B. MacLean, R. William Stones and Steven Thornton

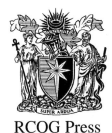

RCOG Press

It was not possible to refer all the material back to the authors or discussants but it is hoped that the proceedings have been reported fairly and accurately.

Allan B. MacLean MD FRCOG
Professor of Obstetrics and Gynaecology, Royal Free & University College Medical School, Royal Free Campus, Rowland Hill Street, Hampstead, London NW3 2PT, UK

R. William Stones FRCOG
University Department of Obstetrics and Gynaecology, The Princess Anne Hospital, Coxford Road, Southampton, SO16 5YA, UK

Professor Steven Thornton MRCOG
Department of Biological Sciences, University of Warwick, Coventry CV4 7AL, UK

First published 2001

ISBN 1 900364 52 2

DECLARATION OF INTEREST

All contributors to the Study Group were invited to make a specific Declaration of Interest in relation to the subject of the Study Group. This was undertaken and all contributors complied with this request. Dr Crowhurst is a consultant for Sims Portext plc; Dr Fernando is a clinical adviser to Sims Portex plc; Dr Foster is on the Medical Advisory Board of the National Vulvodynia Association; Mr Kennedy is a consultant to Oxford Natural Products and to the American Endometriosis Association; Professor Li Wan Po does occasional consulting for various companies with an interest in analgesics; Mr Stones is a scientific adviser for the UK Endometriosis Society; Professor Thornton is a consultant for Glaxo SmithKline, Ferring Pharmaceuticals UK, IBAH and Cytocell; Mr Whorwell is an expert adviser to the pharmaceutical industry on irritable bowel syndrome.

Published by the RCOG Press at
The Royal College of Obstetricians and Gynaecologists
27 Sussex Place, Regent's Park
London NW1 4RG, UK

Registered Charity No. 213280

RCOG Press Editors: Lesley Simon and Sophie Leighton
Cover designed by Geoffrey Wadsley
Printed by FiSH Books, London

Contents

SECTION 9: RECOMMENDATIONS

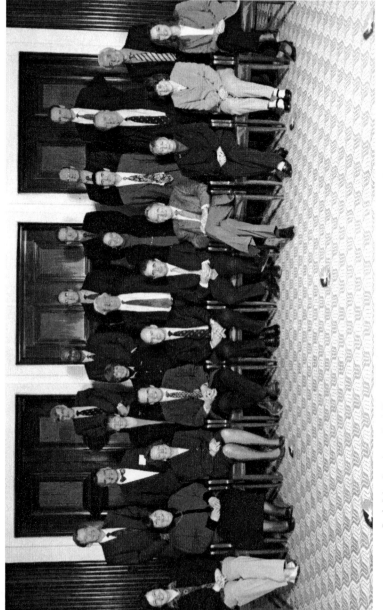

Back: John Crowhurst, Rosh Fernando, Stephen Kennedy, Toby Newton-John, Adrian Tookman, Tim Overton
Middle: John Steege, David Foster, Yvonne Coldron, Victoria Grace, Chris Sutton, Karen Berkley, Peter Whorwell, Martin Lees, Alex Peters
Front: Angela Barnard, Edith Hillan, Beverly Collett, Steven Thornton, Allan MacLean, William Stones, Richard Beard, Kathleen Vits, Nancy Fletcher, Amanda Smith

Participants

Mrs Angela Barnard
The National Endometriosis Society, 50 Westminster Palace Gardens, Artillery Row, London, SW1P 1RL, UK

Professor Richard W. Beard
Hospital of St John and St Elizabeth, 60 Grove End Road, London NW8 9NH

Professor Karen J. Berkley
Program in Neuroscience, Copeland Street, Florida State University, Tallahassee FL 32306-1270, USA

Mrs Yvonne Coldron
Academic Unit for Musculoskeletal Disease, Department of Biochemistry and Immunology, St George's Hospital Medical School, Cranmer Terrace, London SW17 0RE, UK

Dr Beverly J. Collett
Pain Management Centre, Leicester Royal Infirmary Maternity Hospital, Infirmary Square, Leicester, LE1 5WW, UK

Dr John A. Crowhurst
Department of Anaesthesia, Queen Charlotte's and Hammersmith Hospitals, Area C, Level 1, Hammersmith Hospital, DuCane Road, London, W12 0HS, UK

Dr Roshan Fernando
Consultant Anaesthetist and Honorary Senior Lecturer, Department of Anaesthesia, Royal Free Hospital, London NW3 2QG, UK

Mrs Nancy Fletcher
National Childbirth Trust, Alexandra House, Oldham Terrace, Acton, London W3 6NH

Dr David C. Foster
University of Rochester Medical Center, 601 Elmwood Avenue, PO Box 668, Room 2-4446, Rochester, NY 14642, US

Dr Victoria Grace
Dean of Arts, Department of Gender Studies, University of Canterbury, Private Bag 4800, Christchurch, New Zealand

Professor Edith M. Hillan
Faculty of Nursing, University of Toronto, 50 St George Street, Toronto, Ontario, M5S 3H4, Canada

Mr Stephen H. Kennedy
Clinical Reader in Obstetrics and Gynaecology, University of Oxford, John Radcliffe Hospital, Oxford, OX3 6BN, UK

Dr Martin M. Lees
Consultant Obstetrician and Gynaecoloigst (Retired), Royal College of Physicians, 9 Queen Street, Edinburgh, EH2 1JQ, UK

Professor Alain Li Wan Po
Centre for Evidence-based Pharmacology, School of Life & Health Sciences, Aston University, Birmingham, B4 7ET, UK

Professor Allan B. MacLean
Professor of Obstetrics and Gynaecology, Royal Free and University College Medical School, Royal Free Campus, Hampstead, London NW3 2PT, UK and Convener of Study Groups, Royal College of Obstetricians and Gynaecologists, UK

Dr Toby Newton-John
Eastman Dental Hospital, 256 Gray's Inn Road, London, WC1X 8LD, UK

Mr Timothy G. Overton
Consultant Obstetrician and Gynaecologist, Norfolk and Norwich University Hospital NHS Trust, Brunswick Road, Norwich, NR1 3SR

Dr Alexander A.W. Peters
Academisch Ziekenhuis Leiden, Albinusdreef 2, Postbus 9600, 2300 RC, Leiden, the Netherlands

Ms Amanda Smith
Integrative Psychotherapist, Pelvic Pain Clinic, Obstetrics & Gynaecology Department, Northwick Park Hospital, Watford Road, Harrow, HA1 3UJ, UK

Professor John F. Steege
University of North Carolina, CB No. 7570 Mac Nider, Chapel Hill, NC 27599-7570, USA

Mr R. William Stones
University Department of Obstetrics and Gynaecology, The Princess Anne Hospital, Coxford Road, Southampton, Hampshire SO16 5YA, UK

Professor Christopher J.G. Sutton
Professor of Gynaecological Surgery, University of Surrey and Consultant Gynaecologist and Director of Minimal Access Therapy Training Unit, Royal Surrey County Hospital, Guildford, Surrey, UK

Professor Steven Thornton
Department of Biological Sciences, University of Warwick, Coventry, West Midlands, CV4 7AL, UK

Mr Adrian Tookman
Palliative Care, The Royal Free Hampstead NHS Trust, Pond Street, Hampstead, London, NW3 2QG, UK

Dr P.J. Whorwell
Consultant Gastroenterologist, University Hospital of South Manchester, Education and Research Centre, Wythenshawe Hospital, Southmoor Road, Wythenshawe, Manchester M23 9LT, UK

Additional contributors

Erica A. Bakkum
Academisch Ziekenhuis Leiden, Albinusdreef 2, Postbus 9600, 2300 RC, Leiden, the Netherlands

Bart W.J. Hellebrekers
Academisch Ziekenhuis Leiden, Albinusdreef 2, Postbus 9600, 2300 RC, Leiden, the Netherlands

Nicholas Levy
Specialist Registrar, Department of Anaesthesia, Royal Free Hospital, London NW3 2QG, UK

Felicity Plaat
Lead Consultant Obstetric Anaesthetist, Queen Charlotte's and Chelsea Hospital, DuCane Road, London, W12 0HS, UK

Susan A. Selfe
Lecturer Practitioner, School of Nursing and Midwifery, University of Southampton, Southampton, Hampshire, SO16 5YA, UK

Anne Shortliffe
University of North Carolina, CB No. 7570 Mac Nider, Chapel Hill, NC 27599-7570, USA

Manu Vatish
Department of Obstetrics and Gynaecology, Walsgrave Hospital, Clifford Bridge Road,Walsgrave, Coventry, West Midlands CV2 2DX, UK

Kathleen Vits
Physiotherapy Department, The Princess Anne Hospital, Coxford Road, Southampton, Hampshire, SO16 5YA, UK

Wei Ya Zhang
Centre for Evidence-based Pharmacology, School of Life & Health Sciences, Aston University, Birmingham, B4 7ET, UK

Krina T. Zondervan
MRC Training Fellow in Bioinformatics/Epidemiologist, Wellcome Trust Centre for Human Genetics, University of Oxford, Roosevelt Drive, Oxford OX3 6BN, UK

Preface

To dedicate the 41st Study Group of the RCOG to pain may suggest that despite the 150 years that have elapsed since James Young Simpson administered ether for the delivery of a woman with obstructed labour and John Snow gave chloroform analgesia to Queen Victoria for the birth of Prince Leopold we don't yet know it all. How often do we recoil with dismay upon reading a lengthy referral letter describing a patient with pelvic or vulval pain? Many clinicians can manage pain by identifying pathology, finding a name or giving a diagnosis; in the absence of such features, our understanding of pain and its mechanisms remains vague and naïve.

Our Study Group comprised a stimulating mixture of scientists, clinicians, psychologists, other health professionals and two lay members. We traversed neural pathways, examined viscero-visceral interactions and discussed the interplay between the body (soma), the mind (psyche) and our socio-cultural environment. We debated whether every obstetrician and gynaecologist should be better trained in an understanding of psychology and psychotherapeutic methods, or whether it was better to include psychologists in our pain clinics. We agreed that the first impressions given to the patient in the secondary care situation are important, but how do you schedule a clinic to facilitate a difficult and prolonged consultation? How do you avoid investigator bias, according to who sees the patient first? Should there be identified multidisciplinary clinics with acknowledged experts with reputations in laparoscopic surgery or nerve blockade?

There are areas of pain management specific to the vulva, the postoperative patient with adhesions and the patient with cancer. The roles of anaesthetist and palliative-care physician have provided skills and a multimodal approach.

More than 50% of pregnant women experience musculoskeletal pain – pain is such a common symptom in pregnancy that it is sometimes difficult to view it seriously. Yet the acute abdominal pain brings serious sequelae if diagnosis or management are delayed. In labour, management of pain is delegated to the midwife or the anaesthetist, but it is sobering to reflect on the thoughts of Nancy Fletcher of the National Childbirth Trust, representing our patients, clients or consumers. Pain might be viewed as a positive feature, part of the transition to motherhood. If we, as staff, feel discomfort by witnessing pain, and distress at the noise, how should we respond? Are we being paternalistic by thinking we are protecting against harm? Maybe we have more to learn – this book is a good place to start.

Allan B. MacLean
R. William Stones
Steven Thornton

SECTION 1

GENERAL BACKGROUND TO UNDERSTANDING PAIN

Chapter 1
James Young Simpson and pain relief

Martin M. Lees

Introduction

Although my brief is to discuss James Young Simpson and pain relief I would initially like to comment on the nature of pain.

In his book, *On the Edge of the Primeval Forest*, Albert Schweitzer wrote as follows: 'The fellowship of those who bear the mark of pain. Who are the members of this fellowship? Those who have learned by experience what physical pain and bodily anguish mean belong together all the world over; they are united by a secret bond. One and all they know the horrors of suffering to which man can be exposed and one and all they know the longing to be free from pain. He who has been delivered from pain must not think he is now free again and at liberty to take up life just as it was before entirely forgetful of the past. He is now "a man whose eyes are open" with regard to pain and anguish and he must help to overcome these two enemies (so far as human power can control them) and to bring to others the deliverance which he has himself enjoyed. The man who with a doctor's help has been pulled through a severe illness must aid in providing a helper such as he has had himself for those who otherwise could not have one'.[1]

We could spend the entire duration of this book discussing the nature of pain but the first challenge we meet is that we find great difficulty in defining pain and second, if we assume that there is such an entity, then doctors categorise it largely as being physical or mental in origin. During the last three decades there has been a different approach to pain, some of which has come from a greater understanding of the pathophysiology of its origin and much of which has come from a change in the attitude of society towards pain.

Of course we have to deal not only with acute pain but also with chronic pain and to take account of those rare individuals who never experience pain.

If, however, we allow for great differences in the definitions of pain, perhaps the general attitude of science and society can best be summarised by Leriche, who has given the following concept of pain: 'In the suffering patient the pain is like a storm which hardly admits of assessment once it is over. While it is present the patient is beside himself quite beyond all capability of analysing it unless on the contrary he fixes his attention altogether on his suffering. And there you are, powerless to understand distress in the face of this abyss into which you cannot descend, which you try unsuccessfully to picture to yourself, impressed by something of great severity that you would like to be able to alleviate touching lightly with your hand the region of pain, surprised that you can feel nothing and yet at times by your touch even exciting dreadful recurrent spasms of pain'.[2]

Perhaps the greatest advance in our understanding of pain has come from the work of my old teacher, Hans Kosterlitz, who should, I believe, have been awarded the Nobel Prize for the outstanding work which he carried out on the discovery of the endorphins.[3,4] His elegant demonstration, not only of endorphin release but also of the encephalins and dynorphins, has allowed us much greater understanding of the problems which are faced in the causation and appreciation of acute and chronic pain.

Women and birth in society

Although nowadays the majority of women in Western society can choose when to have their children, lack of control over their own fertility has resulted in childbearing as a constant process and this was referred to by another old teacher of mine, Sir Dugald Baird, who in his celebrated lecture, *A Fifth Freedom*, described 'the tyranny of excessive fertility'.[5] In addition, women were considered to be inferior to men and even in the 13th century women were viewed as being biologically imperfect. Labour was presented as a frightening and painful ordeal when a woman was subjected to the whole birth process and to the rough skills of the attendant midwife.

In the past, women were delivered at home among family and friends and among these were individuals who increased the mothers' fears with tales of obstetric disaster and pain experienced by those who had delivered previously.

The degree of pain that an individual suffers during the birth process, whether real or induced by fear, has been inseparable from childbirth. The Romans named it *poena magna*, the great pain. Unfortunately there was little done to alleviate pain because pain in childbirth was regarded as the natural punishment for Eve's sin in the Garden of Eden. Several authorities refer to Euphame MacCalzean who was burned at the stake on Edinburgh's Castle Hill on 25 June 1591.[6,7] Some tell the story that Euphame MacCalzean asked for relief of pain in labour and it is claimed that analgesia in labour was damned on this account.[8] Keys even believed that she was buried alive and that the time was not right for the acceptance of anaesthesia.[9]

The truth of the matter is that Euphame MacCalzean had practised witchcraft, had committed adultery with her son-in-law and had conspired to murder the King; it was for these reasons that she was sentenced to death.

The length of labour, on average, today is around 12 hours and few labours are allowed to continue for more than 20 hours on account of concerns for the fetus. In the past, however, protracted labours took place, often with a total lack of understanding of the possible causation. Even with the advent of forceps, which allowed the delivery to be effected more rapidly, there was considerable damage inflicted by the unskilled attendant, usually a midwife. Lisbeth Burger, a midwife, described the birth at which she and the father had to hold down the mother while the doctor performed the forceps delivery. 'The groaning and whimpering of the mother dominated everything in the room, the jerking and shaking of her tortured body after all that pulling and levering, holding and bleeding, the child finally emerged from the mother's lap torn and haemorrhaging. Exhausted to death the poor mother lay back against the cushions'.[10]

Surgery and anaesthesia

It is horrifying to think that even at the beginning of the 19th century operations were performed in the patient's home. The surgeon would arrive with three or four assistants to hold the patient down during the operative procedure. There are gruesome accounts given of elective surgery performed with minimal premedication. Fanny Burney, in 1811, gave a detailed graphic description of her mastectomy, which was performed with possibly a wine cordial containing laudanum as a premedication.[11] Another notable account of the endurance of a surgical procedure without anaesthesia came from Professor George Wilson who, in a letter to Sir James Young Simpson, described his mid-thigh amputation. His report is so graphic as to be worthy of personal reading.[12] Most people at that time endured their surgery with little more than alcohol prior to operation.

What made it possible for individuals such as Burney and Wilson to have survived these dreadful assaults lies, I think, in the release of endorphins during the acuteness of the episode. This is supported by the work of Beecher in 1946, in which he reported that among seriously wounded soldiers questioned within 12 hours of receiving their wounds in battle 25% reported only slight pain and 32% reported no pain at all, even when major wounds had been sustained.[13]

Table 1.1. Operations performed in the Royal Infirmary of Edinburgh 1830–34

	1830–31	1831–32	1832–33	1833–34
Lithotomy	2	5	11	10
Lithotrity	0	0	0	1
Amputations	15	3	13	29
Excision of head of humerus	0	1	0	0
Excision of elbow joint	0	0	1	4
Ligature of common iliac artery	1*	0	0	0
Ligature of external iliac	0	0	0	1
Ligature of femoral artery	4*	0	0,	0
Ligature of brachial artery	0	0	1	1
Hernia	3	2	2	4
Tumours	2	0	2	0
Excision of mamma	1	4	2	7
Excision of testicle	0	0	1	3
Excision of upper jaw	2	0	1	0
Excision of lower jaw	0	0	1	1
Trepan	1	0	0	2
Tracheotomy	0	0	2	0
Extirpation of eye	0	0	1	0

The cases of ligature of artery marked by asterisks were performed to check secondary haemorrhage; the others were for aneurysm.

From: Answers by the Managers of the Royal Infirmary of Edinburgh to Questions transmitted to them by the Committee appointed by the House of Commons to enquire into the state of Medical Practice and Education 1843.

Table 1.2.   Memorandum of articles etc., to be in readiness for the operation of excision of a bladder calculus

A heavy table; table for dressings; pillows, blankets and sheets; binders, sponges, lint compresses and bandages, towels, oil, ice, syringe, ligatures, warm and cold water, wine and water, warm barley-water, basins, blood-catcher, coat.

Arrangement of patient

Assistant adjusts head, secures the feet. Two at shoulders. Staff introduced. Assistant hold it straight; then to the right; then carried the handle down; retains it until ordered, touching the stone.

Instruments

Staff-knife, pointed knife, Cooper's knife, probe, pointed bistoury, gorget, scoop, sound, tenaculum, cannula, needles and forceps.

Preparations

The patient, well-purged the day before, early in the morning of the operation should have a good injection. After this has operated, a string must be tied on the penis four hours before the operation to retain the urine. The hair must have been well-shaved. Laudanum injected, 120 drops to the cup.

Operation

Tighten skin, take knife. Incision of four inches deep above. Cut transversus, avoid rectum, feel bulb, touch staff, lay bare staff. Introduce probe-knife flat, and push into bladder. Observe urine. Cut gently towards ischium, following knife with the forefinger into the bladder. Enlarge if necessary. Scoop or forceps introduced. Staff withdrawn, first touch stone. Carry forceps along staff to stone, finger in the wound, finger in the rectum. Search stone, low down. Withdraw downward. Dressing, lint in wound. Patient untied.

From: Answers by the Managers of the Royal Infirmary of Edinburgh to Questions transmitted to them by the Committee appointed by the House of Commons to enquire into the state of Medical Practice and Education 1843.

In 1829 the Royal Infirmary of Edinburgh had several surgeons with great reputations on its staff. However, only a few operations were performed and this is illustrated in Table 1.1. Table 1.2 shows the articles to be used for the excision of a bladder calculus. For these procedures alcohol and morphine were used as pre-operative pain-reducing agents.

Into this scene stepped James Young Simpson, born in Bathgate in West Lothian in 1811. He was the youngest of the village baker's eight children. His mother died when he was only nine years of age but he seemed to be extremely bright and at the age of 14 he left school and entered the University of Edinburgh to study medicine.

Simpson was appointed to the Chair of Midwifery at the age of 28 years and later went on to become physician to the Queen in Scotland, President of the Royal College of Physicians of Edinburgh, and was awarded a Baronetcy in 1866 and the Freedom of the City of Edinburgh in 1869. He had several other major achievements in medicine but these have now become overshadowed by the chain of events which occurred late in 1847.

By the beginning of the 19th century Humphry Davy and Michael Faraday had begun to demonstrate the properties of nitrous oxide as a means of inducing anaesthesia.[9]

It was after a public demonstration of the effects of nitrous oxide that Crawford Long considered the possibility of administering ether to a patient and in 1842, using ether, Long removed a small tumour from the neck of a friend.[9] Horace Wells, William Morton and Charles Jackson carried out work that established ether as being an agent which would allow major surgery to be performed on a patient who was under its influence.[9] In 1846 Professor James Millar, at the University of Edinburgh, received a letter from his teacher, Robert Liston, the Professor of Clinical Surgery at University College London, in which he stated that he had amputated a leg at the thigh while the patient was under the influence of ether.[14]

James Young Simpson, who was a real opportunist, immediately visited Liston in London and brought back the essential knowledge of how to administer ether, although it was not used for a major surgical operation in Edinburgh until the beginning of January 1847. James Young Simpson conceived the idea of using ether to relieve labour pain and used it for the first time on a patient with obstructed labour in January 1847.

Syme, the Professor of Surgery in Edinburgh, was a great opponent of ether and used to say that 'the smart use of the knife is a powerful stimulant and it is much better to hear a man bawl lustily than to see him sink silently into the grave'.[14] Despite his opposition to the use of ether, Syme subsequently used it with an apparatus devised by James Young Simpson.[15]

Although Syme claimed that patients were more likely to die if anaesthesia was used, these criticisms were made as a result of the general mortality associated with limb amputations in the years prior to anaesthesia, as demonstrated in Table 1.3. The criticisms were later refuted by Simpson, as shown in Table 1.4.

Although Simpson had devised a better method for administering ether, he met a chemist, David Waldie, by chance in Edinburgh, who suggested to him that chloroform would be a better agent with which to achieve the same effect because of its less irritant properties. Simpson and some friends tested the effects of chloroform on themselves and found it to be a potent agent. Simpson used it for the first time in labour in the management of Jane Carstairs, the daughter of a doctor, whom he safely delivered on 8 November 1847.[14]

Consequences of chloroform administration

There was considerable debate about who should take credit for the use of chloroform for pain relief in labour and there was an acrimonious correspondence between Simpson and Waldie.

There were great ethical and religious objections from Dr Petrie, a Liverpool doctor who considered anaesthesia to be a breach of medical ethics and stated that it was an act of cowardice to avoid pain. The clergy also had very strong views about the use of chloroform, although it is interesting that these comments were verbal statements. Last year Roger Maltby, Professor of Anaesthesia at the University of Calgary, researched the written evidence for the religious statements against chloroform for pain relief in labour and could find none (Personal communication, Roger Maltby).

In the USA, Charles Meigs could not understand why chloroform should have a place since he thought that its use was unnatural.[14]

Doctors such as Syme were in longstanding correspondence with Simpson against the use of chloroform but I believe that the years of 1846, with the introduction of ether, and 1847, with the introduction of chloroform, paved the way for a complete shift in opening up possibilities for pain relief in those patients undergoing elective surgery or in childbirth.[14]

Table 1.3. General mortality of amputations of the limbs in various centres in the years before anaesthesia

Hospital or Authority	Amputations (n)	Deaths (n)	Average mortality	Period in which operations performed
Civil Practice				
Liverpool Infirmary	43	3	1 in 14.33	1834 to 1836
(Mr Halton)			11.66	22 years
Liverpool Northern Hospital	96	18	5.33	1824 to 1843
Edinburgh Infirmary	61	31	1.96	3.25 years
Glasgow Infirmary	276	100	2.76	1794 to 1839
Glasgow Infirmary	155	47	3.29	1841 to 1846
Six Scottish Hospitals	24	3	8.0	1842
Newcastle Infirmary	229	54	4.24	
Royal Berkshire Hospital	27	5	5.4	1838 to 1845
Chester Infirmary	21	9	2.33	1838 to 1841
University College Hospital	66	10	6.6	1835 to 1841
Guy's Hospital	36	4	9.0	1843 to 1845
Great Britain (Mr Philips)	233	53	4.39	
Collected from various Journals				
(Mr Phillips)	308	76	4.05	
Notes of various Surgeons (Mr Phillips)	107	28	3.82	
Total of British Practice	**2046**	**524**	**1 in 3.9**	
Massachusetts General Hospital	67	15	1 in 4.46	
Pennsylvania Hospital	79	22	3.59	
America (Mr Phillips)	95	24	3.95	
Total American Practice	**241**	**61**	**1 in 3.95**	
Germany (Mr Phillips)	109	26	1.419	
France (Mr Phillips)	203	47	4.31	
Hotel Dieu	35	17	2.05	1840 to 1842
Hotel Dieu	178	1104	1.71	1836 to 1842
Hospitals of Paris (Malgaigne)	552	300	1.84	1836 to 1841
Paris (Gendrin)	63	23	2.73	1834
Paris (Dupuytren)	59	15	3.93	
Total of Continental Practice	1199	532	1 in 2.25	
Total of Civil Practice	3486	1117	1 in 3.12	
Military Practice				
Army at Algiers	63	17	1 in 3.71	1837 1840
Baron Percy	82	6	15.33	
New Orleans	52	12	4.33	
Naval Action of June 1, 1794	60	8	7.5	
Bombardment of Algiers	59	24	3.45	
British Army in Peninsula	842	289	2.91	
British Army in Thoulouse	100	31	3.22	
Other Military Records (Alcock)	74	6	12.33	
British Legion	109	55	1.98	
Total of Military Practice	**1451**	**448**	**1 in 3.23**	
Total of Civil and Military Practice	**4937**	**1565**	**1 in 3.15**	

From: Fenwick *Monogr J Med Sci* 1848;**8**:238.

Table 1.4.   Mortality of amputation of the thigh, leg and arm

Reported	Cases (n)	Deaths	Deaths (%)
Parisian hospitals	484	273	57
Glasgow hospitals	242	97	40
General collection (Phillips)	1369	487	35
British hospitals (Simpson)	618	183	29
Etherised patients	302	71	23

From Simpson J Y *Edinb Monogr J Med Sci* 1848;**8**:707.

Chloroform really only gained acceptance in 1853 when John Snow used chloroform at the delivery of Queen Victoria. Although chloroform later developed a bad reputation as a result of occasional deaths from its use, these were infrequent and in Edinburgh there were none in the first six years of its administration.[14]

It is appropriate that Simpson should take the palm for the introduction of chloroform anaesthesia for use in labouring patients. One of the serious consequences, however, was that it allowed more barbaric vaginal obstetric manoeuvres to be performed and encouraged abdominal surgery at a time when infection was still rife.

As a result of the development of chloroform anaesthesia in elective surgery Simpson was visited in 1869 by the celebrated Siamese twins, Chang and Eng Bunker, who were born in the same year as Simpson and had spent a lifetime together earning a living by exhibiting themselves as freaks. Although Chang and Eng themselves had no desire to be surgically divided from each other, some of their relatives had become anxious that they should be separated if it were possible to do so and particularly since chloroform anaesthesia had been introduced they thought that this might be possible and that Simpson could make arrangements for it.

The twins were joined by a band extending from the xiphisternum to the umbilicus with doubtful contents, although Simpson thought that there might be a diverticulum of peritoneum within it which might contain bowel.

Simpson confirmed the findings of Bolt in 1830 in which Bolt gave asparagus to Chang one day and four hours later detected its presence in Chang's urine but not in the urine of Eng. Simpson gave Eng potassium iodide to swallow and was able to demonstrate its presence in Eng's urine but not in the urine of Chang. Despite these observations, Simpson decided not to recommend surgery because he was unsure of what was contained in the band joining the twins but it is interesting that the separation of Siamese twins became a possibility as a direct result of the introduction of chloroform anaesthesia.[16]

Other forms of surgery also became possible. In the field of gynaecology the use of ovariotomy became a reality.

Considerations for the management of pain in obstetrics and gynaecology in the future

Since the watershed year of 1846–47 many developments have taken place in the field of anaesthesia, in particular for the management of pain in labour and in different types of gynaecological pain.

At the beginning of the 20th century 'twilight sleep' was introduced in the USA using morphine and scopolamine. This followed the use of opium, chlorohydrate, cocaine and other agents, all of which had limited benefit. Twilight sleep was used a great deal until a maternal death occurred in 1915; although unassociated with these drugs it really ended their popularity.

Gynaecological pain is seldom acute but is more of a chronic nature. The principal techniques and agents used to relieve pain in the field of obstetrics and gynaecology are multiple although the understanding of the pathophysiology of pain is incomplete.

Regional anaesthesia is one of the important developments that have taken place. Gradual refinement of these techniques will lead to even greater relief of pain in labour and of postoperative pain and discomfort.

It is clear that in the attitude of not only undergraduate students and doctors in training and but also in established doctors there is a disregard for the entity of pain and it is incumbent upon us to become increasingly aware of the fact that pain is produced at a psychological as well as physical level. It appears that the more sophisticated we become in our society the more dangerous it is that we fail to understand the way to incorporate our appreciation of pain into the practice of medicine.

I believe that, in terms of chronic pain and its relief, pain clinics are helpful but only partly so and the most important element in the attempt to relieve pain arises when the clinician becomes so involved with the patient and the relief of that pain that first of all there is a realisation of the factors which are causative, be they physical or psychological or both, and that we can learn from those who have undergone terrible experiences and overcome them. It is important that certain principles should be considered in terms of ethics and their imperatives and these have been well summarised in a paper by David Roy on the relief of pain and suffering in all of its spheres.[17]

There have been many attempts to quantify pain although this is so difficult to achieve. Even the sophisticated McGill–Melzack pain questionnaire does not really give an adequate assessment of the degree of pain experienced, either acutely or chronically.[18]

Whatever its degree or its locus, all pain is experienced within the brain, exemplified mainly by phantom limb syndrome. It is that apparently simple fact that we must remember when we think of the words of Simone Weil. At the entrance of the Centre for Reproductive Biology in Edinburgh is a plaque marking the opening of that Centre by her. At the time she was President of the European Parliament. As a former prisoner in Auschwitz she writes:

'Affliction is an uprooting of life, a more or less attenuated equivalent of death made irresistibly present to the soul by the attack or immediate apprehension of physical pain. If there is complete absence of physical pain there is no affliction for the soul because our thoughts can turn to any object. Thought flies from affliction as promptly and irresistibly as an animal flies from death. Here below, physical pain and that alone has the power to chain down our thoughts.'

She actually states that every true affliction of the soul roots itself in the pain-filled human body. Weil writes:

'Affliction is anonymous before all things; it deprives its victims of their personality and makes them into things. It is indifferent; and it is the coldness of this indifference, a metallic coldness, that freezes all of those it touches right to the depths of their souls. They will never find warmth again. They will never believe any more that they are anyone.'[19]

These words from a remarkable lady carry deep meaning for all of us. One of the reasons that I think this study group carries with it the possibility of fundamental considerations of the difficulties for obstetrics and gynaecology in relation to pain is that we must learn to impart understanding to our undergraduates and to our trainees, and indeed to ourselves as so-called mature clinicians, that chronic pain with its varying degrees presents a challenge which few of us can match. The anguish of acute pain can be relieved, not only by pharmacological agents but most of all through an understanding of the psychological factors that are so involved in the production of pain and in those mechanisms through which it can be overcome.

The legacy of James Young Simpson is that through the introduction of chloroform anaesthesia, he was able, at a stroke, to relieve the misery of acute and intense pain experienced by women in labour. Furthermore, the possibility of elective and emergency surgery became a reality.

At the beginning of this chapter I spoke of Albert Schweitzer and his writings on the appreciation of pain. I would like to end with another quotation from his autobiography.

'Whoever among us has through personal experience learned what pain and anxiety really are must help to ensure that those who out there are in bodily need obtain the help which came to him. He belongs no more to himself alone; he has become the brother of all who suffer. On the "brotherhood of those who bear the mark of pain" lies the duty of medical work.'[20]

References

1. Schweitzer A. *On the Edge of the Primeval Forest*. London: Adam and Charles Black; 1953.
2. Leriche R. *The Surgery of Pain*. London: Baillière, Tindall and Cox; 1939.
3. Kosterlitz HW, Hughes J. Peptides with morphine-like action in the brain. *Br J Psychiatry* 1977;**130**:298–304.
4. Kosterlitz HW, Terenius LY. *Pain and Society*. Wenheim: Verlag Chemie;1980.
5. Baird D. A fifth freedom. *BMJ* 1965;**5471**:1141–8.
6. White AD. *A History of the Warfare of Science with Theology in Christendom*. New York: Appleton & Son; 1898.
7. Ellis ES. *Ancient Anodynes*. London: Heinemann; 1946.
8. Shepherd DAE. Analgesia in labour becomes respectable. *American Society of Anesthesiologists Newsletter*, September 1997.
9. Keys TE. *The History of Surgical Anesthesia*. New York: Schumans's; 1945.
10. Burger L. *Birzig Jahre Storchantante: aus dem Tagebuch einer Hebamme*. Breslau; 1936. p. 20–21.
11. Hemlow J. *et al.*, editors. *The Journals and Letters of Fanny Burney*, 12 Vols. Oxford: Clarendon Press; 1972–1984. p. 596–616.
12. Simpson M. Letter from Dr George Wilson to Professor J Y Simpson. In: *Simpson the Obstetrician*. London: Gollancz; 1972. p. 146–8.
13. Beecher HK. Pain in men wounded in battle. Relationship of significance of wound to the pain experienced. *JAMA* 1956;**448** (161):1609–13.
14. Simpson M. *Simpson the Obstetrician*. London; Gollancz; 1972.
15. Syme J. On the use of ether. *Monogr J Med Sci* 1847;8:74.
16. Simpson JY. A lecture on the Siamese and other Viable United Twins. *BMJ* 1869;139–41.
17. Roy DJ. Relief of pain and suffering: ethical principles and imperatives. *J Palliat Care* 1998;**14**:2.
18. Melzack R. The McGill Pain Questionnaires: major properties and scoring methods. *Pain:* 1975;**1**:277–99.
19. Weil S. *Waiting for God*. 1957; translated by Emma Craufurd. New York: G.P. Putnams & Sons, 1951. p. 118.
20. Schweitzer A. *Out of my Life and Thought: An Autobiography*. New York: Allen & Unwin; 1933.

Chapter 2

Chronic pelvic pain: sociocultural perspectives

Victoria Grace

Introduction

Since the early 1970s medical approaches to pain, especially chronic pain, have been challenged by an enticement to address the social and cultural dimensions of pain in addition to those dimensions familiar to biomedicine and psychology. In this chapter I want to address the broader question of what a focus on sociocultural perspectives in relation to pain might mean – what is the salience of the social and the cultural for understanding pain, and how should we approach such a study? To do this I take chronic pelvic pain as a case study, in the context of this symposium on pain in obstetrics and gynaecology. It is my expectation, however, that the observations and arguments I make may well be relevant to other chronic pain conditions experienced by women, discussed in this book.

I will present three distinct ways of characterising the significance of sociocultural perspectives:

1. Sociocultural as context of pain (biomedical model)

2. Sociocultural as factor, or component, of pain (biopsychosocial model)

3. Sociocultural as co-producer of pain (biocultural model).

My argument is that the biopsychosocial model (Figure 2.1) has gone some of the way to address the problem of the exclusion of the psychosocial inherent to the biomedical

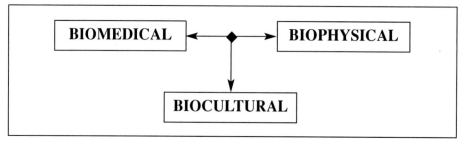

Figure 2.1. Biophysical model of pain, indicating interrelationship between dimensions

model. Following the work of David Morris,[1] I argue, however, that a biocultural model is necessary not only to recast the problems still apparent in the biopsychosocial model, but also to integrate fully the cultural facets of the experience of pain. Without understanding and addressing the sociocultural dimensions of women's chronic pain, we will fall short in our attempts to grapple with these conditions.

Background: the problem of chronic pelvic pain

In the early 1990s I conducted research on women's use of the health services in New Zealand for chronic pelvic pain. Between one quarter and one third of women consulting health professionals experienced a whole cluster of interrelated problems.[2,3] Most of these problems could be traced, in theoretical terms, back to the dualistic assumption of the body and the mind existing as two entirely distinct domains. This dualism is at the root of the familiar chronic pain 'story' where the patient goes to the doctor with pain, the doctor investigates but nothing is found, it appears from a biomedical diagnostic view that nothing is wrong, the patient thinks 'I'm neurotic', and there is a subsequent loss of self-confidence. Feeling undermined and demeaned, the patient keeps battling to have the 'real cause' diagnosed, or adopts an inward resignation to being some kind of mysteriously neurotic, somatising individual for whom, importantly, nothing can be done.

As part of this research I studied, from a social science perspective, the medical, psychiatric and psychological literature on 'chronic pelvic pain without organic pathology' from the late 1940s to the early 1990s. I noted what was then, in my view, one of the most significant developments in the Anglo-American literature in relation to this issue[4] – a paper published in 1991 by John Steege and colleagues called *Chronic pelvic pain in women: toward an integrative model.*[5] In this paper the authors were critical of the practice of 'ruling out' organic disease, or of judging whether or not there is sufficient tissue damage to explain the pain, a practice that they claimed 'is really the product of thinking about pain in Cartesian either/or fashion'.

By the latter half of the 1990s, evidence of a general consensus emerged in the literature on chronic pelvic pain and the problem of an absence of identifiable pathology. There was broad agreement that it is problematic to assume the absolute distinction of body and mind; that it is problematic to place to the fore the search for biomedically identifiable pathology as the benchmark for ascertaining the cause of the pain; that chronic pelvic pain is multifactorial, and that an integrative conceptual model should guide medical investigation and intervention. Chronic pelvic pain cannot be approached through a unidimensional biomedical framework, but must include reference to the psychological, behavioural, social and, at the limit, cultural dimensions.

The question to be addressed here is: how have these multidimensional and inclusive agendas been progressed and what paradigm(s) might best serve this new approach?

The biomedical model

Chapman, Nakamura and Flores[6] characterise the biomedical sensory neuro-physiological model of pain as one asserting that nociception, transmission of noxious signalling, modulation and sensory registration of pain are biologically predetermined processes. They state that the biomedical concept of pain involves:

1.   Transduction of tissue trauma into neural signals

2.   Transmission of such signals to the dorsal horn of the spinal cord and from there to the thalamus

3.   Central registration of the sensory information in somatosensory cortex.

It is the modulation of signals as the information is transmitted that provides the basis for the mechanism for pain relief. Pain from injury to neurological pathways is also recognised in biomedicine and is called neuropathic pain.

From the viewpoint of the biomedical model, chronic pain in the absence of identifiable pathology, or tissue trauma, remains an enigma; it will be assumed that the pathological originating site of the tissue damage has yet to be identified, as pain is precisely a sensory experience resulting from tissue damage, or other noxious stimuli.

For the biomedical model, those dimensions which cannot be identified in objective, somatic, biological terms, such as social factors, cultural constructs or subjective experience, are by definition external to the model, and not immediately relevant to the core business of explaining pain and developing treatment methods. The psychological and sociocultural domains become the *context* in which pain is experienced, responded to and treated; the *context* in which patients come to terms with pain, catastrophise about it, reinforce or ignore it, make use of health care, find ways to cope and support themselves financially, and so on. Similarly, pain can be disabling and have a serious effect on the functioning of society through lost productivity of the workforce and through resources needed for drugs for treatment and for health practitioners' consulting time.

Thus the sociocultural dimensions of pain are of peripheral interest or importance to the biomedical model. In the case of chronic pelvic pain, these dimensions might, for example, concern modes of doctor–patient interaction, insisting on the importance of the gynaecologist dealing sensitively with a negative diagnostic finding. A positive diagnostic finding is 'proof' that the patient is 'not nuts'. Improved and sustained networks of social support and education of family members might better enable the sufferer to find positive and constructive methods of living with chronic pain when curative treatments are not available.

A biomedical model that is firmly grounded in the Cartesian dualism of body and mind, object(ive) and subject(ive), will obviously not cast its fundamental assumptions as problems to investigate. Therefore, those medical scientists and practitioners who are advocating the need for an integrated approach to chronic pelvic pain are clearly looking toward a model that can accommodate the subjective-psychological, the social and the cultural within its explanatory framework. The dominant trend has been to turn to the biopsychosocial model.

The biopsychosocial model

Although conditioned by the slightly earlier biopsychosocial thinking of authors such as Melzack and Casey,[7] the biopsychosocial model was first formally conceptualised by George Engel in the 1970s.[8] He was convinced the time was ripe for a rigorous challenge to a biomedicine that could not integrate the role of psychological and social factors into its explanatory framework. Illness, he argued, represents a complex interaction of biological, psychological and social influences. The interaction between these components might comprise a linear, cause–effect relationship or it might involve more complex feedback systems with each component affected by, and affecting, each other. This concept of a reciprocal determinism enables this model to postulate that biological, psychological and social factors influence each other. Weisberg and Keefe note that, in their view, the biopsychosocial model is particularly relevant to the understanding of chronic pain, 'because, in the case of persistent pain, many opportunities exist for biological, psychological, and social factors to influence pain'.[9]

In addition, the biopsychosocial model proposes that a chronic pain state, for example, is adaptive and evolutionary, in the sense of continually changing over time as adaptations are made to the changing biological, psychological and social circumstances encountered. Chapman, Nakamura and Flores[6] therefore characterise the current biopsychosocial model as comprising 'integrated action' (a model of pain that integrates the three elements of biology, psychology and social factors), 'reciprocal determinism' and evolution.

The question remains, is this model an adequate response to the problems encountered in relation to chronic pelvic pain? The limits of the biomedical model for addressing chronic pelvic pain indicated a need for an integrated model, but does the specific formulation of the biopsychosocial model fulfil the requirement of a rigorous critique and transformation of the dualistic ontology of the Cartesian split between body and mind, objective and subjective?

The conceptualisation of the biopsychosocial model retains a vigorous distinction between its three domains. They remain clearly bounded: the biological with its academic specialisation, the psychological and the social with theirs. The key task, therefore, is one of articulating the 'relationships', the 'interrelationships' or the 'interactions' between these discrete domains. This is indeed the focus of considerable research activity. This formulation, I argue, is not the way to resolve the problem of the dualistic structure, but is rather another, somewhat more sophisticated, way of working within its terms. In other words, the dualistic split between the body (objective) and mind (subjective) remains; what has been added is a requirement to articulate their interaction. (See Grace[10] for a full discussion of these issues.)

Following on from this concern is the observation that the arrows between the components of the model appear to represent directions of influence, or even causation, but the question of *how* these causal processes in fact take place is curiously side-stepped. The epistemological assumptions underpinning the model cannot deal with this question of *how*, except by referring somewhat vaguely to 'mechanisms'. A number of authors writing in the chronic pelvic pain field have commented on what I suggest is the symptom of this problem; for example, Howard writing in 1996 states that 'at this time no single theory or model has given an adequate explanation of why some women [with a history of sexual abuse] develop chronic pelvic pain'.[11] Chapman, Nakamura and Flores[6] draw a bold conclusion in this regard: 'Although the current biopsychosocial framework has enabled providers to identify more factors that contribute to chronic pain, it deals in broad generalities and offers no explanation of how psychosocial factors affect the brain and the body'.

Commenting on contemporary trends in modern medicine, Levin and Solomon[12] are convinced that the shift to systems-theoretical and information-processing models of thinking is indeed significant, but they question whether this shift does in fact reflect a major break with the mechanistic thinking of the previous paradigm. On the contrary, they contend that these developments are, in reality, attempts to adapt the old paradigm of mechanisms (objectivist thinking) to the newly articulated complexities. Functional explanations are still conceived in mechanistic terms.

Where the biopsychosocial model is employed in the literature on chronic pelvic pain, there is a tendency for the psychological and social components to be cast as reactive to pain and not integral to the experience of pain. As Chapman, Nakamura and Flores[6] note with respect to the model more generally, biological factors are most important in initiating, continuing, and modulating pain in the acute stage. 'Psychological factors come into play by shaping the individual's understanding of resulting physiological cues and determining the patient's consequent behaviour'.

The types of concern outlined here appear to be alluded to by some authors writing in the medical literature on chronic pelvic pain. There are, for example, quite a number of cautious references to the 'subjective' aspects of pain, but there is no 'subject' in their analyses, and no permissible access to such a thing. There are approaches to psychology, sociology and anthropology where the formation of subjectivity is understood through the study of language and meaning, and where the interpretation of meaning should be *understood* through interpretive theoretical discourse, and not *explained* solely through sequential juxtapositions of variables. Medical sociologist, David Armstrong, argues that the biopsychosocial model, rather than opening a dialogue between the critical, interpretive social sciences and biomedical science, instead appropriates the psychological and social by recasting them in the objectivist and reductionist terms of a biomedically based biopsychosocial alliance.[13]

Chapman and colleagues write that the biopsychosocial model extends and enhances medical approaches to chronic pain, but that in fact 'it does not integrate smoothly with the knowledge base on pain in medicine'.[6] They claim that in fact it remains for the biomedical and psychosocial domains to be integrated. They propose a perspective that focuses on consciousness and pain as a means to resolve some of these problems and effect a more integrated relationship between the biomedical and psychosocial approaches. David Morris has articulated the basis for a 'biocultural model' for understanding pain that also claims to go beyond the limitations discussed.[1,14] I will consider the key elements contained in such approaches from the point of view of the problems of chronic pelvic pain.

Towards a biocultural model

'Pain is not just a stimulus that is transmitted over specific pathways but rather a complex perception, the nature of which depends not only on the intensity of the stimulus but on the situation in which it is experienced and, most importantly, on the affective or emotional state of the individual. Pain is to somatic stimulation as beauty is to visual stimulus. It is a very subjective experience.' (Allan Basbaum, Professor of Anatomy and Physiology, University of California, Santa Cruz.[15])

Earlier I characterised the biocultural model as one in which the sociocultural might be conceptualised as co-producer of pain; not as the context of pain (biomedical model), nor as a discrete factor interacting with other factors in a multifactorial model of linear causal relationships (biopsychosocial model), but as integral to pain. If the distinctions we call biological, psychological, social and cultural are not conceptualised as dichotomously constructed domains, then we need different conceptual tools to understand and depict how they simultaneously traverse and co-produce, or co-create, one another. From this standpoint, it is not possible to understand or explain facets of one domain in isolation from the others.

Patrick Wall, who several decades ago was one of the originating authors of the influential gate-control theory of pain processes, proposed in 1999 that the sensation of pain is the consequence of our brain analysing the situation in terms of what action would be appropriate. In other words, perceiving pain cannot be separated from the behavioural, historical and sociocultural phenomenon of action. Furthermore, he wrote that 'the feeling of pain coincides with changes in every part of the body and in a distributed pattern in parts of the brain'.[16]

David Levin (philosopher) and George Solomon (MD) have analysed paradigmatic shifts in the history of Western medicine. They situate the features of the biomedical model (and arguably the biopsychosocial model where it follows the biomedical model) as characteristic of 'modern medicine', the paradigm of medicine that has been dominant in the era of modernity, beginning with the 16th-century Renaissance but more particularly in the subsequent transformations of 18th-century Europe. They argue that 'postmodern medicine' of our contemporary era is now undergoing a potential shift in paradigm. Late modern medicine, they suggest, is increasingly approaching the body as a self-regulatory system whose functioning is dependent on, and inseparable from, the larger world 'and which consequently can exist only in continuous, psychologically mediated interaction with a complex field of social, cultural, historical, and environmental conditions'.[12]

Levin and Solomon[12] focus particularly on developments in the field of psychoneuroimmunology to demonstrate how medicine can now represent the body as a psychosomatic unity integrated into its environments, and only now through this work can medicine begin to articulate the networks of causal correlations implied by this representation. This new body of medicine cannot be represented as a 'substance' but rather 'as a system of intercommunicatively organised processes, functioning at different levels of differentiation and integration'. This view, they argue, is supported by increasing evidence of a new concept of disease whereby diseases occur in a 'communicative field, a world, of social, cultural and historical influences: influences which the proprioceptive body processes as meanings'. In this sense they insist that the individual body is also a social body and must be approached as one that is inseparable from the social and cultural life of populations. This of course gives a new and broadened understanding of epidemiology.

This inseparability still implies the salience of distinctions between the bio/psycho/socio/cultural domains, but not in absolute terms. This in turn suggests a different set of assumptions about the methods needed to understand causal processes. Instead of linear causal relationships understood in mechanical terms between discretely bounded and identified phenomena, a phenomenon specific to one domain is understood to emerge from the interactivity of the whole.

To return to the question of understanding chronic pain, David Morris proposes a biocultural model that is arguably commensurate with the requirements of the broader approach described by Levin and Solomon. In a vein similar to Levin and Solomon, Morris[1] states that the future is likely to see a new multidimensional medical model that 'encompasses the intersecting physiologic, emotional, cognitive, and social aspects of pain', whereby pain is 'a complex perceptual experience that continues to change as it passes through culture, history, and individual consciousness'. Morris summarises his biocultural model in four points:

1.   Pain is more than a medical issue and more than a matter of nerves and neurotransmitters.

2.   Pain is historical, psychological and cultural.

3.   Meaning is fundamental to the experience of pain.

4.   Minds and cultures (as makers of meaning) have a powerful influence on pain, for better or worse.

Pain, according to these postulates, has its roots in human culture and consciousness. The term 'culture' is used to invoke the significance of fundamental meanings and values that structure and construct our lives as social beings; meanings and values that underpin the institutions of a society in often contradictory and conflicting ways. The significance of 'consciousness' becomes apparent as the focus shifts to the central role of (cultural) meanings. Numerous authors arguing for the role of culture in pain emphasise that pain is perception, that perception is embodied, that embodiment is historically, socially and culturally situated; and indeed pain is perceived by a conscious being. Consciousness, according to Chapman, Nakamura and Flores 'is an emergent property of a self-organising nervous system, and pain is an aspect of consciousness'.[6] They state that consciousness research makes use of the concepts of decentralised, dynamic, nonlinear, self-organisation processes and complexity. As noted above, these concepts potentially enable the types of inclusive conceptualisations necessary to an integrated approach to chronic pain.

The National Academy of Sciences Institute of Medicine's 1987 report on *Pain and Disability* concluded that there is no objective measure of pain, and that such a concept will always elude medicine. The authors of the report assert that the experience of pain is inseparable from personal perception and social influence.[17] As Wall argues, it is not intelligible to separate an objectively conceptualised event called the sensation of pain from subjective processes of perception, emotion and meanings. As indicated above, emergent understandings of somatic symptoms are viewed within medicine as occurring within a communicative field of social, cultural and historical influences, which the body processes as meanings. The importance of meanings is paramount in a biocultural model of pain.

Morris asserts quite simply that 'meaning is intrinsic to human pain'. By this he means that pain implies continuous processes of conscious and nonconscious interpretation. But he is quick to insist that meaning is never external to pain, never something 'added on': rather, human pain does not exist apart from meaning. 'Meaning helps constitute it'.[18] Morris acknowledges of course that drugs can relieve some kinds of pain while ignoring questions of the meanings of pain, but it does not follow that meanings somehow go away. They may be circumvented, and this action may undermine effective treatment in some cases of chronic pain.

According to Morris, it is precisely chronic pain conditions that highlight the need for a biocultural model, as current research demonstrates how chronic pain eludes the medical clinician who attempts to understand it through tissue damage alone.[19] While valuing medical knowledge about nociception, a biocultural model holds that pain, as perception, is so entangled with meanings associated with our emotional, psychological and cultural experience that an adequate model must enable an understanding of pain, not just in terms of how pain is created in the nervous system, but, to use

Morris's words: 'at the complex point where biology and culture intersect'. Morris finds support for the shift towards a biocultural model of pain in redefinitions of pain within medicine that recognise the role of emotion in pain, which is viewed as subjective, in cross-cultural studies demonstrating how pain, is clearly experienced differently by peoples in different cultures (indeed, chronic pain is not ubiquitous),[20] and in psychological studies and research on pain beliefs.

Pain is of course experienced by an individual and, in this sense, pain is subjective. But the subjective nature of pain perception is not an annoying variable to be ignored in the search for objectively verifiable generalities. A biocultural model views individual subjectivity as never entirely unique and singular, as individuals exist only within the intersubjective framework of specific cultural milieux, which shape and constrain individual psychological processes and thus play a role in pain. To understand, and presumably treat, a person's pain is to take account of the meanings, beliefs, values and social institutional context of that experience. These are sociocultural phenomena. As Levin and Solomon[12] point out, rejecting the dualisms of body and mind also implies the rejection of the dualisms of body and environment, and individual and population.

The observations of numerous authors in a diversity of fields appear to be converging on the salience of the key elements of what Morris has termed a 'biocultural model' for understanding pain. How such a model might be elaborated is less clear. It is clear that we are dealing with phenomenal complexity, and there is a need to develop appropriate methods, epistemological postulates and theoretical tools of analysis before a coherent empirical research programme might be articulated. This is indeed a challenge.

The biocultural model and chronic pelvic pain

Qualitative research in 1991 on women's use of the health services in New Zealand for chronic pelvic pain revealed the extent to which meanings associated with chronic pain were central to their experience of consulting general practitioners and gynaecologists.

Women were recruited for six discussion groups, or 'focus groups', in cities and large urban centres. Three of the groups were organised through the local endometriosis support group, two by a local women's health group, and one by the staff of a pelvic pain clinic at a major public women's hospital. Each group had between five and seven members, and the discussions took, on average, 90 minutes. As the participants had already received a full briefing on the background to the research and its aims, I began the discussion by inviting women to talk about their experiences of chronic pelvic pain and of using the health services for their condition. The discussion was tape-recorded and subsequently transcribed.

Analysis of this material revealed the extent to which the dualism of body and mind, organic and non-organic, structured the medical encounter for chronic pelvic pain, and how it also structured women's responses to that encounter. The classic story of the patient with chronic pain was clearly evident as a theme traversing these transcripts: if no pathology was 'found' on diagnostic investigation, or if women were not examined for diagnostic purposes, there was the implication, first, that 'there was nothing wrong' and second, that it must be somehow, mysteriously 'psychological,' which was interpreted as 'neurotic', 'crazy', 'loony', 'nuts', and importantly, nothing further was suggested or pursued to deal with the pain, which of course remained.

At the same time, there was a strongly and repeatedly expressed desire for having an understanding of the pain. This search for understanding and the social meaninglessness of pain without medically identified pathology, was the most distinct and robust theme underpinning the detail of the discourse analysed in the discussions. In part, this search was motivated by action: to 'know' what was wrong would help the sufferer orient meaningfully to dealing with the pain. But more integral to the structural facets of the discourse was the need to literally *make the pain meaningful* in a way that serves to situate the woman in relationship to her entire psychosocial world. Without this, her world progressively diminished, her self-confidence became undermined, and she experienced greater isolation from those previously close to her, through her and their inability to make sense of her somatically experienced distress, and their possible incredulity at its 'realness'.

A systematic analysis of the transcripts revealed the following pattern:

- **Anguish of meaninglessness, and the social alienation that accompanies this**

'If I'd had a name to what I had, it would be completely different…'
'It was sheer hell [before name] living 17 years day in and day out with the pain…'
'Why am I so tired? Why am I like that? Why is this?'
'One of the hard things that I found was just having pain for so long and not knowing what the hell it was…'
'What's wrong with me?'
'Maybe it's all in my mind?'
'I asked the doctor, am I crazy?'
'…being cast as neurotic by my family, and probably my doctor…'
'…that is the saddest part about it. You block yourself off from your husband, your child, your family, because I kept thinking, my god, there's no name for this, what the hell…'
'…it's a very sad, isolated type of thing…'
'You're on your own with the pain.'
'I just put up with the pain.'
'It's like being in a hopeless situation. There is no solution. There's nothing you can do.'
'There's absolutely no reason why I should have that pain.'
'…and I have a lot of questions; so many questions…'
'I couldn't get a doctor to believe me…'
'That's when [no name] I really started to withdraw from anybody, friends, family. Absolutely withdraw… and I cried and cried and cried when he said, on a pelvic exam, that he suspected endometriosis.'

- **Meanings of others compounded the meaninglessness and the alienation**

'…you are a sensitive type of woman…'
'…you shouldn't take things too seriously…'
'…they just think, she's off again…'
'They said it was just tiredness and tension; that I needed to get away.'
'The word was that, I need to get busy and stop thinking about myself so much.'
'I was just told it's all in my head, and stop fretting.'
'You know, to actually even consider to make up this kind of pain.'
'She said you have to put up with it; to get rid of the stress that was going on in my life.'

'These [words] eat away your confidence in wondering what sort of strange person you are...'

'Perhaps I am sort of neurotic... emotional, uptight.'

'I really felt as if I was being judged by the private hospital team.'

'I felt dirty... the gynaecologist came in and said he's aspirated the area and sent it away to be tested for transmitted disease. I couldn't wait to have a shower and wash it all away; to wash me away.'

'I was questioning him... I really wanted to know what I looked like inside, if it was that bad, and what had caused it. He said he didn't know what it was, but it made him bloody pleased he wasn't a woman.'

If the postulates of a biocultural model do render the complexity of the phenomenon of chronic pain more accurately, then establishing a dominant explanation of pain as only physical does actively create a cultural meaninglessness of pain. Morris comments that the medical construct of pain may help to explain the despair felt by many patients whom medicine cannot relieve of their pain. What is evident in the pattern above is in fact an entire set of cultural meanings around pain; meanings that reflect a lay appropriation of the predominant medical view. Pain is a signal or symptom of damage to bodily tissue; it is essentially meaningless. Once pathology is identified and diagnosed, this establishes the originating site of pain within the body, thus legitimising its existence, and establishing the patient as victim of some pathological process. If pathology cannot be 'found', there is no culturally legitimate way of understanding or explaining the pain. Instead there is the alienating implication of malingering, or being 'neurotic'.

- **Diagnosis ('name') ends search for meaning, but creates another form of meaninglessness**

'It [endometriosis] was finally diagnosed...'

'I could hardly take it in after the diagnosis...'

'They gave it a name, but that was about it. I don't know what caused it.'

'I found I had endometriosis, and in a way I was really pleased. I thought, thank goodness, there is really something wrong with me. Then I thought, "what is it? Will I die?" They didn't know anything about it.'

'I've never quite known what the diagnosis is...'

'I more or less took it because the doctor was telling me to do that.'

'And they sent me for another scan, and they followed that by doing a vaginal scan this time. And it showed up. I still really don't know what it's all diagnosed as... anyway, they want to take out my ovaries as well as the womb.'

'I haven't really been told what I've got... I've got some veins that are swollen.'

'It's actually a very alone person's disease.'

'[After name] I still didn't know what the hell was wrong with me...'

'He didn't know how to explain it...'

'I wasn't much the wiser again.'

'He knew exactly what was wrong with me...'

'Can they work out why you keep having cysts?'

'I didn't get better after that...'

'Even then, the specialists don't seem to know anything though, do they.'

'He said, we'll have to give you an op, a hysterectomy... and to me that was, you've got a sore thumb, we'll cut your arm off, just to me...'

'It's not so much being described what was wrong with me, but what I can do about it.

The only option I had was to take the drug, the other option I was given was having children.'

'I thought I was just waiting for an operation to have it cut out and then it would be fine.'

'They say now I've had my surgery, I'm supposedly well.'

'And within a month of the operation I was in the pain again, that the operation was supposed to have stopped.'

'He didn't explain anything. You are the one experiencing it, and you don't know. And that's what angers me, is that we don't know what they do to us.'

'Maybe... you can't question all those medical practices and that, but you can't cut a person to pieces to find things...'

The yearning for a diagnosis and the relief of finally receiving a 'name' for the pain did not in fact entirely fulfil the desire for understanding. The immediacy of the relief appeared to be most systematically related to the legitimising effect: 'there is something wrong with me'.

A further project would be necessary to probe into the nature of the meanings sought and yet frustrated through a diagnostic label. The postulates of the biocultural model would suggest the radical failure of a medical diagnostic label to address or engage the more fundamental questions of cultural meanings and beliefs that the woman has in many cases lived with and endured for many years. Some of these meanings are evident in the transcripts.

•   Meanings of pain

'I personally think they just don't realise that you can have the pain without having much perhaps visibly wrong with you. They really have no idea.'

'I felt I deserved to be told what was wrong with me... I'd been sick for a very long time.'

'It [anti-inflammatory drug] still does not release pain.'

'You have to be a pretty strong person to have endo for 25 years and be told that you're crazy by everybody and still survive life.'

'Sometimes emotions are covered up and you can hardly express how you feel...'

'I found that they thought I was a raving lunatic too – I think people who do that have not suffered enough...'

'I'm wondering if your pain stopped when you actually decided to hell with the lot of them, you're going to do something different?'

'Now when I do get pain it's sort of self-inflicted...'

'I take care of myself now...'

'I thought I was dying...'

'I wanted to die. I really did.'

'I have been suicidal many times with this pain.'

'The thing that gets me desperate is, "what's our future?" How much longer can we go on with this?'

'I asked her [doctor] why have I got this? What have I done to deserve it? And I have suffered a lot of sexual abuse as a child and she felt that the abuse had a lot to do with my having endometriosis. That's just me, and I actually feel that that's a part of it for me.'

'And I, just a continued pain, and I, then I've been through some periods of sexual abuse, and rape...'

'Pain is different for everyone.'

'It's something women have to put up with...'

'There's something... a thought I'd like to pursue in the future, but I wonder whether there's any connection with child sexual abuse in any way with endo, and not that it necessarily be a cause, but... a trauma to that pelvic area.'

'Those pains, though, I just remembered I, everything for me, everything that happened in here was pain until I dealt with sexual, you know, child sexual abuse and rape... this [genitals/pelvis] was for men or child molesters or whatever else to use, and I carried it around with me, it was something I carried around with me, so that everything that happened there was pain.'

'Perhaps because of the femininity side of things... female OK, but the femininity side I've never accepted... My mother was, you know, her place was in the home, and she wasn't allowed to work, and she was an abused woman, and I was sort of brought up with those feelings in the family.'

'We women, we're responsible for so much and, with our families and all the rest of it...'

'And my mother had ovarian cancer, and that was the big thing in the back of my mind.'

'It makes you wish you just had sons.'

'You are very angry with the pain because it means that you have missed out again [not conceiving].'

'There's a great grieving for women who have small children... that long-term grieving that you'll never get back those lost years.'

'Certainly in my illness now the spiritual healing is so crucial to whatever, it just eases.'

'[He said] I think you're going to have to have your hysterectomy, and I want to take out your ovaries. And that's baldly what it is. I have no support, I have no, I've got thousands of questions I want to ask someone, who am I to ask? I can't find out... I'm having to face it, that I'm going to have this operation. And to me it's major. It's not just the ordinary hysterectomy, it's taking the ovaries which is going to affect my whole body... and I identify myself as a woman sexually. I haven't had children. Some women express it through their womb, some of them express it through their breasts. Every woman is different, as how she identifies as being a woman. And they're going to take away anything that I, they're going to take away how I feel, and so I'm going to be a nothing. And I need, I think I need to talk it out with someone... that's what pain does to you, you become a nothing.'

As Morris notes, 'we continue to endow pain with meanings while believing incorrectly, incoherently, that pain is meaningless' furthermore 'we need to understand that pain is meaningless only when we believe it is meaningless, in which case we have only provided one more example of how pain always wraps itself in meaning'.[1]

In the selection of quotes above we see a number of ways in which women position themselves in a discourse on their own pain: as a long-suffering person being wrongly subjected to the punishing power of 'they' who can deliver or withhold what almost seems to be a judgement; as someone who can take control; a positive discourse of a person of strength and character who has survived, rendering pain a trial of endurance; where the experience of suffering has endowed them with some important human quality; fears of inheritance of disease (and the meanings surrounding 'inheritance'); that pain is subjective and specific; fears about death; wishing for death; and most significantly, where the trauma of childhood sexual abuse is implicated in the pain. There is suggestive evidence here that the cultural meanings of gender are central to the apparent 'meaninglessness' of women's (unexplained) pain in the pelvic area.

The writing of the Canadian medical doctor Nellie Radomsky provides further insight into the potential significance of these possibilities. Radomsky reflects on her clinical work with women suffering from pain; pain in many different sites of the body. Her book has the title *Lost Voices – Women, Chronic Pain and Abuse*.[21] She was disturbed by the number of women who came to her with chronic pain that was unexplained in biomedical terms, and she was prompted to become acutely aware of the limits of the biomedical model in responding to these conditions. Her empathy led her to talk with her women patients in ways that enabled her to understand not only how their pains were made meaningful through stories of abuse but also how women's own meanings were radically silenced in the contemporary cultural framing of pain.

In referring to these connections it is important to be mindful of the epistemological caution that interpretation of a meaning does not imply the postulation of a 'cause'. To suggest that understandings of pain in gynaecology should involve understandings of cultural meanings surrounding gender does not imply a recourse to the kind of oppressive therapeutics evident in the (pseudo)psychoanalytic theory of Anglo-American psychiatry in the early to middle years of the 20th century. This is a delicate line to open up because the devastating sense of hopelessness that surrounds the notion that 'they think I'm neurotic' is a legacy of precisely this kind of intervention. The biocultural model is radically opposed, epistemologically and ontologically, to any suggestion of imposing an inappropriate 'theory' about 'women's nature'. Rather, what I understand is suggested is the importance of the woman herself being assisted to explore the meanings of her pain and to interpret these meanings in relation to the broader cultural world in which they are situated, and through which they become intelligible.

This is why Morris applauds the employment of psychologists in multidisciplinary pain clinics today, and why he can see a role for the involvement of specialists in cultural anthropology, women's studies, philosophy, history, or literature. Such scholars, he submits, may be well-trained to help interpret the meanings with which patients and cultures have endowed the experience of pain, and to generate understandings of how pain is socially and culturally constructed. Especially pertinent to pain in obstetrics and gynaecology is the way in which pain is interpreted and reinterpreted in the cultural context that constructs meanings of masculinity and femininity, and particularly in relation to sexuality. Women are more likely than men to experience a variety of recurrent and chronic pains, to report more severe levels of pain, more frequent pain, and pain of longer duration.[22] If pain is inseparable from the meanings we attribute to it, then cultural constructs of gender have to be significant to understanding chronic pain in gynaecology. As Morris points out, it is unclear what it means to be a woman today suffering from pain of uncertain origin. It is clear, however, that beliefs about gender differences continue to affect clinical decisions concerning pain.[18]

Conclusion

I have argued for the importance of a biocultural model as a means to transform some of the problems currently plaguing the biomedical approach to chronic pelvic pain. There are innumerable avenues to explore in the process of preparing the ground for rigorous and systematic research of chronic pain in accordance with a biocultural model. Promising leads are opening up in numerous fields, including consciousness research, and theories of memory. The complexity of such a comprehensive, interdisciplinary research programme is bewildering, but the fact that it is currently being 'thought' is more than a beginning.

References

1. Morris DB. Pain and its meaning: a biocultural model. In: White AH, Schofferman JA, editors. *Spine Care* (Vol. 1). St Louis, MO: Mosby; 1995. p. 496–508.
2. Grace VM. Problems women patients experience in the medical encounter for chronic pelvic pain. *Health Care for Women International* 1995;**16**:509–19.
3. Grace VM. Problems of communication, diagnosis and treatment experienced by women using the New Zealand health services for chronic pelvic pain. *Health Care for Women International* 1995;**16**:521–35.
4. Grace VM. Mind/body dualism in medicine: the case of chronic pelvic pain without organic pathology. *International Journal of Health Services* 1998;**28**:127–51.
5. Steege JF, Stout AL, Somkuti SG. Chronic pelvic pain in women: toward an integrative model. *J. Psychosom. Obstet & Gynaecol* 1991;**12**:3–30.
6. Chapman CR, Nakamura Y, Flores LY. Chronic pain and consciousness: a constructivist approach. In: Gatchel RJ, Turk DC, editors. *Psychosocial Factors in Pain. Critical Perspectives.* New York: The Guilford Press; 1999. p. 35–55.
7. Melzack R, Casey, KL. Sensory, motivational, and central control determinants of pain: a new conceptual model. In: Kenshalo D, editor. *The Skin Senses.* Springfield IL: Thomas; 1968. p. 423–43.
8. Engel GL. The need for a new medical model: a challenge for biomedicine. *Science* 1977;**196**:129–36.
9. Weisberg JN, Keefe, FJ. Personality, individual differences, and psychopathology in chronic pain. In: Gatchel RJ, Turk DC, editors. *Psychosocial Factors in Pain. Critical Perspectives.* New York: Guilford Press; 1999. p. 56–73.
10. Grace VM. Pitfalls of the medical paradigm in chronic pelvic pain. *Baillière's Clinical Obstetrics and Gynaecology* 2000;**14**:525–39.
11. Howard FM. The role of laparoscopy in the evaluation of chronic pelvic pain: pitfalls with a negative laparoscopy. *Journal of the American Association of Gynecologic Laparoscopists* 1996;**4**:85–94.
12. Levin DM, Solomon GF. The discursive formation of the body in the history of medicine. *Journal of Medicine and Philosophy* 1990;**15**:515–37.
13. Armstrong D. Theoretical tensions in biopsychosocial medicine. *Soc Sci Med* 1987;**25**:1213–18.
14. Morris DB. *The Culture of Pain.* Berkeley, CA: University of California Press; 1991.
15. Basbaum AI. Unlocking the secrets of pain: the science. In: Bernstein E, editor. *Medical and Health Annual.* Chicago: Encyclopaedia Britannica; 1987. p. 84–103.
16. Wall P. *Pain. The Science of Suffering.* London: Weidenfeld and Nicolson; 1999.
17. Osterweis M, Kleinman A, Mechanic D, editors. *Pain and Disability: Clinical, Behavioral, and Public Policy Perspectives.* Washington DC: National Academy Press; 1987.
18. Morris DB. Sociocultural and religious meanings of pain. In Gatchel RJ, Turk DC, editors. *Psychosocial Factors in Pain. Critical Perspectives.* New York: Guilford Press; 1999. p. 118–31.
19. Roy R. *The Social Context of the Chronic Pain Sufferer.* Toronto: University of Toronto Press; 1992.
20. Good AD, Brodwin PE, Good BJ, Kleinman A, editors. *Pain as Human Experience: An Anthropological Perspective.* Berkeley, LA: University of California Press; 1992.
21. Radomsky NA. *Lost Voices – Women, Chronic Pain and Abuse.* New York: Harrington Park Press; 1995.
22. Unruh AM. Gender variations in clinical pain experience. *Pain* 1996;**65**:123–67.

Chapter 3

Multiple mechanisms of pelvic pain: lessons from basic research

Karen J. Berkley

One message that this chapter will attempt to convey is that the way in which a clinician or scientist conceptualises how the body creates pain can influence diagnosis, treatment and research strategies. Current conceptualisations of pain mechanisms are for the most part derived from the nearly 350-year-old drawing by René Descartes, made familiar to most of us in many articles by Wall and Melzack, in which fire on the foot activates a pathway to the brain that interacts via the pineal gland with the soul–mind. With respect to pelvic or visceral pain, this Cartesian derivation is evident in the diagram, shown in Figure 3.1A, which is modified from that published in 1948 by Kinsella in *The Mechanism of Abdominal Pain*.[1] What is interesting about Kinsella's diagram is (a) its focus on the fact that visceral afferents do indeed exist (they had just been discovered at that time), (b) that the visceral afferents converge on spinal neurons with afferents from the body wall (skin and muscles), and (c) that the 'mind,' depicted as a cloud above the brain, influences visceral sensation by activating descending paths from the cerebral cortex to the spinal cord.

The fascicular (or pathway) view

While Kinsella's diagram may now seem amusing, modern traditional views have in fact not changed much. Figure 3.1B presents a diagram of pain mechanisms similar to that which is currently provided in most clinical and basic science textbooks. This diagram implies that the 'mind' *is* the brain (not a cloud outside it), and shows that reciprocal spinal-cord-to-brain and brain-to-spinal-cord pathways for pain and pain modulation involve multiple routes rather than single lines up to and down from the brainstem and cortex. Furthermore, the pathway for touch perception and the pathway for visceral control are for the most part separate from the pathway for pain. This pathway conceptualisation has been dubbed the 'fascicular' view.[2] For its pain pathway, primary afferent fibres convey information about peripheral noxious stimulation to the spinal cord. For touch, primary afferent fibres convey information about gentle tactile stimulation to the dorsal column nuclei (as well as in the spinal cord). For visceral control, primary afferent fibres convey information about events occurring in viscera to the solitary nucleus (and spinal cord).

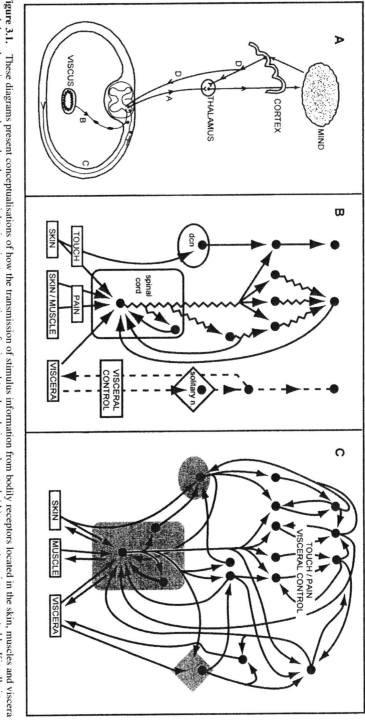

Figure 3.1. These diagrams present conceptualisations of how the transmission of stimulus information from bodily receptors located in the skin, muscles and viscera to and through various central neural pathways might give rise to perceptions of pain and touch and visceral control; (A) represents a view promoted by Kinsella in 1948[1] to call attention to two features important for understanding pelvic pain: the existence of visceral afferents and the influence of the 'mind', shown as a cloud above the brain (modified from Kinsella's[1] Figure 10); (B) represents the currently popular and traditional pathway, or fascicular view, in which different pathways of information flow are invested with different perceptual functions; dcn, dorsal column nuclei; solitary n., solitary nucleus; (C) represents a dynamic distributed ensemble view in which the many perceptions of pain and touch arise from the overall balance of activity that results as co-operatively controlled stimulus information flows through all three primary afferent recipient areas (the solitary and dorsal column nuclei and the spinal cord dorsal horn) into a dynamic brain; (B) and (C) are modified and updated from reference 16; see text for further details

The experience of pain is thereby created when a noxious or pathophysiological stimulus (i.e. a stimulus that threatens or actually produces damage) in skin, muscle, or a visceral organ activates a specific class of peripheral neural receptors called 'nociceptors' that convey their information to the spinal cord from whence the information is relayed through a series of neural structures to reach the cerebral cortex. To account for the fact that reported pain experiences vary despite similar peripheral stimuli, an additional rheostat-like 'pain modulatory' control mechanism exists that involves the ability of neurons in various parts of the brain to decrease or increase neural activity in the spinal cord via descending fibres.

Sensitisation

Although this traditional view can be a useful one, it requires peripheral bodily pathophysiology (that is, a noxious stimulus) for pain to occur. Thus, a problem arises for painful conditions, particularly chronic ones, when no peripheral tissue or organ pathophysiology can be found, forcing consideration of other, solely central nervous system (CNS) -derived mechanisms for explanation. One such mechanism is the concept of 'sensitisation.' Sensitisation can happen peripherally and/or centrally.

Peripherally, primary afferent fibres that supply various bodily structures have specific response properties. The receptive fields of single afferents usually cover small areas and their responses are organ-specific and modality-specific. The result is the existence of a huge array of peripheral sensory afferents supplying different bodily tissues with different response characteristics. Lists of these afferents fill long tables in specialised textbooks.[3] Under a number of conditions, however, the response properties of the afferents can change.[4] For example, trauma or injury sensitises certain afferents (mainly C-fibres) so that they develop the ability to respond to some stimuli to which they were previously insensitive, or respond more vigorously to those stimuli. Injury can also reduce the responses of some of them.

Sensitisation also occurs in spinal cord neurons, a process called 'central sensitisation'.[5,6] In it, a noxious event in peripheral bodily tissues triggers, by means of several molecular processes, a long-lasting sensitisation of recipient neurons in the spinal cord. This spinal sensitisation can, in some cases, continue for a long time after the initial provoking peripheral pathophysiology has healed. The result is either that incoming information which normally would not activate the spinal neurons (i.e. an innocuous or gentle stimulus) now does so, or that incoming noxious information is of even greater effectiveness in activating the spinal neurons. This now highly popular mechanism is under intense scrutiny, involving on the one hand debates on whether, or how much, or for how long, continued noxious stimulation is necessary to maintain the central sensitisation and, on the other hand, what molecular actions are involved both in peripheral body tissues and spinal cord that could be a target for the development of new analgesics.

Consequences of the fascicular view for clinical strategy

Although this three-part fascicular conceptualisation of pain mechanisms (i.e. the existence of a discrete pain pathway, descending modulation, peripheral and spinal cord sensitisation) has been quite useful for stimulating basic research, particularly into new analgesic agents that influence the activity of spinal neurons, and for incorporating the idea that the mind (brain) can modulate pain experience, it ties the perceptual experience of pain to noxious (pathophysiological) events that occur peripherally in bodily tissues. Thus, nociceptors are often referred to as '*pain* receptors,' as if activity in these stimulus-transducing neural receptors is invested with the pain perception beforehand, and the functions of the CNS ascending and descending components of the '*pain* pathway' are simply to bring pain into consciousness and to modulate the pain intensity.

One clinical consequence of this fascicular view is that it encourages dichotomisation of both diagnosis and treatment. Diagnosis is centred on the search for peripheral pathophysiology located in the region where patients localise most of their complaints. Therapy is then likely to be directed separately on the one hand towards suspected peripheral pathophysiology using drug or physical therapies, *or* on the other hand towards psychosocial processes using the more diverse situational interventions (see Table 3.1). The two types of therapy would be used together only when the

Table 3.1.   A growing list of therapies for pain[1]

Drugs	Somatic interventions	Situational approaches
Primary analgesics	***Simple***	***Self***
NSAIDs	Heat/cold	Education
Acetaminophen	Exercise	Meditation
Opioids	Massage	Diet
	Vibration	Art, music, poetry, performing arts
Other analgesics, adjuvants	Relaxation	Sports, gardening, hobbies
α2-adrenergic agonists		Humour
β-adrenergic antagonists	***Minimally invasive***	Aromatherapy
Antidepressants	Physical therapy	Religion
Anticonvulsants	Traction	Pets
Anti-arrhythmics	Manipulation	
Calcium channel blockers	Ultrasound	***Patient and clinician***
Cannabinoids	TENS	Co-education
Capsaicin	Acupuncture	Attitude
Corticosteroids	Local anaesthetic infiltration	Clinical setting and arrangement
COX-2 inhibitors		
GABA$_B$ agonists	***Invasive***	***Interactive***
Serotonin (5-HT) agonists	Radiation therapy	Hypnosis
Sex steroid hormones	Dorsal column stimulation	Biofeedback
Sodium channel blockers	Nerve blocks	Support groups
Antihistamines, laxatives	Neurectomy	Advocacy groups
Neuroleptics	Local ganglion blocks	Networking
Phenothiazines	Sympathectomy	Self-help groups
	Rhizotomy	
Routes	DREZ lesions	***Structured settings***
Topical, transdermal	Punctate midline myelotomy	Group therapy
Oral, buccal, sublingual	Limited myelotomy	Family counselling
Intranasal, inhalation	Commissural myelotomy	Job counselling
Vaginal, rectal	Cordotomy	Cognitive therapy
Intramuscular	Brain stimulation	Behavioural therapy
Intraperitoneal	Brain lesions	Psychotherapy
Intravenous		Multidisciplinary clinic
Epidural, intrathecal, spinal		Hospice
Intraventricular		

[1] Modified and updated from reference 7. COX, cyclo-oxygenase; DREZ, dorsal root entry zone; GABA, γ-aminobutyric acid; NSAIDs, nonsteroidal anti-inflammatory agents; TENS, transcutaneous electrical nerve stimulation.

patient's pain seemed not to match properly its presumed pathophysiology. While successful for some patients, this dichotomous approach becomes difficult to apply towards many of the musculoskeletal and visceral pain conditions, particularly those involving the poorly understood problems of referred pain with associated muscle and skin hyperalgesia, that are so much more prevalent in women than men.[7]

Basic research findings

Prompted by this clinical problem and by basic and clinical research findings in the past 20 years, a different conceptualisation of the mechanisms of bodily perception, including pain, is now emerging. With respect to pelvic pain, some of these new data, mainly from rodents, but some from women, are discussed below.

Specificity and plasticity of afferent information

Responses of peripheral afferent fibres in the hypogastric, pelvic and pudendal nerves that supply the female rat's pelvic organs convey remarkably detailed, precise and both organ- and modality-specific information to the CNS.[8,9] For example, fibres in the pelvic nerve that respond to mechanical stimulation of the vagina do not respond to stimulation of the bladder or colon; those that respond to stimulation of the bladder do not respond to stimulation of the vagina or colon, etc. Fibres that respond to steady pressure on one part of the vaginal wall are unlikely to respond to gentle stimuli that move across the same part of the vaginal wall or to steady pressure on a different part of the vaginal wall. None of the pelvic nerve fibres responds to stimulation of perineal muscles or skin; such responses are the province of pudendal nerve afferents. Under a number of conditions, both normal and pathological, these response properties change. Thus, the response sensitivity of some fibres changes with the normal fluctuations of the rat's ovarian cycle.[10] Furthermore, trauma, injury and inflammation can sensitise these afferents.[9] Thus, the response properties of peripheral afferents are plastic, not static. However, despite this plasticity, the response properties still remain precise and specific. For example, sensitised fibres that respond to vaginal stimulation still would *not* respond to colon or bladder stimulation (unless the bladder or colon stimulus was strong enough to stimulate the vagina indirectly).

Divergence and convergence

What is surprising is that, despite this specificity of response properties of peripheral afferent fibres, information from pelvic organs *diverges* and is delivered to widespread regions in the spinal cord many segments rostral and caudal to its segments of entry[11] where it then *converges* with information arriving from other tissues.[12] Thus, it would not be at all unusual to find a neuron located in, say, the dorsal horn of an upper lumbar segment of the spinal cord that responded to gentle tactile stimulation of the foot, pressure on a leg muscle, and distension of the vaginal canal *and* distension of the colon.[13]

New clues and conceptual leaps

The initial discovery of convergence many years ago led to the development in 1965 of the gate control theory,[14] a concept that forced us to face the fact that CNS-driven *perceptions* resulted from how the nervous system controlled the relative effectiveness of different types of converging incoming *information*. This theory had a revolutionary impact on clinical practice by providing a mechanism within the spinal cord that could help explain the lack of correspondence between the existence and intensity of a noxious stimulus and the existence or intensity of the pain experience. Descending influences from many parts of the brain together with converging incoming information could help 'gate' and modulate spinal cord neurons to influence what information reached the brain. However, this conceptualisation still tied the perception of pain to an incoming noxious stimulus, with the decision about pain being made in the spinal cord and then brought to consciousness by activation of pain pathways ascending from the spinal cord to the brain.

Subsequent evidence has added a series of clues to expand our understanding of the significance of divergence and convergence to pain, and thereby to change our conceptualisation of pain mechanisms. Here are four of the clues.

Descending influences

The first clue comes from examining what happens to the convergent responses of spinal neurons after the spinal cord has been transected to remove descending brain influences. As predicted by gate control theory, those properties change dramatically. After the spinal cord is transected, many more convergent responses emerge, some responses change from inhibition to excitation (and vice versa), and the effectiveness of stimulation for activating neurons is dramatically modified.[15] Such changes reveal the huge, varied, but mostly inhibitory, influences descending from many different parts of the brain on the responses of spinal neurons.

Involvement of dorsal column nuclei and solitary nucleus

While this result may not be unexpected given the previous discussion, a related second clue is the truly startling discovery that the somato-visceral and viscero-visceral convergence observed in the spinal cord also occurs in both the *dorsal column nuclei* and the *solitary nucleus*.[16-19] Again, similar to the spinal cord, response properties in these other two entry regions are influenced by systems descending to them from more rostral brain structures.[20,21] These results were startling because, as discussed above and shown in Figure 3.1B, neurons in the dorsal column nuclei are supposed to be the recipients of primary sensory afferents that respond to gentle tactile stimulation of the skin, and thus are considered responsible for the perception of touch. Similarly, neurons in the solitary nucleus are supposed to be the recipients of information only from visceral stimulation and therefore to be involved only in the control of visceral function.

Widespread divergence, convergence and interactions throughout brain

The third clue comes from the fact that information from neurons in the spinal cord, dorsal column nuclei and solitary nucleus is delivered from these three regions to each other, as well as to a large number of locations in the brain which themselves interconnect.[17,22-24] This extensive divergence, extensive consequent convergence and extensive interconnectivity within the brain together have important consequences. One consequence is that it is likely that 'central sensitisation' is not limited to the spinal cord, but occurs as well in many parts of the brain.[6] Indeed, such a situation, sometimes referred to as the brain's (in addition to the spinal cord's) 'pain memories' or 'pain traces,' has been reported clinically.[25] Thus, electrical stimulation in the thalamus can reproduce pains in patients who have long since recovered from the peripheral injury that initiated their pain. For example, Nathan[26] reported that thalamic stimulation (being performed for a movement disorder) reproduced a patient's prior toothache, while Lenz and colleagues,[27] under similar circumstances, reported reproduction of the patient's angina (without cardiac abnormalities). Another consequence of the extensive divergence, convergence and interconnectivity is the enormous potential they provide for interactions of information derived from somatic and visceral structures with other sensory structures (eyes, ears, nose, etc.) on neuronal responses throughout the entire brain.

Studies of neural mechanisms for other perceptual realms

The fourth clue involves consistent findings from research on neural mechanisms underlying perceptions other than pain, such as vision, audition, olfaction, movement and somatosensation. This sophisticated research has shown that, instead of pathways, perceptual processes involve 'dynamic distributed ensemble networks'. These networks encompass components throughout the entire nervous system that change continuously with experience across the lifespan, and the molecular mechanisms underlying the changes are remarkably similar to those that underlie learning.[28-32] One consequence of this view is that many parts of the nervous system are engaged when an individual experiences pain. A second is that the ensemble that determines pain in one individual may differ from that which determines pain in another individual, even under circumstances that would seem virtually identical for the two individuals. A third is that within a given individual there probably exist multiple pain ensembles that are uniquely associated with different pains, and those ensembles change with that individual's accumulating experiences across their lifetime. The former two situations have already been reported in brain-imaging studies of humans in pain,[33-35] and there are hints supporting the third.[36]

The dynamic ensemble view

Together, these new research findings have led to a conceptualisation of pain mechanisms that differs considerably from the fascicular view. As shown diagrammatically in Figure 3.1C, this view attempts to incorporate the fact that it is through divergence and convergence of ever-changing information that networks of interconnected neurons within the CNS create various bodily perceptions. It begins with the premise that pain perception, rather than being simply a direct consequence of a noxious stimulus, is an experience created by the entire nervous system that takes into account information arriving from all sources in context with previous and contemporary circumstances to motivate the individual for self-protective action. In it, pain perception at any moment is a consequence of any of a number of possible ensembles of central neuronal activity distributed throughout the CNS. Such pain-relevant activity ensembles are derived from moment-to-moment by the many co-operative controls momentarily exerted on how information about bodily stimuli (skin, muscles, viscera) flows from the periphery not only throughout the spinal cord, but through the dorsal column nuclei and solitary nuclei into an active and dynamic brain whose control processes are being continually updated by experience in all sensory realms. Thus, it is the entire nervous system that creates pain, in light of its past learning, when the current situation demands focused self-protection from harm.

Consequences of the dynamic ensemble view for training, diagnosis and therapy

This emerging view of pain mechanisms encourages scientists and clinicians to develop different perspectives both for the study of pain mechanisms and for clinical strategies for diagnosis and treatment. What follow are a few examples relevant to clinical practice.

Remote central sensitisation and remote referred pain

The vast extent of divergence and convergence of information from widespread areas of the body on neurons in the spinal cord, dorsal column nuclei and solitary nuclei provides a substrate for central sensitisation to extend into neural regions associated with body segments more remote from the original site of pathophysiology than would be predicted from the fascicular conceptualisation. For example, this newly appreciated situation creates the possibility that muscle tenderness in, say, the shoulder could actually reflect some prior nociceptive event in, say, the uterus. While this idea may at first seem far-fetched, it does in fact have some research support. Thus, Giamberardino and colleagues[37] compared skin and muscle pain thresholds in the abdomen (left and right), thigh (quadriceps area) and upper arm (deltoid area) across the menstrual cycle in women with and without severe dysmenorrhoea. Given that the presumed source of dysmenorrhoea involves strong uterine contractions and that uterine viscerotomes are mainly in the upper lumbar segments, the investigators expected that muscle and skin pain thresholds would be reduced in dysmenorrhoeal compared with non-dysmenorrhoeal women only at the abdominal test sites (regions of uterine referral) and only perimenstrually (times when the uterus is contracting strongly). Instead, the dysmenorrhoeal women showed a generalised muscle (but not skin) hyperalgesia; that is, they had significantly lower muscle pain thresholds at all four sites throughout the menstrual cycle. The investigators also observed a significant enhancement of the cyclicity of both muscle and skin pain thresholds.

There are many potential clinical implications of dysmenorrhoea's spatial (generalised muscle tenderness) and temporal (enhancement of cyclical pains) influences. Because dysmenorrhoea is so common, clinicians may not think to ask patients about the severity of their dysmenorrhoea or to consider how such dysmenorrhoea could influence the patient's current diagnosis and therapy. One example relates to fibromyalgia, which has been reported to co-occur frequently with dysmenorrhoea.[38,39] Thus, it could be of value when examining fibromyalgia patients, to enquire about their menstrual discomforts. If severe, treatment directed specifically at the dysmenorrhoea might eventually be of significant benefit for the fibromyalgia. Another example relates to tension headaches, which are associated with pericranial tenderness.[40] There is a strong tendency for these head pains to occur perimenstrually in some women.[40] Here again, for those patients with severe dysmenorrhoea, pre-emptive (i.e. just before the premenstrual phase) drug and other treatments (see Table 3.1) for their dysmenorrhoea could be of value not only in reducing their dysmenorrhoeal pains but also in preventing their headaches.

Influence of pathophysiology in one visceral organ on physiology of another

In addition to providing a substrate for *viscero-somatic* interactions such as those discussed above between pelvic organs and muscle or skin, the divergence –convergence mechanisms provide a substrate for *viscero-visceral* interactions. In this regard, it is well known that the urinary, gastrointestinal and reproductive tracts are normally co-ordinated so that their functions do not conflict. For example, micturition and defaecation inhibit each other, and are themselves both inhibited during copulation.[41,42] In animal studies, functional co-ordination between the colon and bladder,[43,44] and between the bladder and uterine cervix[45] involves input to the spinal cord from these organs and output from the spinal cord to these organs via the hypogastric and pelvic nerves.[9,13,15,42,46]

The existence of such physiological viscero-visceral interactions raises the issue of how pathophysiology in one pelvic organ influences the functions of other pelvic organs, whether or not the other organs are healthy. The few studies in women that have been directed specifically at this issue indicate that such influences could be profound. Thus, it is well documented that dysmenorrhoea or endometriosis, interstitial cystitis, irritable bowel syndrome, migraine and tension headaches, temporomandibular joint disorder and fibromyalgia frequently co-occur in various patterns.[39,40,47-49]

Studies in animals and humans support and extend the concept of potentially profound viscero-visceral interactions in the clinical setting. Thus, for example, *bladder* inflammation in rats can produce *vaginal* hyperalgesia (Figure 3.2A) or reduce the rate of *uterine* contractions (Figure 3.2B). Similarly, pain behaviours associated with artificial ureteral stones are increased in rats that had previously been subjected to surgical induction of abdominal endometriosis by partial hysterectomy and autotransplantation of endometrium on upper abdominal mesenteric cascade arteries.[50,51] Importantly, however, in the same study it was also shown that the pain behaviours associated with the ureteral stones were *decreased* in rats in whom the same surgical procedures had been performed, but who had received autotransplantation of fat instead of endometrial tissue.

The potential implications of these viscero-somatic and viscero-visceral interactions for future clinical training, diagnosis and therapy (particularly in cases of chronic pain) are profound. For example, the studies on rats described above[50,51] prompted a clinical study, in which it was found that in women who suffered from repeated ureteral calculi, the presence of dysmenorrhoea was associated with an increase in the number of pain

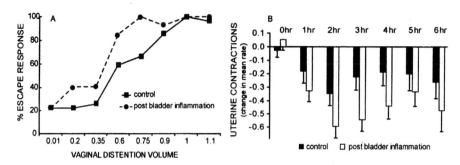

Figure 3.2. Examples of viscero-visceral interactions in laboratory rats: influence of bladder inflammation on vaginal sensitivity (A, increased sensitivity) and uterine contractility (B, decreased contractions); (A) shows that the percentage of trials that a rat escaped different volumes of vaginal distension increased when the rat was retested several days after that rat's bladder had been mildly inflamed with a solution of turpentine in olive oil; (B) shows how the mean rate of uterine contractions in urethane-anaesthetised rats (no. of contractions/5 min) changed over a six-hour period after infusion into the bladder of either saline or turpentine in olive oil; note that the rate of bladder contractions was decreased significantly more after the turpentine infusion than after the saline infusion

crises and a vastly changed cyclical pattern of those crises.[52] The rat study also raised the issue of whether certain visceral pathophysiologies (e.g. partial hysterectomy) might promote a reduction in crises evoked by ureteral calculi (i.e. 'silent' ureteral calculi).

The existence of these viscero-visceral and viscero-somatic interactions forces us to recognise and incorporate into clinical practice new knowledge that pain symptomatology may more frequently than we now realise reflect pathophysiology in organs remote in time and space from the current complaints and, perhaps even more importantly, that pathophysiology in one organ may *mask* as well as exaggerate symptoms of pathophysiology arising from another. For the immediate future, such recognition should encourage gynaecologists and obstetricians to work together more closely with clinicians in other specialties (e.g. gastroenterologists, urologists, cardiologists, rheumatologists, neurologists, dentists, physical therapists and, of course, psychologists and psychiatrists). Cross-specialty postgraduate training, either through coursework or greater clinical co-operation and consultation, could prove of great benefit in this regard.

Deliberate polytherapy

Table 3.1 lists a vast, growing array of drugs/drug routes (left column), somatic manipulations (middle column) and situational adjustments (right column) that can be used to relieve pain. What seems surprising when confronted with such a huge and hopeful table is why so much pelvic pain remains intractable. Part of the reason may relate to the clinician's (and patient's) implicit or explicit conceptualisation of pain mechanisms. Such conceptualisations influence not only how the clinician gathers data from patients but also how both the clinician and patient make use of the items in the table to devise treatment strategies.

It is likely that most clinicians, patients and even basic scientists assume that pain is brought about by a mechanism that looks something like the diagrams in Figure 3.1A or B. That is, they most probably assume that there are 'pain stimuli' which activate a 'pain pathway' in the CNS whose intensity can be amplified or attenuated by a variety of circumstances. Such a Cartesian, fascicular view reinforces traditional clinical approaches in which information is gathered mainly about the patient's most pressing morbid condition (e.g. pain in the pelvis), and treatment consists of the application of one, or only a few, of the therapies listed in the table that is known to 'work' for that type of pain condition. An extension of this strategy would be to add psychological treatments in those situations when no pathophysiology of bodily tissues can be found and when the pain is of long-standing with failure to respond to single therapies (e.g. 'chronic pelvic pain without pathology').

In contrast, some clinicians and patients are beginning to appreciate, or have implicitly adopted, a conceptualisation something like the dynamic ensemble diagram in Figure 3.1C. These individuals understand that both the quality and the location of pains are learned perceptions that are created by an ever-changing nervous system. Such pains are created not by a current noxious stimulus (i.e. pathophysiology) but by activity in that person's nervous system, which has learned and continues to modify the conditions important for evoking experiences that give rise to self-protective behaviours. Such a dynamic, holistic view fosters more active co-operation between the patient and clinician, allowing the gathering of more complete information about the patient's past history, current life situation and troublesome symptoms so that the patient and clinician can together develop a strategy of deliberate polytherapy. Such deliberate polytherapy means that therapies such as those listed in Table 3.1 would be combined; for example, two from the left-hand column, three from the middle column, several from the right-hand column. Such combinations could then be changed if the items chosen were found to be insufficiently effective or as the patient's condition or life situation changes. In this scenario, the patient and clinician are active partners in the diagnostic process as well as in the creation of a treatment strategy. Such a scenario does not necessarily require more than one clinician in the partnership, if that clinician has had adequate cross-specialty training and access to consultations from other specialists when necessary. Importantly, this approach has now been successfully adopted by some gastroenterologists for the diagnosis and treatment of women with functional bowel disorders.[53]

Conclusions

It appears that a new conceptualisation of pain mechanisms is becoming evident from basic and clinical research. This conceptualisation suggests that pain is derived from the ever-changing, diverging and converging information about bodily events that influence multiple brain structures, thereby giving rise to dynamic multiple ensembles of individually unique activity patterns in the brain that change during life. Such a conceptualisation encourages the realisation that pain is a complex collection of multiple, learned perceptions that change over time and that motivate individuals to take appropriate self-protective action. With respect to pelvic pain in the clinic, this view encourages us to appreciate more fully the potential interacting influences between organs and to develop more substantive interactions between clinical specialties, both in training and during practice. Perhaps more importantly, this view encourages deliberate adoption of a partnership relationship between patient and clinician, both to improve diagnosis and to enhance the creation of specific polytherapeutic strategies tailored to that patient.

Acknowledgements

The work from the author's laboratory discussed in this chapter was supported by grant NS11892 from the National Institutes of Health, USA.

References

1. Kinsella VJ. *The Mechanism of Abdominal Pain*. Australia: Angus and Robertson; 1948.
2. Berkley KJ. On the dorsal columns: translating basic research hypotheses to the clinic. *Pain* 1997;**70**:103–7.
3. Willis WD, Coggeshall RE. *Sensory Mechanisms of the Spinal Cord*, 2nd edn. New York: Plenum Press; 1991.
4. McMahon SB, Koltzenburg M. Novel classes of nociceptors: beyond Sherrington. *Trends Neurosci* 1990;**13**:199–201.
5. McMahon SB, Lewin CR, Wall, PD. Central hyperexcitability triggered by noxious inputs. *Curr Opin Neurobiol* 1993;**3**:602–10.
6. Coderre TJ, Katz, J, Vaccarino AL, Melzack R. Contribution of central neuroplasticity to pathological pain: review of clinical and experimental evidence. *Pain* 1993;**52**:259–85.
7. Berkley KJ, Holdcroft A. Sex and gender differences in pain. In: Wall PD, Melzack R, editors. *Textbook of Pain*, 4th edn. Edinburgh: Churchill Livingstone; 1999. p. 951–65.
8. Peters LC, Kristal MB, Komisaruk BR. Sensory innervation of the external and internal genitalia of the female rat. *Brain Res* 1987;**408**:199–204.
9. Berkley KJ, Robbins A, Sato Y. Functional differences between afferent fibers in the hypogastric and pelvic nerves innervating female reproductive organs in the rat. *J Neurophysiol* 1993;**69**:533–44.
10. Robbins A, Sato Y, Hotta H, Berkley KJ. Responses of hypogastric nerve afferent fibers to uterine distension in estrous or metestrous rats. *Neurosci Lett* 1990;**110**:82–5.
11. Sugiura Y, Terui N, Hosoya Y. Difference in distribution of central terminals between visceral and somatic unmyelinated (C) primary afferent fibers. *J Neurophysiol* 1989;**62**:834–40.
12. Pomeranz B, Wall PD, Weber WV. Cord cells responding to fine myelinated afferents from viscera, muscle and skin. *J Physiol Lond* 1968;**199**:511–32.
13. Berkley KJ, Hubscher CH, Wall PD. Neuronal responses to stimulation of the cervix, uterus, colon and skin in the rat spinal cord. *J Neurophysiol* 1993;**69**:545–56.
14. Melzack R, Wall PD. Pain mechanisms: a new theory. *Science* 1965;**150**:971–8.
15. Wall PD, Hubscher CH, Berkley KJ. Intraspinal modulation of neuronal responses to uterine and cervix stimulation in rat L1 and L6 dorsal horn. *Brain Res* 1993;**622**:71–8.
16. Berkley KJ, Hubscher CH. Are there separate central nervous system pathways for touch and pain? *Nature Med* 1995;**1**:766–73.
17. Berkley KJ, Hubscher CH. Visceral and somatic sensory tracts through the neuroaxis and their relation to pain: lessons from the rat female reproductive system. In: Gebhart GF, editor. *Visceral Pain, Progress in Pain Research and Management*, Vol. 5. Seattle: IASP Press, 1995. p. 195–216.
18. Hubscher CH, Berkley KJ. Responses of neurons in caudal solitary nucleus of female rats to stimulation of vagina, cervix, uterine horn and colon. *Brain Res* 1994;**664**:1–8.
19. Hubscher CH, Berkley KJ. Spinal and vagal influences on the responses of rat solitary nucleus neurons to stimulation of uterus, cervix and vagina. *Brain Res* 1995;**702**:251–4.
20. Marino J, Canedo A, Aguilar J. Sensorimotor cortical influences on cuneate nucleus rhythmic activity in the anesthetized cat. *Neuroscience* 2000;**95**:657–73.

21. Van Eden CG, Buijs RM Functional neuroanatomy of the prefrontal cortex: autonomic interactions. *Prog Brain Res* 2000;**126**:49–62.

22. Albe-Fessard D, Berkley KJ, Kruger L, Ralston HJ III, Willis WD Jr. Diencephalic mechanisms of pain sensation. *Brain Res Rev* 1985;**9**:217–96.

23. Berkley KJ, Scofield SL. Relays from the spinal cord and solitary nucleus through the parabrachial nucleus to the forebrain in the cat. *Brain Res* 1990;**529**:333–8.

24. Berkley KJ, Guilbaud G, Benoist J-M, Gautron M. Responses of neurons in and near the ventrobasal thalamic complex of the rat to stimulation of uterus, cervix, vagina, colon and skin. *J Neurophysiol* 1993;**69**:557–68.

25. Nathan PW. Pain traces left in the central nervous system. In: Keele CA, Smith R, editors. *The Assessment of Pain in Man and Animals*. Edinburgh: Livingstone, 1962. p. 129–34.

26. Nathan PW. Pain and nociception in the clinical context. *Philos Trans R Soc Lond B Biol Sci* 1985;**308**:219–26.

27. Lenz RA, Gracely RH, Hope EJ, Baker FH, Rowland LH, Dougherty PM, *et al.* The sensation of angina can be evoked by stimulation of the human thalamus. *Pain* 1994;**59**:119–26.

28. Deadwyler SA, Hampson ER. The significance of neural ensemble codes during behavior and cognition. *Ann Rev Neurosci* 1997;**20**:217–44.

29. Nicolelis MA, Fanselow EE, Ghazanfar AA. Hebb's dream: the resurgence of cell assemblies. *Neuron* 1997;**19**:219–21.

30. Fausto-Sterling A. *Sexing the Body*. New York: Basic Books; 2000.

31. Bateson P, Martin P. *Design for a Life*. London: Jonathan Cape; 1999.

32. Ghazanfar AA, Nicolelis MAL. The structure and function of dynamic cortical and thalamic receptive fields. *Cerebral Cortex* 2001;**11**:183–93.

33. Davis KD, Kwan CL, Crawley AP, Mikulis DJ. Functional MRI study of thalamic and cortical activations evoked by cutaneous heat, cold, and tactile stimuli. *J Neurophysiol* 1998;**80**:1533–46.

34. Ingvar M, Hseih J-C. The image of pain. In: Wall PD, Melzack R, editors. *Textbook of Pain*, 4th edn. Edinburgh: Churchill Livingstone; 1999. p. 215–34.

35. Gelnar PA, Krauss BR, Sheehe PR, Szeverenyi NM, Apkarian AV. A comparative fMRI study of cortical representations for thermal painful, vibrotactile, and motor performance tasks. *Neuroimage* 1999;**10**:460–82.

36. Apkarian AV. Functional magnetic resonance imaging of pain consciousness: cortical networks of pain critically depend on what is implied by 'pain'. *Curr Rev Pain* 1999;**3**:308–15.

37. Giamberardino MA, Berkley KJ, Iezzi S, deBigotina P, Vecchiet L. Pain threshold variations in somatic wall tissues as a function of menstrual cycle, segmental site and tissue depth in non-dysmenorrheic women, dysmenorrheic women and men. *Pain* 1997;**71**:187–97.

38. Ostensen M, Rugelsjoen A, Wigers SH. The effect of reproductive events and alterations of sex hormone levels on the symptoms of fibromyalgia. *Scand J Rheumatol* 1997;**26**:355–60.

39. Naliboff BD, Heitkemper MM, Chang L, Mayer EA. Sex and gender in irritable bowel syndrome. In: Fillingim R, editor. *Sex, Gender, and Pain: From the Benchtop to the Clinic*. Seattle: IASP Press, 2000. p. 327–54.

40. Holroyd KA, Lipchik GL. Sex differences in recurrent headache disorders: overview and significance. In: Fillingim R, editor. *Sex, Gender, and Pain: From the Benchtop to the Clinic*. Seattle: IASP Press; 2000. p. 251–79.

41. Kock NG, Pompeius R. Inhibition of vesical motor activity induced by anal stimulation. *Acta chir Scand* 1963;**126**:244–50.

42. McMahon SB. Sensory-motor integration in urinary bladder function. In: Cervero F, Morrison JFB, editors. *Visceral Sensation. Progress in Brain Research*, Vol. 67. Amsterdam: Elsevier Science Publishers; 1986. p. 245–53.

43. Bouvier M, Grimaud JC. Neuronally mediated interactions between urinary bladder and internal anal sphincter motility in the cat. *J Physiol Lond* 1984;**346**:461–9.

44. Bouvier M, Grimaud JC, Abysique A. Effects of stimulation of vesical afferents on colonic motility in cats. *Gastroenterology* 1990;**98**:1148–54.

45. Cheng C-L, Man C-P, deGroat WC. Effects of capsaicin on micturition and associated reflexes in rats. *Am J Physiol* 1993;**265**:R132–R138.

46. deGroat WC. Anatomy of the central neural pathways controlling the lower urinary tract. *Eur Neurol* 1998;**34** (Suppl.1):2–5.

47. Alagiri M, Chottiner S, Ratner V, Slade D, Hanno PM. Interstitial cystitis: unexplained associations with other chronic diseases and pain syndromes. *Urology* 1997;**49**(Suppl.5A):52–7.

48. Berkley KJ. Female pain versus male pain? In: Fillingim R, editor. *Sex, Gender, and Pain: From the Benchtop to the Clinic*. Seattle: IASP Press, 2000. p. 373–81.

49.   Bradley LA, Alarcón GS. Sex-related influences in fibromyalgia. In: Fillingim R, editor. *Sex, Gender, and Pain: From the Benchtop to the Clinic*. Seattle: IASP Press; 2000. p. 281–307.
50.   Giamberardino MA, Affaitati G, Lerza R, Vecchiet L, Berkley KJ. The impact of painful gynecological conditions on pain of urological origin. *Society for Neuroscience Abstracts* 1999;**25**:143.
51.   Giamberardino MA, Berkley KJ, Affaitati G, Lerza R, Vecchiet L. Influence of endometriosis on pain behaviors and muscle hyperalgesia induced by a ureteral calculosis in female rats (personal communication, with permission).
52.   Giamberardino MA, deLaurentis S, Affaitati G, Lerza R, Lapenna D, Vecchiet L. Modulation of pain and hyperalgesia from the urinary tract by algogenic conditions of the reproductive organs in women. *Neurosci Lett* 2001; **304**:61–4.
53.   Naliboff BD, Chang L, Munakata J, Mayer EA. Towards an integrative model of irritable bowel syndrome. *Prog Brain Res* 2000;**122**:413–23.

Chapter 4

General background to understanding pain
Discussion

Discussion following Dr Lees' paper

Sutton: Could you comment on the extraordinary physical resemblance between James Young Simpson and Lawson Tait?

Lees: I have seen Lawson Tait's portrait, which Robert Keller had in our department throughout the whole of his reign as Professor. I must say, I agree with you that they do bear a great resemblance. I showed what is purported to be James Young Simpson's young portrait, but I honestly do not think it is. In the College of Physicians in Edinburgh is another portrait that resembles James Young Simpson and I am not sure but I believe somebody made a mistake. Andrew Calder, our present Professor, has that original painting on his wall but I have put doubt in Andrew's mind. As far as Lawson Tait is concerned, I am sorry, I have nothing to add about the resemblance.

Sutton: It is just that Lawson Tait lived with James Young Simpson and used to assist him in a great number of his operations and many people believe that he was the illegitimate son of James Young Simpson. It is interesting because, at the time when Lawson Tait was born, there was no record of births in Scotland because of a feeling of antidisestablishmentarianism. Many people believe that he is the illegitimate son. I brought it up because the resemblance is absolutely amazing.

Lees: I am indebted to you for raising this. I know it is often said that Simpson had several illegitimate children but unfortunately I have not been able to pursue that in a more detailed way. Now that you have raised it I will look into it more closely.

Crowhurst: I wonder if you could tell me something to which I have not known the answer. When Queen Victoria gave birth to Prince Leopold in 1853, Snow gave her the chloroform on one of the Queen's own silk handkerchiefs, I understand, but was Simpson actually the obstetrician? He did have a royal appointment, did he not?

Lees: He was not the obstetrician at her delivery – Snow was that person. As you know, he was really an anaesthetist by that time. Of course, 'pukka' anaesthetists did not exist, but Snow was really in the vanguard of it all. The delivery of Victoria was easy: she was highly multiparous and there was nothing to it. I do not mean to offend the ladies present or to offend you as an anaesthetist, but I believe it was simple. The main feature of it is that it put the seal on the use of this as an anaesthetic agent. Before that there was such acrimony and the debate as to whether it was David Waldie – or was it Simpson? – still goes on. The obstetrician could have been anyone. It was not anything to which they attributed any value – as usually is the case.

Discussion following Dr Grace's paper

Foster: Speaking from the home of George Engel and the biopsychosocial model, I want to raise some questions about the practicality of the biocultural versus biopsychosocial models. I have had personal experience watching some of my colleagues who have been trained under the biopsychosocial model evaluate a patient on their first visit and take somewhere between an hour and a half and two hours. Generally it included a fairly non-directive interview where you had the patient draw out their own conclusions from their life's experiences. When it comes to pain, I believe that this type of model has some attractive qualities, but when it comes to the general clinical care of patients, even chronic pain patients, other than incorporating other individuals who have expertise in that area, would there be any recommendations in our training of medical students and residents in how they approach patients using a biocultural model in contrast to a biopsychosocial model?

Grace: It may be premature to try to think about ways in which the idea of a broader biocultural model might be implemented in clinical circumstances. The way I was presenting it was more a matter of thinking about it at the level of the broader paradigm of our understanding of chronic pain. That is not to say that I do not believe that in practical terms there are ways in which we could implement such a model, but a good deal of research and work would need to be done before the means to do so would become apparent.

I deliberately did not want to set up what I was saying so as to suggest that this model might be mutually exclusive of the others. There is certainly some really important work going on within the biopsychosocial model. It was more a matter of looking critically at some of the possible limitations or problems that are emerging there or some ways in which that model may not have fulfilled the promise that it originally appeared to have.

Beard: I entirely endorse Dr Grace's biocultural approach as a practical one because that is what you find with women who have had chronic pain for a very long time; there is an interaction between the biomedical and the biopsychosocial and you cannot short-cut that. There is a tendency, in gynaecology particularly, because we are all under so much pressure from the amount of time we have, to try to limit the length of consultation. However, with patients who have pelvic pain you really have to make them feel – and feel yourself – that time is not the issue. Certainly, with the interactive work that we have done between myself on the biomedical side and our counsellors, who are the biopsychosocial side, we have found that this type of evaluation may take anything up to two to three hours. I am afraid that you must take that long with people who have had pain for as long as these women have had.

Berkley: With respect to Dr Foster's question and your answer about how to apply things, don't you think that some of this is already under way? There have been two things recently. There was a wonderful study published in *Pain* about a year ago out of Israel.[1] This was an assessment of pain in an Israeli hospital on the edge of the Bedouin desert. They had Bedouin parturients and Israeli parturients but all the clinicians were Israeli. Both groups had to evaluate their pain and the women were all at 8.5 on a scale of 10. Then the clinicians evaluated the Bedouins and the Israelis. They evaluated the Israelis at 8.5 but they evaluated the Bedouins at about 4.5, I think. That is a direct set of data that speaks to the issue of cultural context.

The other set of studies dealt with how one could implement protocols that would help practitioners care for patients in different cultures. The studies were reviewed in the context of a labour ward.[2] I cannot remember who did it but the study was most impressive because they had little handbooks. First, you cannot assume that an individual is going to represent her culture, but these are some of the cultural norms you might want to anticipate for this group versus another group versus another group – things like whether it is good to drink water or not. Some cultures say 'yes, you should be hydrated', others say no. Pushing a woman to hydrate herself might be much more outrageous for one culture than another. In a sense, that kind of thing incorporates your model, does it not? It brings into the clinic some sort of background information that might be helpful and some kind of sensitivity to the fact that you may not be looking at patients in the same way. There must be other situations like this.

Grace: Possibly. The studies to which you are referring quite clearly show ways in which women from different cultural groups appear to report on and experience pain very differently. Indeed, it would be the case that the phenomenon of chronic pain is not necessarily a ubiquitous phenomenon. Certainly, that evidence is there in a number of different contexts.

In talking about the question of 'culture' in the biocultural model, it is important not only to characterise it in terms of what are obviously distinct differences between 'cultural' groups but rather more to be aware of the ways in which the values, the meanings, the understandings of embodiment of self, individuality and subjectivity and so on are different across a number of different contexts, and these may or may not differ within a particular cultural grouping. So it is not only referring to 'culture' in that narrower sense of 'cultural difference', but in the broader sense of values, meanings, understandings of the relationship between mind and body, the social meanings of illness and so on.

On the question of the extent to which this kind of model may be in practice already and be being incorporated into clinical applications already, I am not so sure about that. Certainly there will be instances where something that strikes one as being very obviously a particular cultural understanding will be taken into account in the doctor–patient interaction in the way in which understandings are conveyed and interpreted and understood. In terms of the deeper, more paradigmatic level of conceptualising pain and understanding pain, what it actually means, how it can be treated and so on, from the literature that I have read on chronic pelvic pain, which is all that I am able to comment on, I am not aware that that is the case. It was interesting to hear Professor Beard talking about the work that he is doing but I do not know the extent to which that is in the literature. Would it be right to say that if it is happening it is relatively recent?

Smith: In reply to that, as a psychotherapist working in a pelvic pain clinic, I can say that in pretty much all psychotherapy training we have specific modules on cultural issues and cultural differences. When we are working with women, as part of the assessment we are trained to look at all these issues and to be aware of cultural issues. In psychotherapy training it is pretty well embedded now to be aware that there are cultural differences, just as there are differences between the sexes and people's sexuality, to be aware of differences including cultural differences. Working in north London in the NHS we are constantly faced with a multicultural mix of clients, so it is very much integrated into the assessment process.

In reply to Dr Foster, I believe that it can be integrated into medical training about counselling skills and understanding of different cultures as part of the assessment process.

Newton-John: One final point on culture. We have been talking about patient culture. I wonder to what degree there is also 'clinician culture' in terms of understanding these issues. The idea is that the doctors in the clinic do the biomedical bit and then we allied health professions do the biopsychosocial bit. It seems to represent the dichotomy that Dr Grace talked about. Culture works in both directions.

Grace: It certainly does. The question that you raise is an important one to do with clinician culture as well. I think the 'biocultural model' is as relevant to clinicians' understandings as it is to patients' understanding. I believe that it would be a mistake to pick up on the 'cultural' aspect of David Morris's model purely in terms of ethnicity or cultural difference, but rather more to focus on the broader sets of understandings, which may vary considerably within one cultural grouping or on the other hand may be similar across cultural divisions. On the dichotomy you refer to and the way of bridging that gap, I do not know. For myself, as someone who does not have a natural science, medical background, I could see ways in which we could have a discussion across some pretty entrenched boundaries with respect to conceptualisations of pain. The more that those kinds of boundaries can be breached the better we will enable interdisciplinary understanding. So that rather than the way the biopsychosocial model tends to be constructed, with these discrete domains that remain separate and are then related in an 'additive' sense, we can envisage the prospect of some form of transformation of our understanding mutually by virtue of these kinds of conversations; that is the most productive potentially.

Discussion following Professor Berkley's paper

Collett: What do you think is going to be important with regard to the work that is going on concerning genetic differences between people in pain perception?

Berkley: Jeffrey Mogil, in Canada, is one of the prime players in this field. He has made an extraordinary career out of finding differences in different strains of rats in their nociception, in their responses to noxious stimuli. He has found genetic loci that might help explain some of these differences in responsiveness.[3] The main outcome measure he uses is the response to tail stimulation. He finds very different responses in the different groups, some of which are different between sexes. The group has also found sex differences and genetically linked sex differences in certain types of analgesic responses.

The testing that has been done has been done at a given moment in time so that you have a measure at one moment of a latency and intensity of some kind of behavioural measure. What happens over time? Do these statistical differences that show up between strains or specifically bred groups of animals show up under different circumstances? Jeff is clever enough to understand this and he realises that it may not hold up over time, as the animal develops a history of nociceptive information-inducing experiences over that animal's lifetime.

At the last Society for Neurosciences meeting they put together an extraordinary study. A very clever MD PhD student of his found this industrial strength, literally cross-correlation type of statistical analysis program that is used for analysis in industry of various kinds of outcomes and put it to work against the data that Dr Mogil had collected for the last six to eight years with the same output measure.[4] He had about 100 000 data points on this tail response and he could look across for the sources of variance in this from time of year, sex, age of the animal, experimenter and strain of the animal. The answer? The biggest source of variance – 100% – was the experimenter who was testing the animal.

These sorts of data do not throw out the genetic approach but they indicate that we are not born with different nociceptor sensitivities. They may change over time, and are in the eye of the beholder. Jeff Mogil's whole career has been spent developing this genetic idea, yet he understands very well and has taken it to heart.

Steege: I just had the fascinating experience of spending a day with our mutual friend and colleague, John Slocomb in Colorado. He and I have been friends for years and yet have differed dramatically in how we think about pain. We had the experience of examining the same six patients in the course of a day. Then I learned first-hand the role of the experimenter in interpreting the data coming in. We were hearing the same histories and doing the same examination two minutes apart and yet arriving at rather different conclusions.

Berkley: That is astonishing. Did you come up with the same treatment strategies? [No.] That is really scary. But, although it is a terrible thing to say, there is more than one way to skin a cat. What the data from the brain work suggest, not only in the field of how does the brain make pain but also how does the brain create perception in general in the sense of oneself in general, is that there is not necessarily one right way to produce pain. You may be just as right or wrong as John Slocomb. So there is hope in that.

On your first comment about treating one organ to affect what seems to be a problem from another organ: that is very real. You may see someone with severe dysmenorrhoea and you find a subclinical bladder problem. You treat the bladder problem and the dysmenorrhoea goes away. That is a possibility to keep in the back of one's mind.

References

1.   Sheiner EK, Sheiner E, Shoham-Vardi I, Mazor M, Katz M. Ethnic differences influence care giver's estimates of pain during labour. *Pain* 1999;**81**:299–305.
2.   Weber SE. Cultural aspects of pain in childbearing women. *J Obstet Gynecol Neonatal Nurs* 1996;**25**:67–72.
3.   Mogil JS, Yu L, Basbaum AI. Pain genes? Natural variation and transgenic mutants. *Annu Rev Neurosci* 2000;**23**:777–811.
4.   Chesler EJ, Wilson SG, Lariviere WR, Mogil JS. Something in the air: laboratory environment interactions with organismic influences on thermal nociception. *Soc Neurosci Abstr* 2000;**26**:1141.

SECTION 2

PAIN AND PAIN RELIEF

Chapter 5

The pharmacology of pain and analgesia

Alain Li Wan Po and Wei Ya Zhang

Introduction

Pain is one of the most common symptoms of disease and it is not surprising that analgesic agents are among the most widely prescribed drugs. Despite the development of a whole array of novel analgesic agents, pain is often intractable and frustrating to control for both patient and carer. However, this again is understandable because pain is such an important protective mechanism for alerting the body to noxious stimuli that blocking one pain pathway leads to the predominance of another. Thankfully, however, in the majority of cases, pain can be adequately controlled and often completely cleared with the wide range of analgesic agents available. Understanding the pharmacology of pain and analgesia provides a basis for the rational prescribing of analgesic agents and optimum pain relief. The objectives of this chapter are (i) to provide a broad overview of the pharmacology of the well-established analgesics in the light of new research and historical hindsight, (ii) to discuss novel targets for analgesics, and (iii) to look into the future with respect to potential new analgesics.

Pain mechanisms

Sensory fibres which carry pain-inducing signals from the skin and internal tissues to the spinal cord are of two kinds: (i) myelinated Aδ fibres, with conduction velocities in the range 5–30 m/s and (ii) smaller unmyelinated C fibres, 0.2–2.0 m/s. Most of the latter are polymodal nociceptors, which respond to a wide range of stimuli. The C fibres are themselves subdivisible into those that express receptors for glial cell-line-derived neurotrophic factor (GDNF) and which terminate deep in the substantia gelatinosa of the spinal cord and those that terminate in the dorsal horn and synthesise peptides such as substance P and express the nerve growth factor (NGF) receptor. The free nerve endings of the Aδ fibres act as receptors which respond to intense pressure and heat, while those of the C fibres respond to chemical stimuli. Irrespective of the stimuli, the pain receptors become more sensitive in the presence of prostaglandins.

Repetitive firing enhances the response to a given noxious (hyperalgesia) or normally innocuous (allodynia, touch-evoked pain) stimulus.[1,2] The types of signals conveyed by the different fibres and the normal and pathological responses usually associated with them are shown in Figure 5.1. Pain fibres from the viscera and from the skin may synapse with the same second-order neurons and in such instances, pain from one location (e.g. viscera) may be perceived as originating from another region (e.g. skin) and is said to be referred pain.

Aδ and C fibres enter the spinal cord via the dorsal root to synapse with second-order neurons in the dorsal horn. The axons of the second-order neurons ascend to the brain as the spinothalamic tract. Impulse traffic along the tract is modulated by descending projections which terminate at spinal segmental interneurons or at the synapse between the first- and second-order neurons (Figure 5.1).

Types of pain

Pain is often classified as transient, acute or chronic. Transient pain is in response to activation of the pain receptors in the absence of tissue damage. This provides an

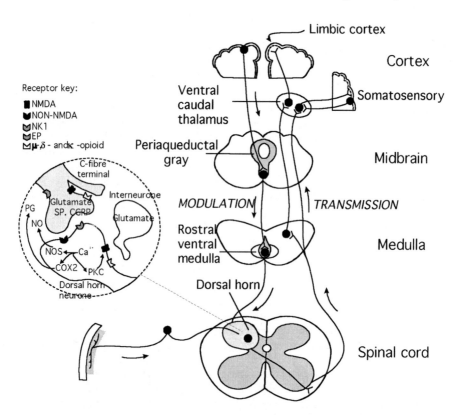

Figure 5.1.   Pain transmission and modulation and potential sites of action of analgesic compounds

alerting mechanism for the body to avoid injury. Acute pain follows tissue injury, which may alter the response of the nociceptors, their central connections and the autonomic system in the region. The pain resolves spontaneously and usually before complete spontaneous healing of the causative injury occurs. Chronic pain is usually triggered by an injury or disease but is perpetuated by other factors. The ability of the central nervous system to change function (plasticity) in response to tissue or nerve damage provides a challenge to both clinician and investigator. Analgesics usually provide relief for acute pain but are often inadequate for chronic pain.

Pharmacological interventions

The pain sensation may be reduced or abolished pharmacologically by:

- Lowering the sensitivity of the pain receptors (e.g. mild analgesics and local anaesthetic agents)

- Interrupting nociceptive signals in sensory nerves (e.g. opioids, local anaesthetics)

- Suppressing transmission of nociceptive impulses in the spinal cord (e.g. opioids)

- Altering the emotional response to pain (e.g. anxiolytic agents and tricyclic antidepressants).

Analgesics

The opium poppy (*Papaver somniferum*) was probably the first truly effective analgesic to be discovered and it, of course, remains in the form of morphine, the analgesic *par excellence* for severe pain in terminal diseases. Accounts of the drug can be found in ancient Egyptian, Greek and Roman documents. Three centuries ago, John Jones (1645–1709),[3,4] gave a detailed account of the effects of the herb. In particular, he described vividly the 'most agreeable, pleasant and charming sensation…like a most delicious and extraordinary refreshment of the spirits…a pleasant ovation of the spirits, serenity, etc. as we find after a competent measure of generous wine *ad hilaritatem*', from taking moderate doses of the drug. He was also careful to report that after a period of heavy opium use, 'great and intolerable distresses, anxieties and depressions of spirits, which in a few days commonly end in a most miserable death, attended with strange agonies, unless men return to the use of opium, which soon raises them again, and certainly restores them'.

Morphine, the active ingredient of opium, was isolated by Friedrich Sertürner, a German pharmacist, in 1805.[5-7] His work led to the identification and isolation of a whole host of plant alkaloids, which were to revolutionise the practice of therapeutics and lay the foundation of modern pharmacology. With the widespread use of morphine and opium, it soon became clear that the problems highlighted by John Jones (mood elevation followed by depression and leading to addiction) meant that opium and morphine, were not ideal for chronic use. The narrow therapeutic index (safe and effective dose range) of morphine, was also highlighted by both Jones[3] and Sertürner.[6]

Elucidation of the mode of action of morphine began with the suggestion that specific opiate receptors existed (Table 5.1). This led to the identification of opiate receptors[8] and of an endogenous compound in the brain, which acted as an agonist at those sites.[9,10] This led to the identification of enkephalin[10] and subsequently to three main types of opioid receptors (δ (DOR or OP_1), κ (KOR or OP_2) and μ (MOR or OP_3) and other endogenous ligands[11] (enkephalins for the δ receptor and dynorphins for the κ receptor). Morphine has a preference for the μ receptor. Morphine analgesia is preserved in mice deficient in KOR and DOR genes[12] and it appears that the respiratory depression associated with morphine is also mediated through the μ receptor.[13] Morphine withdrawal is abolished in MOR-deficient mice and attenuated in KOR-deficient mice.[13] These findings suggest that while some selectivity can be achieved to separate the beneficial effects from the adverse effects of morphine, complete separation is unlikely.

The opioid receptors are distributed widely in the central nervous system. Work in the late 1990s suggests that opioid-like receptors are also found in peripheral tissues and these receptors contribute to the analgesic effects of morphine.[14] Although the clinical value of this peripheral action is still being debated[15] there is increasing evidence that it may be important in inflamed tissues. Opioid-containing immune cells migrate preferentially to inflamed sites to release β-endorphin for pain relief. This recruitment is thought to be initially selectin-mediated and anti-selectin treatment abolishes the peripheral opioid analgesia.[16]

The full complexities of morphine analgesia and of the endogenous opioid system are still being unravelled with the help of new animal pain models and novel biotechnological techniques. The participation of the opioid system in the mechanism of action of nonopioid agents and in the placebo effect have for example yielded many surprises (see below). Within the spinal cord, the release of peptides and glutamate causes activation of a whole array of receptors. These act in concert to induce a state of spinal hypersensitivity. Three broad classes of glutamate receptors are known: metabotropic receptors, N-methyl-D-aspartate (NDMA) and α-amino-3-hydroxy-5-methyl-isoxazolepropionic acid (AMPA) receptors. It is the NDMA receptor that has attracted most attention in pain research. Ketamine blocks the NDMA receptor but its nonselectivity leads to adverse psychomimetic effects which limit its clinical use and the search is on for more selective agents.

Table 5.1.   Some highlights of research on morphine pharmacology

1973	Identification of stereoselective morphine receptors Pert C, Snyder SH, 1973[8]
1975	Identification of endogenous ligands for opioid receptors Hughes J et al., 1975[10]
1980	Identification of three major subtypes of opioid receptors (δ,κ and μ) Kosterlitz HW, Paterson SJ, 1980[11]
1994	Opioid receptor-like receptor identified Mollereau C et al., 1994[49]
1995	New endogenous opioid peptide identified (Orphanin FQ or nociceptin) Meunier JC et al., 1995[50] and Reinscheid RK et al., 1995[51]
1996	Demonstration that analgesic and addictive effects of morphine largely mediated through the μ receptor Matthes HWD et al., 1996[13]
1998	Identification of nocistatin, an endogenous peptide which may play a role opposite to nociceptin in pain transmission Okuda-Ashitaka et al., 1998[52]

The duality of drug action

As with ketamine, morphine illustrates well the trade-off that needs to be made in relation to the benefits and harm which follow the use of therapeutic agents. Recognition of this duality of drug action and the development of novel methods of chemical synthesis led to attempts over a century ago to develop synthetic drugs with more favourable benefit–risk profiles than morphine. The semi-synthetic diacetyl ester of morphine, branded as Heroin, was introduced in 1898, as such a compound by Friedrich Bayer and Company of Germany. As history would tell us, that claim was highly optimistic. Although without heroin, palliative care physicians would be deprived of one of the most useful drugs, heroin addiction remains a major problem for society at large. Fear of patients becoming addicted to the opiates led to widespread suboptimal use of the opiates, even in situations where dependency was not a problem, as in the management of terminal cancer pain. Work on developing opioids with improved selectivity of action through selectivity of effect on opioid receptors, as described above, continues. The following discussions will show that the development of new analgesics, centring on improving the clinical profiles of lead analgesic compounds to increase efficacy and reduce adverse effects, has also been applied to other analgesic compounds. In essence, much of drug development centres on separating the dose–response curves for beneficial and adverse effects through structural modification of a lead compound (Figure 5.2).

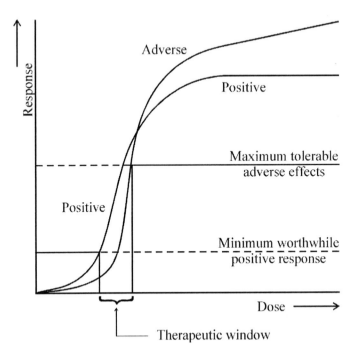

Figure 5.2. Example of dose–response curve for beneficial and adverse effects

Different analgesics

It is still common to classify analgesics as minor (mild) analgesics and major (potent) analgesics. With the development of a whole host of newer analgesics and better definition of the profile of the older analgesics, this classification is less helpful than it first appears. For example, the opioids, which are highly effective in nociceptive pain, are less so in neuropathic pain with little associated inflammation. Hybrid classification systems are therefore more often used.

Aspirin and the salicylates

The history of aspirin should perhaps start with the willow bark (*Salix* spp., particularly *S. fragilis*; Salicacea), used by Hippocrates for women giving birth, described by Galen as an antipyretic and anti-inflammatory,[17] and promoted by Dodoens in 1595 as an analgesic.[18] Interest in the tree was renewed as a result of the Reverend Edward Stone's suggestion[19] that it was a possible substitute for the expensive Cinchona bark (source of quinine) for treating patients with malarial fever (agues). His suggestion was based on the fact that willow bark was as bitter as Cinchona and it grew well in marshland where agues abounded (application of the doctrine of signatures). The bark's bitter taste was used as a surrogate measure for potency of different species of the willow bark.[20,21]

The active ingredient, salicin, was isolated from the willow bark in 1826[22] and subsequently from species of the meadowsweet (*Filipendula ulmaria*, previously known as *Spirea ulmaria,* Rosaceae). The drug was used as an officially recognised antipyretic and analgesic for over 100 years thereafter.[23] Recognition that salicin was converted to salicylic acid when exposed to air and following ingestion led to the latter's clinical evaluation, not only as an antipyretic but also as a substitute for phenol. It was argued that salicylic acid would be less toxic to tissues on the erroneous postulate that it would act as a slow-release form of phenol.[20,24] Widespread use of salicylic acid, as an internal antiseptic, soon followed. Its use in typhoid led to confirmation of its antipyretic activity, which was also shown in rheumatic fever and rheumatoid arthritis. The large doses required for the latter, soon led to recognition of salicylic acid's adverse gastrointestinal effects. Aspirin, first synthesised in 1853, was identified as a potential candidate by the pharmaceutical division of the Bayer company. The head of the pharmacology division thought that the drug might be cardiotoxic and rejected it. Independent testing rescued the drug,[24] which went on to become the most widely used drug until being overtaken by paracetamol.

Nitric oxide, which is involved in numerous biological functions, exerts a gastro-protective effect and nitro-aspirin derivatives, which act as nitric oxide donors, are being developed as safer alternatives to the parent drug.[25]

Paracetamol

Paracetamol (acetaminophen) was the result of a search for an antipyretic superior to phenacetin and safer than aspirin. The drug was discarded following first investigations in 1893 because of the mistaken belief that it caused methaemoglobinaemia. Luckily, subsequent workers showed that phenacetin was rapidly metabolised to paracetamol and was an effective analgesic.[26] Paracetamol was first marketed in 1953 as being safer for children and those with gastric ulcers than aspirin. These claims have stood the test of time, particularly in the light of the association of aspirin with Reye's syndrome in the paediatric population. Despite the long history of use of paracetamol, its mechanism of action is still largely unknown, although there is increasing evidence that central mechanisms are important.[27] The endogenous opioid pathway seems to be involved and there may be synergism between effects at spinal and supraspinal sites.[28]

Ibuprofen

The discovery of ibuprofen was a major development in the history of analgesic drug development. It resulted from a search for an alternative to corticosteroids, which was also more effective and safer than aspirin in the high doses required for the treatment of rheumatoid arthritis. Ibufenac was one of the more promising agents to emerge from modification of the aspirin molecule but it was unfortunately found to be hepatotoxic. Luckily work persisted on other phenylalkanoic acids and ibuprofen emerged as an effective and relatively safe analgesic and antipyretic (Figure 5.3).[29,30] Today, ibuprofen is the third most widely prescribed analgesic in the world. In dysmenorrhoea it is probably the best drug available to date.[31]

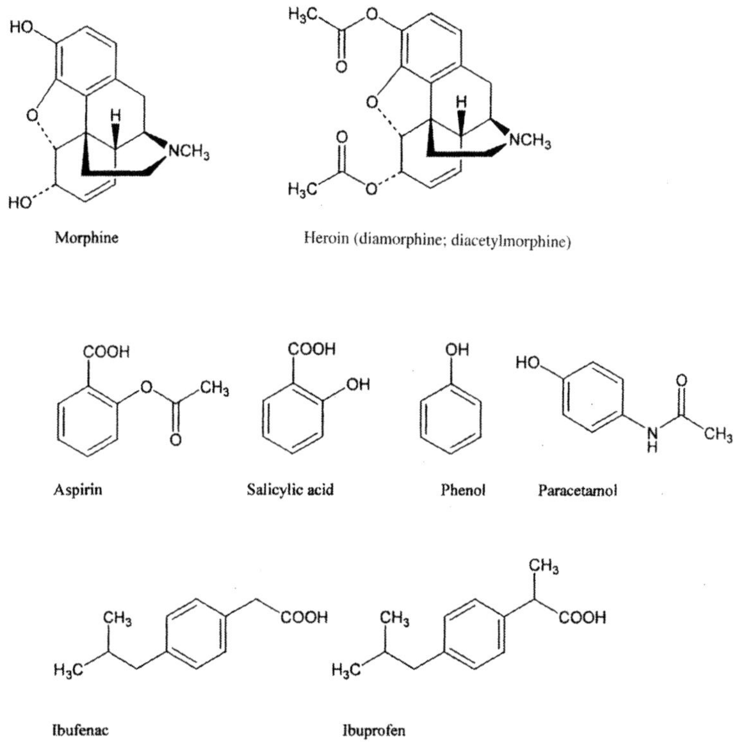

Morphine

Heroin (diamorphine; diacetylmorphine)

Aspirin

Salicylic acid

Phenol

Paracetamol

Ibufenac

Ibuprofen

Figure 5.3. Structures of selected analgesic compounds

Aspirin and other nonsteroidal anti-inflammatory drugs (NSAIDs) such as ibuprofen exert their anti-inflammatory and analgesic effects by inhibiting cyclo-oxygenase (COX) and hence prostaglandin formation.[32] Two isoforms of COX have been identified, a constitutive (COX-1) and an inducible (COX-2) form. Much of the early development work aimed at developing better alternatives to ibuprofen has focused on eliminating its adverse gastrointestinal adverse effects. Although more than 20 similar compounds have since reached the market, none had any better gastrointestinal safety profile[33] until the introduction of the highly selective COX-2 inhibitors, celecoxib and rofecoxib. Two large-scale studies[34,35] have shown that the risk of serious gastrointestinal adverse effects is approximately halved when compared with non-selective NSAIDs. However, this effect disappears in patients receiving concomitant aspirin for cardiovascular protection.[34] Despite rapid uptake of the highly selective COX-2 inhibitors by clinicians, doubt continues about their true value and, as is often the case, those agents would appear not to be as useful as claimed by the manufacturers.[36]

Novel therapeutic targets

Clearly, a better understanding of pain mechanisms and the development of new animal models for investigating analgesic effects have contributed substantially to the development of new analgesic agents. Furthermore, a number of agents, including some that are well-established, are undergoing structure–activity optimisation in the light of newly recognised molecular targets (Table 5.2).

Table 5.2. Potential targets for new analgesic agents

1.	Glutamate receptor antagonists at
	(i) N-Methyl-D-Aspartate (NMDA)/Glycine receptor
	(ii) α-amino-3-hydroxy-5-methyl-isoxazolepropionic acid (AMPA)/Kainate receptor
2.	Newer opioids
	(i) Selective δ or κ agonists
	(ii) Aminopeptidase and endopeptidase inhibitors
3.	Vanilloid-gated ion channel agonists
4.	NK$_1$ (Substance P) receptor antagonists
5.	Cannabinoids
6.	Selective α-2 adrenergic receptor agonists
7.	5-HT$_1$ agonists
8.	Nitric oxide (NO)
	(i) NO synthetase inhibitors
	(ii) NO donors
9.	Neuronal calcium-channel blockers
10.	Acetylcholine nicotinic acid receptor agonists
11.	Purinergic derivatives
	A1 adenosine receptor agonists
	Adenosine kinase inhibitors
12.	Sodium channel blockers
13.	Cytokine inhibitors
14.	Purinergic P2X3 receptor antagonists

Vanniloid receptor agonists

Capsaicin, the 'hot' component of chillies, has been used in pain-relieving balms for a long time. The traditional explanation for its action has been that of counter-irritancy and details of capsaicin's basic mechanism of action are still being unravelled. Capsaicin has a biphasic action on sensory C fibres. An initial burning sensation is followed by a more prolonged antinociception, possible due to depletion of substance P. Excitation of the primary afferents, by binding of capsaicin to a specific receptor (VR1 or vanilloid receptor 1), is followed by desensitisation of the neurons. The major site of action appears to be in the spinal cord. The pungency and bronchoconstrictive activity of capsaicin appear to be separable from its antinociceptive effects, as is evidenced by the availability of antinociceptive capsaicin analogues with reduced pungency and little bronchoconstrictive activity.[37] To date, use of capsaicin and capsaicin analogues is limited to topical applications for relieving non-specific muscular pain or post-herpetic neuralgia.

NK_1 (substance P) receptor

Substance P is found in abundance in the central nervous system and animal experiments show that antagonists block behavioural responses to noxious stimuli and should reduce pain.[37,38] However, clinical trials in humans have been disappointing. The results suggest that NK_1 receptor antagonists are more likely to be useful as adjuvants to other analgesic compounds than as analgesics in their own right.[39]

The endocannabinoid system

The discovery of cannabinoid receptors is relatively recent[40,41] and two types of cannabinoid receptors have been identified, CB_1 and CB_2. Although CB_1 receptors are found on peripheral neurons and in non-neuronal tissues, they are in particular abundance within the central nervous system. CB_2 receptors occur mainly in immune cells, possibly participating in immunosuppression. However, both CB_1- and CB_2-like receptors are found outside the central nervous system. Endogenous cannabinoid receptor agonists, anandamide and 2-arachidonyl glycerol, synthesised by neurons, activate CB_1 receptors to induce antinociception to both acute and tonic pain. Palmitylethanolamide, released together with anandamide and formed from a common phospholipid precursor, activate peripheral CB_2-like receptors. The CB_1 and CB_2 endogenous ligands act synergistically to reduce pain responses.[42] CB_1 receptors also show a high degree of co-expression with vanilloid (VR1) receptors in neurons and may provide an anatomical basis for the marked combination of VR1-mediated excitation and CB_1-mediated inhibition of nociceptive responses.[43] The precise value of the cannabinoids in clinical pain has yet to be defined.

α_2 adrenoceptor agonists

Clonidine is an α_2 adrenoceptor agonist with a long history of use as an antihypertensive and antimigraine agent. Systemic administration leads to undesirable adverse effects, including sedation and hypotension, making local administration the only clinically useful way of administering the drug. Epidural administration leads to an analgesic action through excitation of receptors located in the dorsal horn of the spinal cord. Although clonidine is considered to be of value as an adjunctive analgesic for severe pain not adequately controlled by morphine or local anaesthetic agents, its clinical applications appear limited and its use is largely experimental so far.[44]

5-HT$_1$ receptor agonists

While the overall mechanism of action of antimigraine drugs is still unclear, the importance of 5-HT$_1$ receptors in causing the syndrome is beyond doubt. Selective 5-HT$_1$ receptor agonists are effective in relieving migraine headache as well as the associated symptoms, including photophobia and nausea. Agents that act at both central and peripheral sites within the trigemino-vascular system, are available but the extent to which centrally acting agents differ from peripherally acting agents is still unclear.[45,46]

Variability in response to analgesics

It is widely accepted that there is wide variation in human response to drugs and this appears to be particularly marked for analgesics. The classical explanation for such variability in drug effects is variation in physiological function arising from genetic and environmental influences as well as from the presence of disease and age-related immaturity in infancy or decay in old age. Indeed, even gender differences in response to κ opioids have been reported.[47] These changes lead to changes in the pharmacokinetics and pharmacodynamics of the drugs and hence to changes in drug effects. The importance of environmental influences is typified, for example, by liver metabolic enzyme inhibition by dietary components such as grapefruit. Over recent years there has been accumulating evidence for non-specific activation of endogenous opioids accounting for some of the response variability to analgesics.[48] In particular, the placebo response and variability in analgesic response to ketorolac was reduced by naloxone injection.[48] These intriguing results re-emphasise the importance of the endogenous opioid system in the experience of pain. The full intricacies of this system and its interactions with other neurotransmitter systems have yet to be fully defined. Moreover another opioid-like receptor system, which participates in the central modulation of pain, has recently been identified. Its natural ligand, orphanin FQ or nociceptin, appears to participate in pain modulation but not respiratory depression.[49-53] This opens up a new avenue for designing selective antagonists with fewer adverse effects than existing compounds.

Conclusion

There has been much effort put into the design of increasingly selective agonists or antagonists at receptors located both within the central nervous system and in peripheral tissues, to control pain. It is perhaps paradoxical that the emerging evidence suggests that for pain control, receptor-selectivity is unlikely to lead to the magic bullet that is sought by both clinician and patient. Perhaps the value of morphine is that it is nonselective and can therefore interrupt several pathways, which lead to the experience of pain, at the same time. It may well be possible that in future combinations of highly selective agents would produce optimum analgesic cocktails. Until then, for chronic pain and for pain associated with symptom clusters, as is often the case in gynaecological conditions, treatment will in many cases continue to involve much trial and error.

References

1. Lullmann H, Mohr K, Ziegler A. *Colour Atlas of Pharmacology*. Stuttgart: Thieme Publishing Group; 2000.
2. Katzung K. *Basic and Applied Pharmacology*. New York: Appleton and Lange; 2000.
3. Jones J. *The Mysteries of Opium Reveal'd*. London: Richard Smith at Angel and Bible without Temple-Bar; 1700.
4. Miller RJ, Tran PB. More mysteries of opium reveal'd: 300 years of opiates. *Trends Pharmacol Sci* 2000;**21**:299–304.
5. Sertürner FW. *Trommsdorff's Journal der Pharmacie* 1805;**13**:234.
6. Sertürner FW. *Gilbert's Annalen der Physik* 1817;**55**:56.
7. Casey AF, Parfitt RT. *Opioid Analgesics: Chemistry and Receptors*. New York: Plenum Press; 1986.
8. Pert CB, Snyder SH. Opiate receptor: demonstration in nervous tissue. *Science* 1973;**179**:1011–14.
9. Terenius L, Wahlström A. Inhibitor(s) of narcotic receptor binding in brain extracts and cerebrospinal fluid. *Acta Pharmac Tox* 1974;**35**(Suppl.1);55.
10. Hughes J, Smith TW, Kosterlitz HW, Fothergill LA, Morgan BA, Morris HR. Identification of two related pentapeptides from the brain with potent opiate agonist activity. *Nature* 1975;**258**(5536):577–80.
11. Kosterlitz HW, Paterson SJ. Characterization of opioid receptors in nervous tissue. *Proc R Soc Lond B Biol Sci* 1980;**210**(1178):113–22.
12. Kieffer BL. Opioids: first lessons from knockout mice. *Trends Pharmacol Sci* 1999;**20**:19–26.
13. Matthes HW, Maldonado R, Simonin F, Valverde O, Slowe S, Kitchen I, et al. Loss of morphine-induced analgesia, reward effect and withdrawal symptoms in mice lacking the mu-opioid-receptor gene. *Nature* 1996;**383**(6603):819–23.
14. Stein C, Yassouridis A. Peripheral morphine analgesia. *Pain* 1997;**71**:119–21.
15. Picard PR, Tramer MR, McQuay HJ, Moore RA. Analgesic efficacy of peripheral opioids (all except intra-articular): a qualitative systematic review. *Pain* 1997;**72**:309–18.
16. Machelska H, Cabot PJ, Mousa SA, Zhanf Q, Stein C. Pain control in inflammation governed by selectins. *Nature Med* 1998;**4**:1425–8.
17. Gross M, Greenberg LA. *The Salicylates. A Critical Bibliographic Review. Monographs of the Institute for the Study of Analgesic and Sedative Drugs*, no. 2. New Haven: Hillhouse Press; 1948.
18. Dodoens R. *A New Herbal or History of Plants*, translated by H Lyte; 1595.
19. Stone E. *Philos Trans R Soc London* 1763;**53**:195.
20. Sneader W. *Drug Prototypes and Their Exploitation*. Chichester: John Wiley & Sons; 1998.
21. James S. *Observations on the Bark of a Particular Species of Willow*. London: J. Johnson; 1792.
22. Mueller RL, Scheidt S. History of drugs for thrombotic disease. Discovery, development, and directions for the future. *Circulation* 1994;**89**:432–49.
23. Martindale. *The Extra Pharmacopoeia*, 23rd edn. London: The Pharmaceutical Press; 1952.
24. Kolbe H. *Arch Pharm* 1874;**5**:445.
24. Mann CC, Plummer ML. *The Aspirin Wars*. Boston: Harvard Business School Press; 1991.
25. Del Sodato P, Sorrentino R, Pinto A. NO-aspirins: a class of new anti-inflammatory and antithrombotic agents. *Trends Pharmacol Sci* 1999;**20**:319–23.
26. Flinn FB, Brodie BB. The effect on the pain threshold of N-acetyl-p-aminophenol, a product derived in the body from acetanilide. *J Pharmacol Exp Therap* 1948;**94**:76–7.
27. Björkman R. Central antinociceptive effects of non-steroidal anti-inflammatory drugs and paracetamol. *Acta Anaesthesiol Scand* 1995;**39**(Suppl.103):2–44.

28.   Raffa B, Stone DJ, Tallarida RJ. Discovery of 'self-synergistic' spinal/supraspinal antinociception produced by acetaminophen (paracetamol). *J Pharmacol Exp Ther* 2000;**295**:291–4.
29.   Nicholson JS. Ibuprofen. In: Bindra JS, Ledimicer D, editors. *Chronicles of Drug Discovery*. New York: John Wiley & Sons; 1982, p. 149–72.
30.   Nicholson J, Adams SS. *Ibuprofen.* British Patent No 971 700 to Boots Pure Drug Company; 1964.
31.   Li Wan Po, Zhang WY. Efficacy of minor analgesics in primary dysmenorrhoea: a systematic review. In: O'Brien S, Cameron I, MacLean A, editors. *Disorders of the Menstrual Cycle*. London: RCOG Press; 2000. p. 260–74.
32.   Ferreira SH. Prostaglandins, aspirin-like drugs and analgesia. *Nature New Biology* 1972;**240**:200–203.
33.   Henry D, Lim L L-Y, Garcia Rodriguez LA, *et al.* Variability in risk of gastrointestinal complications with individual non-steroidal anti-inflammatory drugs: results of a collaborative meta-analysis. *BMJ* 1996;**312**:1563–66.
34.   Silverstein FE, Faich G, Goldstein JL *et al.* Gastrointestinal toxicity with celecoxib vs nonsteroidal anti- inflammatory drugs for osteoarthritis and rheumatoid arthritis: the CLASS study: a randomized controlled trial. Celecoxib Long-term Arthritis Safety Study. *JAMA* 2000;**284**:1247–55.
35.   Bombardier C, Laine L, Reicin A, *et al.* Comparison of upper gastrointestinal toxicity of rofecoxib and naproxen in patients with rheumatoid arthritis. *N Engl J Med* 2000;**343**:1520–28.
36.   Anonymous. Rofécoxib. Un antalgique AINS décevant. *La Revue Préscrire* 2000;**208**:483–5.
37.   Caterina MJ, Schumacher MA, Tominaga M, Rosen TA, Levine JD, Julius D. The capsaicin receptor: a heat-activated ion channel in the pain pathway. *Nature* 1997;**389**:816–24.
38.   Urban L, Cambell EA, Panesar M *et al. In vivo* pharmacology of SDZ 249-665, a novel non-pungent capsaicin analogue. *Pain* 2000;**89**:65–74.
39.   Hill R. NK1 (substance P) receptor antagonists – why are they not analgesic in humans? *Trends Pharmacol Sci* 2000;**21**:244–6.
40.   Mailleux R, Vanderhaeghen JJ. Distribution of neuronal cannabinoid receptor in the adult rat brain: a comparative receptor binding radioautography and *in situ* hybridisation histochemistry. *Neuroscience* 1992;**48**:655–68.
41.   Pertwee RG. Cannabinoid receptors and pain. *Progr Neurobiol* 2001;**63**:569–611.
42.   Calignano A. La Rana G, Gluffrida A, Piomelli D. Control of pain initiation by endogenous cannabinoids. *Nature* 1998;**394**:277–80.
43.   Ahluwalia J, Urban L, Capogna M, Bevan S, Nagy I. Cannabinoid 1 receptors are expressed in nociceptive primary sensory neurons. *Neuroscience* 2000;**100**:685–8.
44.   Patel SS, Dunn CJ, Bryson HM. Epidural clonidine. A review of its pharmacology and efficacy in the management of pain during labour and postoperative and intractable pain. *CNS Drugs* 1996;**6**:474–97.
45.   Ferrari MD, Saxena PR. 5-HT$_1$ receptors in migraine pathology and treatment. *Europ Neurol* 1995;**2**:5–21.
46.   Bateman DN. Triptans and migraine. *Lancet* 2000;**355**:860–61.
47.   Gear RW, Miaskowski C, Gordon NC, Paul SM, Heller PH, Levine JD. Kappa-opioids produce significantly greater analgesia in women than in men. *Nature Med* 1998;**2**:1248–50.
48.   Amazio M, Pollo A, Maggi G, Benedetti F. Response variability to analgesics: a role for non-specific activation of endogenous opioids. *Pain* 2001;**90**:205–15.
49.   Mollereau C *et al.* ORL1, a novel member of the opioid receptor family: cloning, functional expression and localisation. *FEBS Lett* 1994;**343**:42–6.
50.   Meunier JC *et al.* Isolation and structure of the endogenous agonist of opioid receptor-like ORL$_1$ receptor. *Nature* 1995;**377**:532–5.
51.   Reinscheid RK. Orphanin FQ: a neuropeptide that activates an opioid-like G protein-coupled receptor. *Science* 1995;**270**:792–4.
52.   Okuda-Ashitaka E, Minami T, Tachibana S, *et al.* Nocistatin, a peptide that blocks nociceptin action in pain transmission. *Nature* 1998;**392**:286–9.
53.   Breyer MD, Jacobsen HR, Breyer RM. Functional and molecular aspects of renal prostaglandin receptors. *J Am Soc Nephrol* 1996;**7**:8–17.

Chapter 6

The psychology of pain

Toby Newton-John

Introduction

There has long been an awareness of the role of psychological processes in the experience of pain.[1] The ancient use of plants and herbs with no pharmacological value as placebo analgesics, the use of rhythmic drumming and chanting to induce an hypnotic state and the practice of 'pointing the bone' in Aboriginal culture to create intense feelings of pain and discomfort[2] all demonstrate the close interrelationship between psychology and pain. The aim of this chapter is to present a brief overview of contemporary research investigating the influence of psychological variables on pain, both in acute and chronic pain contexts, and to relate this research to particular issues of women's health. Two types of gynaecological pain disorder, vulvodynia and chronic pelvic pain, will be discussed and suggestions for the clinical management of these disorders will be made.

Pain theories

Prior to 1965, much of the medical discourse concerning pain and psychology was based on 17th-century theory. In 1664, the French philosopher René Descartes had proposed that there was a linear relationship between the intensity of a painful stimulus and the amount of observable tissue damage. Massive damage would result in great pain, and minor trauma would lead to minimal discomfort. A report of pain in the absence of tissue damage was not considered to be genuine pain, but a function of psychic disturbance in a biologically normal individual (now termed 'functional' or 'psychogenic' pain).

This dualistic view of pain persisted well into the 20th century, despite the accumulation of overwhelming evidence to the contrary. For example, there are many instances of significant tissue damage in the absence of pain, such as that reported by athletes on the playing field or soldiers on the battlefield; painful conditions such as 'tension' headache or trigeminal neuralgia, which are not associated with tissue trauma; phantom limb pains, in which pain is reported in an area which no longer exists, and so on (see Melzack and Wall[1] for a fuller account of pain anomalies).

However, the publication of the gate control theory of pain[3] legitimised psychological processes as forming an inextricable part of the pain experience – irrespective of the extent of tissue damage. Melzack and Wall said that variables such as mood state, attention, past experience of pain and the meaning of the pain to the individual would all influence the response to pain. The limits of medical science in being able to detect 'all forms of pathology' given the technology available at any one time were also acknowledged. Pain was now a much broader and more complex construct than a correlate of the amount of tissue damage that could be observed. Largely as a consequence of the gate control theory and the research evidence that has accrued to support it, the International Association for the Study of Pain published the following definition of pain: 'an unpleasant sensory *and emotional* experience associated with actual *or potential* tissue damage, or described in terms of such damage' [italics added].[4] This currently accepted definition of pain acknowledges the loose association between pain and injury, and instead recognises the importance of emotional factors in all forms of pain experience.

The contemporary term 'biopsychosocial' refers to the integration of biological, psychological and social factors within the experience of health or illness.[5] When applied to the issue of pain, this model is theoretically consistent with the tenets of the gate control theory. It suggests that biological factors represent only one element of a multifactorial phenomenon termed pain, and that pain should be seen as a dynamic, fluid process rather than an endpoint of nociception, transmission and perception. It is on a biopsychosocial understanding of pain that the remainder of this article is based.

Psychology and gate control theory

Gate control theory posited a number of dimensions of 'descending influence' on pain experience, which may be considered as the precursors to the systematic investigation of psychological influences on pain. There is now an enormous literature documenting these influences,[1,5,6] and the present chapter gives merely a brief overview of this extensive body of research.

Cultural factors are known to influence pain behaviour significantly,[7,8] and the differences between cultures can be startling. For example, there is evidence that headache, which affects as many as 70% of the Western population at least once per month, is almost non-existent in Oriental and African countries.[8] An analysis of cross-cultural nursing assessments revealed significant differences between white Americans of Northern European descent, and Mexican Americans in their expression of pain. Stoicism and tolerance of pain are seen as desirable pain responses among white Americans, whereas the Mexican culture accepts crying out and the expression of strong emotions when in pain.[9] However, there are numerous problems with cross-cultural methodologies when exploring pain differences,[7] not the least of which is the reliance on language to provide the dependent variable. Pain cannot be directly measured, only described, and linguistic nuances represent a major source of error variance. It is never clear whether subjects from different cultures interpret the same instructions in exactly the same way, and whether they intend their responses to the same items to be interpreted by the experimenters in exactly the same way.

Nevertheless, Rollman's review of the cross-cultural pain literature suggests that differences in pain behaviour, where they genuinely exist, are more likely to arise from psychosocial than genetic influences.

An individual's past experience of pain can also greatly affect future responses to painful stimuli. Social learning theory has offered a number of theoretical perspectives on classical and operant conditioning factors in pain, particularly in relation to childhood experiences of injury or disease.[10] It is estimated that 70–90% of all sickness episodes are handled outside the formal healthcare system, and that self-treatment within the family provides a substantial proportion of health care.[11] Hence, the influence of the family on pain is significant. In particular, the modelling of parental responses to injury (and hence vicarious learning from parental attitudes towards pain), has been shown to be an important predictor of later pain experience.[12] For example, Fillingham and colleagues showed that individuals with a family history of chronic pain were significantly more likely to have experienced pain themselves in the past month and to report poorer health, than a matched sample of individuals with no family pain history. Whether for genetic, social learning or other reasons, pain does appear to 'run in families'.[6,11]

Conditioning is another psychological phenomenon that can powerfully influence pain experience. An aversive experience at the dentist can result in the conditioned association of pain and fear with the sound of the drill, the smell of the dental surgery and the sight of white coats and masks. The fact that 45% of dentate adults in the UK report fear as being their most important barrier to dental care attests to the strength of classical conditioning to pain.[13] Operant conditioning is also an important social learning influence on pain and disability, at both acute and chronic ends of the pain spectrum. A child who falls and scrapes a knee will often look up to see if his or her mother is watching before bursting into tears. The promise of a sympathetic maternal reaction can powerfully shape the pain response. Similarly, chronic pain patients with solicitous (overprotective) spouses tend to be significantly more disabled and to report greater pain intensity than patients whose spouses are less overtly sympathetic.[14]

The gate theory hypothesised mood state as an important psychological variable in the response to pain, and this has been reliably shown to be the case. In the classic laboratory experiment, a sample of normal healthy subjects (usually university students) undergo a mood induction procedure, such as completing a bogus examination. Half the sample are given false feedback that they have scored in the bottom 10% for their year; the other half are told that they are in the top 10%. Both groups then rate their current mood state to confirm that the induction has produced an appropriately dichotomised sample ('high mood' versus 'low mood'), and they are then exposed to an identical noxious stimulus. The 'low mood' groups reliably rate the stimulus as significantly more painful than the 'high mood' group.[5] Anxiety also figures strongly in terms of influencing pain experience, as the previously cited data regarding the prevalence of dental fears would attest. Pre-operative anxiety levels have also been shown to predict outcome from cardiac surgery better than a host of clinical variables, including medical status, surgical procedure, pre-operative length of stay, priority of surgery, gender and age.[15]

Beliefs about the capacity to exert control over the painful stimulus, or over the context in which pain is occurring, also influence pain intensity. The success of the patient-controlled analgesia (PCA) system is evidence of this. A comparison of PCA versus the continuous infusion method for administering spinal epidurals found that the level of analgesia was equivalent across the two conditions, but the PCA group required less local anaesthesia and reported higher satisfaction.[16] Ultimately, how one construes pain – the meaning that is attributed to the sensation labelled as 'painful' – determines the behavioural and affective reaction to it. The interpretation of a sudden pain in the chest following a meal as indigestion will result in a quite different set of behaviours and emotions to an interpretation of the same pain as indicating a cardiac arrest. Beliefs about the predictability and controllability of the pain, about the potential threat posed by the pain, and about the individual's resources to respond effectively to the pain, all impact upon the pain experience.

A factor analysis of a well-known pain assessment measure, the McGill Pain Questionnaire,[17] revealed that the questionnaire items clustered into three categories, termed sensory–discriminative, cognitive–evaluative and motivational–affective domains. These three dimensions in many ways encompass the broad spectrum of psychological variables which are relevant to the experience of pain. The individual locates and discriminates the stimulus as painful, the stimulus is actively processed and evaluated against past experience and for current meaning, and these in turn lead to emotional and behavioural reactions to the pain. This chain then becomes cyclical rather than linear, as beliefs and interpretations about the pain influence mood and behaviour, which in turn affect how the individual thinks about the pain.

The overview given above offers something of the complexity and diversity of influences upon pain, and reinforces the importance of the biopsychosocial model when considering pain in any context.

Pain – acute versus chronic

In the majority of cases, pain is a (fortunately) relatively short-lived experience. The injury heals, or the precipitant of the pain is removed from the environment, and the central nervous system returns to normal. However, for a significant minority of pain sufferers, the pain does not ameliorate over time. In perhaps 5–10% of low back pain cases for example, the acute pain becomes chronic pain – generally defined as pain experienced on a daily basis for a period of six months or longer.[4] Chronic pain is the term used to describe long-term, intractable, non-malignant pain conditions, such as arthritis, fibromyalgia, trigeminal neuralgia and the specific conditions of vulvodynia and chronic pelvic pain to be discussed later.

Acute pain is a common, everyday occurrence. It is the most common presenting complaint to general practice,[1] and 7% of adults in the UK attend their general practitioner with low back pain each year.[18] Chronic pain conditions on the other hand constitute an enormous drain on social, economic and personal resources. Often sufferers are unable to remain in paid employment, are frequent users of healthcare services, take high levels of medication, both prescription and over the counter, and experience a great deal of stress within their families and social networks. In this country, it is estimated that when work and production losses are included along with assessment and treatment costs, the total cost of back pain approaches £10.6 billion per annum.[19] Attempts have therefore been made to try to identify which acute pain sufferers are at risk of developing a chronic, disabling pain problem – and psychological factors have also been shown to play an important role in this transition.

Studies have examined patients presenting to primary care with acute pain and then followed them up over the next 6–12 months, in an attempt to determine which characteristics are associated with the development of chronic disability. While clinical factors such as duration of symptoms and the severity of pain account for some of the variance in predicting chronic pain, the strongest predictors are generally psychosocial.[18,20-22] Turk's review of this literature simply states, 'Many studies have demonstrated that demographic and psychosocial factors are better predictors of chronicity than are clinical or physical factors'.[22] The characteristics that have been identified as predictive of chronicity include a premorbid history of psychological problems, current mood disorder, a past history of alcohol or substance abuse, job dissatisfaction and high levels of anxiety or fear avoidance behaviour.[18,20,21] Once again, psychological factors have been shown to be an integral part of the pain experience.

Sex and gender differences in pain

Having discussed some of the more pertinent psychological issues as they relate to pain in all its forms, we can turn to the second topic of this chapter – the psychology of pain as it specifically relates to women. Before doing so, it is important to differentiate between the terms sex difference and gender difference. Sex differences exclusively refer to biological differences between males and females, whereas gender differences refer to the wider issues of how men and women are expected to behave within their cultural and societal contexts. Making a theoretical distinction between sex and gender is straightforward enough; however, in research contexts the two are often difficult to disentangle. For example, it has been found in laboratory studies that when a noxious stimulus is applied and subjects are asked to rate at what point that stimulus becomes 'painful', women tend to report a lower pain threshold than men.[23,24] However, it has also been found that the sex of the experimenter affects such ratings: men will give significantly lower pain ratings (i.e. stimulus is 'not painful') to a female experimenter than to a male, whereas female subjects do not discriminate on this basis.[25] Are the findings demonstrating a difference in pain threshold between males and females therefore reflecting a biological, or sex, difference, or presenting an example of gender stereotyping in which men must appear 'macho' and stoical in front of women? Whatever the case, gender is an influential variable in pain experience.

Women's pain

It is also important to recognise that irrespective of how the experimental variables are manipulated in research settings, women's experiences of pain are fundamentally different from those of men. For women, pain is often a 'normal' aspect of biological functioning as it relates to reproductive cycles. Pain may also be indicative of pathological processes such as endometriosis or ectopic pregnancy that are sex-specific. As Skevington has said 'Intermittent periodic pain is a potentially regular life event for half of the population. Where such pains occur, they create schematic markers, being carefully monitored for a host of social and cultural reasons, as well as those connected with health and wellbeing'.[5] By contrast, men are more likely than women to experience pain from injury, and from acute and chronic life-threatening diseases.[24] Thus, for women, pain conceivably may be a recurrent, benign and non-pathological phenomenon, whereas this is not the case for men.

The two chronic pain conditions that are arguably the most problematic for women, and which have been the subject of most empirical examination, are vulvodynia and chronic pelvic pain. These pain disorders will be discussed in turn, with particular reference to the psychological dimensions of each.

Vulvodynia

Vulvodynia is medically defined by the complaint of chronic vulval discomfort, taking the form of burning and any combination of stinging, irritation, itching, pain, rawness and dyspareunia.[26,27] As is typical of many of the chronic pain disorders, there are often few detectable physical findings with this condition, yet the pain may be provoked by any stimulus that exerts pressure on the vulva.

Research data indicate that women afflicted with vulvodynia are predominantly Caucasian, likely to have had an onset of pain in their mid-twenties and seek treatment in their reproductive years. Known risk factors include early oral contraceptive use, early menses and early first sexual experience.[26,27]

The original conceptualisations of vulvodynia echo the Cartesian dualism discussed in the introduction of this article. The combination of vulval burning in the absence of abnormal physical findings, and the complaint of dyspareunia, were fertile grounds for labelling the disorder as 'psychosomatic'.[28] Investigations into histories of childhood sexual abuse, marital disharmony and other sources of potential psychic conflict were then undertaken in order to confirm the notion that vulvodynia was a nonphysical problem. However, it appears that the incidence of sexual abuse in patients with vulvodynia is similar to that in nonclinical populations.[26,28,29] For example, Stewart and colleagues compared 50 vulvodynia patients with 32 women with identifiable vulval pathology and found no differences in the incidence of childhood physical or sexual abuse.[29] An association between an abusive past history and the development of chronic pain has been made elsewhere, but in relation to pain disorders in general rather than gynaecological pain specifically.[30,31]

Vulvodynia tends to be a long-term disorder and one that is inherently likely to interfere with sexual functioning. It would therefore be expected that significant levels of marital strain would be observed in this clinical population. The data here are equivocal. Although marital conflict has been observed in interviewer observations of women with vulvodynia,[26,32] cross-sectional quantitative studies have found minimal evidence of marital distress in women presenting for treatment.[33] However, in other studies examining marital function in chronic pain patients, a distinct response bias has been detected: only those patients whose relationships are relatively healthy will give consent to take part in research explicitly examining marital satisfaction.[14] This makes interpreting the results of such studies problematic.

Chronic pelvic pain

Chronic pelvic pain is broadly described as pain suffered by women in the lower abdominal area for of least six months' duration, which is not associated with the menstrual cycle or sexual intercourse.[31] It is among the most common of the female pain disorders: a community prevalence rate of 15% in women of reproductive age has been observed,[31] while approximately one-third of patients attending gynaecological clinics rate pelvic pain as their most significant problem.[32] There is an equally poor correlation between pain and observable pathology in this disorder as in vulvodynia, or when pathology is detected its severity is not consistent with the reported pain severity.[34] Even so, the International Association for the Study of Pain continues to distinguish between pelvic pain with pathology and pelvic pain of an apparently gynaecological origin for which no definite lesion can be found.[35]

The psychological characteristics of women suffering chronic pelvic pain have also been explored in a number of studies, again with the objective of determining the underlying psychological cause of their pain. Research designs typically involve comparisons between chronic pelvic pain patients with identified pathology (e.g. endometriosis) and those without; between chronic pelvic pain patients and female chronic pain patients with other pain sites; and between chronic pelvic pain patients and women not reporting pain. The results of such studies confirm the flawed theory on which they are based.[31] Generally, the findings indicate higher levels of psychopathology (depression, anxiety, catastrophising) in chronic pain samples – irrespective of the pain site – than in non-pain groups. This would be expected, given the stressor under which the pain sufferers are living. The differences between those with identified pathology and those without pathology are in terms of somatic preoccupation and disease conviction, with statistically significantly greater disturbance observed in the non-identified pathology groups.[31,36] The greater awareness of bodily sensations and stronger beliefs in the presence of disease has been interpreted as evidence that this group carry an expectation of pain and illness, which predisposes them to developing pain in the absence of pathology.[36]

However, there is further evidence that women suffering chronic pelvic pain often feel dissatisfied and frustrated by their medical consultations, as they are led to feel that their symptoms are 'psychogenic' or otherwise psychiatrically rather than physically based.[37] In such cases surely it would be expected that these women would become more focused on their symptoms and more convinced of the presence of disease, as they are having to try and 'prove' that their pain is valid each time they attend a doctor. Moreover, the observation of a significant correlation between two variables does not demonstrate causality, and cross-sectional research is unable to shed light on an individual's premorbid characteristics.

The evidence presented here concerning vulvodynia and chronic pelvic pain may be seen as reflecting a wider medical discourse on women's illness. It has been suggested elsewhere that within a medical ideology of female frailty, women's disorders are characteristically conceived to be psychogenic in nature.[38] Rather than accepting limitations in current knowledge about the aetiology of chronic pain conditions, and helping to reassure patients about the nature of their problem, it seems that female patients are often made to feel that they are to blame for their disorder.[24,38] Reid and colleagues refer to 'attempts to construct the (female) sufferers' pain as the outcome of thwarted urges or neglected duties of the peculiarly female kind'.[38] Certainly there is evidence that women are significantly more likely to consult a doctor, and to report more symptoms within a consultation, than are men.[39] However, their greater frequency of medical attendance does not fully explain the fact that women vastly outnumber men in referrals for mental health problems.[24] While dualistic notions about 'organic' versus 'psychological' pain persist, these kinds of counterproductive interpretations will continue to occur.

Psychological treatment of chronic pain – the pain management programme

In chronic pain conditions where medical and surgical treatments have little to offer, pain management programmes have been developed in order to combat the effects of living with pain. The essential difference between the pain management approach and the biomedical approach to pain is that the goal of pain management is not to cure or necessarily even to relieve pain. Rather, the aims are to improve fitness, to restore meaningful activity within the patient's daily life and to improve psychological function.

Pain management is ideally delivered as a multidisciplinary package, involving physical therapists, occupational therapists, nurses, medical personnel (typically consultant anaesthetists or rheumatologists) and psychologists. However, irrespective of the specialty, the various components of this kind of intervention are based on established psychological principles of reinforcement, learning theory and cognitive theory. Detailed guidelines of cognitive behavioural pain management programmes are available[40,41] – however, a brief overview of the approach will be given here.

Exercise and stretch programme

Physiotherapy for the chronic pain patient is described as a 'hands off' treatment, as opposed to the more traditional forms of physiotherapy such as manipulation and mobilisation.[42] Here, the patient is given a specific set of stretches and exercises to perform, having first established a baseline level which they can manage without causing a sustained increase in pain. By systematically monitoring the amount that is performed and setting a realistic quota to be achieved each week, the patient can gradually increase his or her exercise capacity. The aim is to break the conditioned association between movement, fear and pain, and it is important that the patient does not feel pushed or coerced into increasing the exercise quota before feeling ready to do so. The phrase 'little and often' describes this physiotherapy approach, as opposed to the 'no pain, no gain' idea which many patients erroneously believe they should be following.

Pacing and activity scheduling

Chronic pain patients commonly report an 'overactivity–underactivity' cycle irrespective of the area affected by pain. On a day when their pain is less intense, they will carry out a great many more activities than usual, in an attempt to recoup the lost time due to their pain. However, this overactivity will inevitably produce a flare-up of pain, resulting in the patient stopping all activity (lying down, returning to bed, taking extra analgesia) until the pain subsides. This continuous cycling from excessive activity to inadequate activity prevents the patient from making any sustained improvement in function. Pacing techniques therefore involve establishing a manageable baseline of activity and spreading this over the course of a day or week. Patients are encouraged to break up prolonged activities such as sitting and standing into smaller units of time, using a stopwatch or kitchen timer as a prompt. As long as the patient does not overextend his or her tolerance for the activity before stopping, a flare-up of pain will be prevented. With the improved fitness and stamina brought about by the exercise component, the tolerance can be gradually extended out over time.

Cognitive therapy

This chapter has already highlighted several kinds of psychological distress, such as fear, anger and low mood, which often impact negatively upon coping with chronic pain. Cognitive therapy first aims to identify the beliefs, assumptions, interpretations and predictions that generate the affective disturbance. Having determined the idiosyncratic cognitive processes which give rise to the emotions, patients are taught methods of modifying their beliefs in order to reduce the associated distress. Attention diversion exercises might also be taught as part of coping skills training.

Relaxation training

Based on the principle that pain evokes muscle tension, and muscle tension in turn exacerbates pain, relaxation methods are commonly used with upper limb pain patients. To be optimally effective, relaxation training should be carried out in an applied fashion, such that patients are taught to use their relaxation skills during active movement (walking, standing, writing), as well as during physically non-active periods. Basic relaxation training may also be enhanced with electromyographic biofeedback applied to the painful areas.[43]

Other pain management treatment components commonly include goal setting, sleep management, assertiveness and communication skills training, medication reduction programmes and vocational counselling. The inclusion of the patient's partner in the pain management programme is an often neglected area of pain treatment, but one that evidence suggests is an important element of the comprehensive treatment package.[11,14] A meta-analysis of 25 randomised controlled trials of cognitive behavioural pain management versus attention placebo or waiting list control conditions demonstrated clinically significant advantages for the treatment condition.[44] Significant effect sizes were obtained in all outcome areas, with particular improvements in positive coping measures and reduced behavioural expression of pain. Studies examining the utility of cognitive behavioural pain management for vulvodynia and chronic pelvic pain have also been favourable,[32,36] although the range of studies is considerably more limited than for heterogeneous chronic pain conditions.

Conclusion

It has been argued in this chapter that although psychological factors have been acknowledged as an intrinsic part of the pain experience since ancient times, their role has often been misconstrued. The false dichotomy between physical and psychological domains that was established in early theories of pain has persisted in many ways until the present day, in both medical and lay circles. And yet, there is a large body of evidence that clearly shows that mind and body are not independently functioning entities, but are closely interrelated in all aspects of pain detection, transmission and perception. Cognition, affect and behaviour are known to share a reciprocal relationship with noxious stimuli in such a way that each exerts some influence upon the other. This was seen to be the case when discussing examples of acute pain, both laboratory-based and naturally occurring, in relation to the transition of acute injury to chronic pain disorder, and in relation to the management of chronic pain itself. In each facet of pain, psychological variables were found to be salient.

However, clinical pain problems do not occur in a vacuum and issues of gender were raised when discussing two pain disorders of women, vulvodynia and chronic pelvic pain. It was argued that the psychological research literature on these pain disorders has been dominated by the kind of Cartesian dualism that the gate control theory sought to render obsolete. Poor methodology and the overinterpretation of results only add to the problems with much of this research. But perhaps even more importantly, it is the pain patients themselves whose suffering is increased by notions of psychogenic pain. Having to justify their complaint in a context of distrust and accusation serves no purpose whatsoever. Given an overriding aim of improving the management of pain, it seems that the beliefs and behaviours of the practitioners in these areas needs as much attention as those of the patients themselves.

References

1.   Melzack R, Wall PD. *The Challenge of Pain*, 2nd edn. Harmondsworth: Penguin; 1988.
2.   Levy G, Levy M. *The Puzzle of Pain*. Roseville: G&B Arts International; 1994.
3.   Melzack R, Wall PD. Pain mechanisms: a new theory. *Science* 1965;**150**:971–9.
4.   International Association for the Study of Pain. Pain terms: a list with definitions and notes on usage. *Pain* 1979;**6**:249.
5.   Skevington SM. Beliefs, images and memories of pain. In: Skevington SM, editor. *Psychology of Pain*. Chichester: John Wiley and Sons;1995. p. 97–130.
6.   Gamsa A. The role of psychological factors in chronic pain. II. A critical appraisal. *Pain* 1994;**57**:17–29.
7.   Rollman GB. Culture and pain. In: Kazarian J, Evans P, editors. *Cultural Clinical Psychology*. Oxford: Oxford University Press; 1998. p. 267–86.
8.   Ziegler DK. Headache: public health problem. *Neurologic Clinics* 1990;**8**:781–91.
9.   Calvillo ER, Flaskerud JH. Review of literature on culture and pain of adults with focus on Mexican Americans. *Journal of Transcultural Nursing* 1991;**2**:81–91.
10. Osborne RB, Hatcher JW, Richtsmeier AJ. The role of social modeling in unexplained pediatric pain. *J Pediatr Psychol* 1989;**14**:43–61.
11. Turk DC, Rudy TE, Flor H. Why a family perspective for pain? *Int J Fam Ther* 1985;**7**:223–34.
12. Fillingim RB, Edwards RR, Powell T. Sex-dependent effects of reported familial pain history on recent pain complaints and experimental pain responses. *Pain* 2000;**86**:87–94.
13. Naini FB, Mellor AC, Getz T. Treatment of dental fears: pharmacology or psychology? *Dental Update* 1999;**September**:270–76.
14. Newton-John TRO, Williams AC de C. Solicitousness revisited: a qualitative analysis of patient–spouse interactions in chronic pain. In: Devor M, Rowbotham M, Wiesenfeld-Hallin Z, editors. *Proceedings of the 9th World Congress on Pain. Progress in Pain Research and Management*. Seattle: IASP Press; 2000. p. 1113–22.
15. Stengrevics S, Sirois C, Schwartz CE, Friedman R. The prediction of cardiac surgery outcome based upon preoperative psychological factors. *Psychology & Health* 1996; **11**:471–7.
16. Curry PD, Pacsoo C, Heap DG. Patient-controlled epidural analgesia in obstetric anaesthetic practice. *Pain* 1994;**57**:125–8.
17. Melzack, R. The McGill Pain Questionnaire: major properties and scoring methods. *Pain* 1975;**1**:277–99.
18. Thomas E, Silman AJ, Croft P, Papageorgiou AC, Jayson MIV, McFarlane GJ. Predicting who develops chronic low back pain in primary care: a prospective study. *BMJ* 1999;**318**:1662–7.
19. Manaidakis N, Gray A. The economic burden of back pain in the UK. *Pain* 2000;**84**:95–103.
20. Croft PR, Macfarlane GJ, Papageorgiou AC, Thomas E, Silman AJ. Outcome of low back pain in general practice: a prospective study. *BMJ* 1998;**316**:1356–9.
21. Klenerman L, Slade P, Stanley IM, Pennie B, Reilly JP, Atchison LE. The prediction of chronicity in patients with an acute attack of low back pain in a General Practice setting. *Spine* 1995;**20**:478–84.

22. Turk DC. The role of demographic and psychosocial factors in transition from acute to chronic pain. In: Jensen TS, Turner JA, Wiesenfeld-Hallin Z, editors. *Proceedings of the 8th World Congress on Pain.* Seattle: IASP Press; 1997. p. 185–213.

23. Robinson ME, Wise E, Riley J, Atchison JW. Sex differences in clinical pain: a multisample study. *J Clin Psychol Med Settings* 1998;**5**:413–24.

24. Unruh, A. Review Article: Gender variations in clinical pain experience. *Pain* 1996;**65**:123–67.

25. Levine FM, De Simone LL. The effects of experimenter gender on pain report in male and female subjects. *Pain* 1991;**44**:69–72.

26. Masheb RM, Nash JM, Brondolo E, Kerns RD. Vulvodynia: an introduction and critical review of a chronic pain condition. *Pain* 2000;**86**:3–10.

27. Jones RW. Vulval pain. *Pain Reviews* 2000;**7**:15–24.

28. McKay M. Vulvodynia. A multifactorial clinical problem. *Arch Dermatol* 1989;**125**:256–62.

29. Stewart DE, Reicher AE, Gerulath AH, Boydell KM. Vulvodynia and psychological distress. *Obstet Gynecol* 1994;**84**:587–90.

30. Linton SJ. A population-based study of the relationship between sexual abuse and back pain: establishing a link. *Pain* 1997;**73**:47–53.

31. Price JR, Blake, F. Chronic pelvic pain: the assessment as therapy. *J Psych Res* 1999;**46**:7–14.

32. Baranowski AP, Mallinson C, Johnson NS. A review of urogenital pain. *Pain Rev* 1999;**6**:53–84.

33. Schover LR, Youngs DD, Cannata R. Psychosexual aspects of the evaluation and management of vulvar vestibulitis. *Am J Obstet Gynecol* 1992;**167**:630–36.

34. Stout AL, Steege JF, Dodson WC, Hughes CL. Relationship of laparoscopic findings to self-report of pelvic pain. *Am J Obstet Gynecol* 1991;**164**:73–9.

35. Merskey H, Bogduk N. *Classification of Chronic Pain.* Seattle: IASP Press; 1994.

36. Glover L, Pearce S. Chronic pelvic pain. In: Mayou R, Bass C, Sharpe M, editors. *Treatment of Functional Somatic Symptoms.* Oxford: Oxford University Press; 1995. p. 313–27.

37. Grace VM. Problems of communication, diagnosis, and treatment experienced by women using the New Zealand health services for chronic pelvic pain: a quantitative analysis. *Health Care for Women International* 1995;**16**:521–35.

38. Reid J, Ewan C, Lowy E. Pilgrimage of pain: the illness experiences of women with repetitive strain injury and the search for credibility. *Soc Sci Med* 1991;**32**:601–12.

39. Mechanic D. Sex, illness, illness behaviour and the use of health services. *J Hum Stress* 1976; **December**:29–40.

40. Williams AC de C, Erskine A. Chronic pain. In: Broome A, Llewelyn S, editors. *Health Psychology: Processes and Applications.* London: Chapman and Hall, 1995. p. 353–76.

41. Hanson RW, Gerber KE. *Coping With Chronic Pain: A Guide to Patient Self-Management.* New York: Guilford Press; 1990.

42. Protas EJ. Physical activity and low back pain. In: Max M, editor. *Pain 1999 – An Updated Review.* Seattle: IASP Press; 1999. p. 145–52.

43. Newton-John TRO, Spence SH, Schotte D. Cognitive-behavioural therapy versus EMG biofeedback in the treatment of chronic low back pain. *Behav Res Ther* 1995;**33**:691–7.

44. Morley S, Eccleston C, Williams AC de C. Systematic review and meta-analysis of randomized controlled trials of cognitive behaviour therapy and behaviour therapy for chronic pain in adults, excluding headache. *Pain* 1999;**80**:1–13.

Chapter 7

Practical psychological approaches to women with pain

Amanda Smith

Introduction

In this paper I will be focusing on practical psychological approaches to women with chronic pelvic pain (CPP), which is pain suffered in the lower abdomen area for six months or more. Women who experience CPP and are referred to a gynaecology department, are usually investigated by laparoscopy. Many of these women, however, are found not to have recognisable pelvic pathology. For example, Gillibrand[1] found pelvic pathology in only 31% of 331 British women with pelvic pain. When pathology is found, its severity does not always correlate well with self-report of pain severity. This has been demonstrated with pelvic adhesions,[2] with endometriosis[3,4] and with pelvic pathology in general.[5] Chronic pain, as a condition in itself, has often left gynaecologists perplexed as to how to manage these women effectively.

In this chapter I will give a brief overview of the evolution of theories and models of pain, over the last century, highlighting the role of psychological factors in these theories. It is important to be clear about which theory of pain is being used at any one time, as this strongly influences the type of approach chosen to treat and manage chronic pain. I will then outline some practical psychological approaches to managing CPP that have developed from these pain theories. Through this I hope to enhance doctors' understanding of the psychological aspects of pain theory and demystify psychological approaches to pain management, so that gynaecologists will start to integrate this approach when managing women with CPP. Throughout this chapter I refer to the clinician as a psychologist; however, this could also be a psychotherapist or a counsellor with a specialisation in pain management.

'Linear causal models' to 'multi-causal models' of pain

Theories of chronic pain and the role of psychological factors in chronic pain have changed and evolved over the last century. For a good review, I strongly recommend two papers by Gamsa.[6,7] In the first of her papers,[6] she highlights how pain used to be viewed in 'linear causal models', where either organic pathology was the cause of pain or, if no organic pathology could be found, then it was believed that the pain was caused by psychological factors, this view was influenced by psychoanalytic theorists. This tendency to attribute pain to *either* organic *or* psychological causes reflected traditional dualistic thinking, splitting the mind from the body.[8,9] This view was predominant from the 1940s to 1970s, and indeed is still held by some practitioners to this day, which unfortunately limits the effective management of women with CPP. Fry and colleagues[10] conclude in their review of the sociopsychological factors in CPP that 'in common with other research into chronic pain conditions, it appears unhelpful to separate this type of pain into "psychogenic" and "organic" categories'.

The 'linear causal model' has now been replaced by 'multi-causal models' of pain, where both physical and psychological factors, which include sensory, cognitive, (thinking) emotional and behavioural factors, are believed to be involved in the phenomena of pain and there is a complex interaction between all of these areas. Due to this, multi-theoretical approaches are needed to manage chronic pain effectively, as I will outline later.

An early example, which influenced the development of interactive models and multi-causal models of pain, is the classic study, carried out in 1946, by Beecher.[11,12] He compared the reactions to pain of soldiers in battle with a comparable number of civilians about to undergo an operation. He found that only one in four soldiers with serious injuries complained of pain severe enough to require analgesics. When compared with the civilians, the soldiers who had severe wounds complained less of pain and required less medication than did the civilians. Beecher suggested that the soldiers experienced less pain as their injuries were invested with positive *meaning*, their injuries provided them with a respectable reason to leave the battlefield and *meant* a return to the safety and security of a hospital. For the civilians, however, their condition *meant* removal from the safety of their home, to the *anxiety* of being in hospital and facing surgery. This study suggested that psychological factors, such as the '*meaning*' of pain can influence the experience of pain.

It was not until 1965, however, that the first comprehensive model of pain was developed that integrated psychological and physiological factors. The model was developed by Melzack, a psychologist, and Wall, a physiologist, and is called the 'gate control' theory of pain.[13] According to this theory, pain phenomena are viewed as consisting of sensory–discriminative, (physical) motivational–affective, (feelings) and cognitive–evaluative components (mental thought processes – a few examples of these include our beliefs, assumptions, expectations, the meaning we place on events, perceptions etc.) The theory proposes that a neural mechanism in the spinal cord acts like a 'gate' that can facilitate or inhibit the flow of nerve impulses from peripheral fibres to the central nervous system. More than any other theory, the gate control theory emphasises the important role of psychological variables and how they affect the reaction to pain. With chronic pain, in particular, successful pain control often involves changing the cognitive–motivational components while the sensory component remains intact. This development brought the psychological study of pain into mainstream research. Since then, further research has shown how somatic input is subjected to the modulating influences of cognitive,[14] affective[15] and behavioural factors,[16,17] before it evokes pain perception.

Cognitive and behavioural approaches

Cognitive theory, which examines cognition or mental thought processes, has now advanced since the 1970s and examines intervening variables such as beliefs, expectations, attributions, meaning, problem-solving, cognitive coping skills, self-statements, self-efficacy, personal control, attention and use of mental imagery. Cognitive strategies attempt to change the way patients 'think' about pain and to increase the patient's feeling of 'control' over all aspects of the problem. Cognitive theorists argue that modification of the patient's beliefs (for example, unrealistic fears about what the pain 'means') will generate changes in both the experience of pain and in maladaptive behaviour. Pain studies investigate the effects of these thought processes on the experience of pain and related problems. For example, thoughts that the pain may be due to cancer, when tests show that it is not, actually increase anxiety and fear, which in turn increase the experience of pain and can also reduce the person's ability to cope effectively. Melzack[20] has suggested that 'cognitive processes are at the forefront of the most exciting new psychological approaches to pain, fear and anxiety'. Behaviour theorists propose that changes in behaviour, for example by monitoring and changing their daily activities by learning 'pacing skills', can modify the experience of pain.

These approaches have been applied to a number of psychologically based problems, such as depression, anxiety, phobias and personality disorders.[21-25] These approaches have also been applied to managing pain.[26-32]

Psychophysiological approaches

Pain research also includes psychophysiological studies, which examine the influence of mental events (thoughts, memories, emotions) on physical changes that produce pain. Gamsa[6] outlines three assumptions that underlie psychophysiological explanations of pain: (i) a relationship exists between identified psychological states (e.g. stress) and physical changes (e.g. increased electromyograph levels, autonomic arousal); (ii) a relationship exists between specified physical changes and pain; (iii) physical changes that are said to precipitate pain, precede the pain. General arousal models propose that frequent or prolonged arousal of the autonomic nervous system, including prolonged muscular contractions, generate and perpetuate pain. Treatments such as electromyograph (EMG), biofeedback and relaxation techniques are designed to decrease levels of muscle tension and autonomic arousal and thereby reduce pain. Theoretical formulations to explain the mechanisms which link abnormal psychophysiological patterns with pain are well summarised.[6,18,19]

Quality of communication between doctor and patient

Psychological mechanisms and interventions occur at each stage of the woman's interaction with the medical profession, starting with her visit to the GP, followed by her meeting with the gynaecologist and nurses and then, if her chronic pain continues, when she is treated as part of an integrated multidisciplinary team and referred for psychological pain management.

Grace[33,34] has highlighted the problems that women face when seeing their doctor about CPP. Over 40% of women left the gynaecological consultation feeling there were aspects of their CPP that they had not discussed. Almost 40% of the women felt that the 'meaning' of the diagnosis was not explained adequately, and 80% of the women who had had surgery for CPP stated that they had not been informed of alternatives to surgery.

The quality of communication between the doctor and patient with CPP has been examined,[35] at the initial consultation and the effect on pain at follow-up ($n = 105$ women aged 17–60 years). Results showed that a favourable patient rating of the initial consultation was associated with complete recovery at follow-up (six months later). For those whose symptoms persisted, factors found to predict continuing pain levels were the initial level of pain, number of functions of daily life impaired, the presence of endometriosis, and the doctor who carried out the initial consultation. Although the mean hostility score was found to be significantly elevated compared with normative data, patient hostility scores and the doctor's level of experience or gender were not significantly associated with continued pain.

A study by Elcombe and colleagues[36] further illustrates the influence of psychological mechanisms on the experience of pain. The researchers carried out a prospective study of 71 women undergoing diagnostic laparoscopy for pelvic pain. They found 47.9% had no pathology, 39.4% had some abnormality but not of clinical significance and 12.7% had what they considered to be significant pathology (endometriosis in four patients, ovarian cysts in two, adhesions in two and pelvic inflammatory disease in one). The women were interviewed before laparoscopy, and after at one week, three months and six months and they evaluated five different types of 'beliefs', held by the women. They found that the women's pain fell rapidly after laparoscopy and remained at a reduced level at the three- and six-month follow-ups. Women with initially high levels of pain reported the greatest pain improvements after laparoscopy. They concluded that diagnostic laparoscopy can have beneficial effects and that these effects appear to be the result of psychological mechanisms. They found that pain improvements after laparoscopy were predicted by two sets of 'beliefs': belief about the pain and the change in each woman's 'evaluation' of the seriousness of her condition. The researchers explain each of these in more detail and suggest that psychological variables may be more important than any factor other than baseline pain to the course of CPP after diagnostic laparoscopy.

Price and Blake[37] have reviewed how the clinical assessment can be a significant part of the therapy and that modification of illness beliefs within a flexible management approach that explicitly considers women's 'need for explanation' may provide the key. They highlight that the biomedical model of management is poorly suited to the effective management of women with CPP and that the problem is probably best understood, managed and explained to patients in biopsychosocial terms.

A multidisciplinary approach – the pelvic pain clinic

For those women who continue to have CPP after laparoscopy, either with or without pathology, and are unable to manage it effectively themselves, an integrated 'pain management' approach is recommended. The approach carried out at the pelvic pain clinic in the Obstetrics and Gynaecology Department at Northwick Park Hospital is an integrated model, which is consistent with the recommendations of the International Association for the Study of Pain (IASP) that chronic pain should involve both medically trained and psychologically trained health professionals.[38]

It should be noted that the pelvic pain clinic is a tertiary referral clinic and so the women referred are a sub-group of women with CPP who have not had a reduction in pain after laparoscopy and have not been helped to date, despite often having seen numerous doctors. Of this sub-group referred to the clinic during 1998, the majority of patients were found to have pelvic congestion (77%).[39] This could be due to the fact that the director of the clinic, Professor Beard, has a special interest in this patient group and/or this particular condition, which is not often identified at laparoscopy. The majority of the women have never been referred for psychological pain management before attending the clinic.

The psychological approach used at the pelvic pain clinic is based on cognitive–behavioural models that incorporate all the elements of Melzack and Wall's gate control model. It is suggested that these patients are lacking the necessary coping skills to manage a pain condition effectively. Hence, psychological pain management and stress management involves a full assessment of psychological factors and coping mechanisms and continuing sessions involve teaching these coping mechanisms combined with counselling for the various psychological issues that may be limiting them in effectively managing their condition.

Integrated multidisciplinary team model

The woman will first see the doctor for an assessment and be referred for all the necessary medical investigations, such as a laparoscopy, ultrasound scan and venogram. Once all the results are complete the women will be given their diagnosis and relevant treatment. Treatment involves (i) medication if necessary and (ii) cognitive–behavioural pain and stress management. They will then return to the doctor at five months for a follow-up review of progress. Alongside this, they have access to a help-line five days a week, staffed by the clinical nurse specialist who is available for support and to answer any questions they may have. The nurse also runs a support group, fortnightly, which all patients can attend.

Number of sessions

The women are asked to attend a minimum of four sessions of psychological pain and stress management and informed that there is initially a maximum of ten sessions. They see the same therapist for each session, to enable a relationship to build up and for continuity of treatment. Towards the end of these sessions, if it is felt that she would benefit from further sessions, then a set number can be re-contracted, for example four or eight. The assessment session is 90 minutes, and continuing sessions are usually of one hour. Follow-up sessions are booked at three months and six months. Sessions are usually monthly, although they can be more frequent. If the woman would like her husband to attend, this is encouraged. Likewise, if she would rather attend alone this is also acceptable.

Confidentiality

The patient is informed that confidentiality is within the team. This allows open communication between the psychologist and team, consisting of the gynaecologist managing her case and the nurse manager. If there is a particular issue that the woman does not want the gynaecologist or nurse to know, or is not ready for the team to know about, then the psychologist will discuss this with the woman and respect her need for confidentiality. Psychologists, psychotherapists and counsellors are bound by their respective governing organisation's codes of ethics and practice.[40-42] These specify that the patient's right to confidentiality must be respected. As confidentiality is within the team, this has to be made clear to them at the beginning of psychological therapy. In my experience, the woman is usually happy for the team to be aware of the relevant emotional, cognitive, or behavioural factors which may be affecting her management of the pain. With regard to the gynaecologist writing to her GP, if there are any sensitive emotional issues that come from the psychological therapy, it is the responsibility of the gynaecologist to discuss these with the woman and obtain her permission for these to be disclosed to her GP.

Assessment questions, education and continuing management

This illustrates a selection of the main questions asked, particularly during the assessment phase. Each question builds on the other and draws out more relevant information, which can be pieced together throughout the therapy and used to determine future interventions. The following ten areas are covered: diagnosis; understanding of their condition and the pain; when the pain started; description of the pain; what makes the pain worse; what has been found to reduce it; emotional factors in current life events; personality type; emotional factors in the past and childhood.

Diagnosis?

This helps the psychologist establish if they are working with someone with CPP due to visible pathology, such as endometriosis or adhesions etc., or a functional disorder such as pelvic congestion and the irritable bowel syndrome, or CPP of unknown origin.

Understanding of their condition, and understanding about the pain?

This helps to assess the woman's level of understanding about the condition and whether she needs more information. It also draws out her beliefs and assumptions about the cause of her pain, including her anxieties and fears, which we know increase the experience of pain. From this information the psychologist will be able to determine how much further 'education' is needed about the condition and about chronic pain itself, which will be carried out either during the assessment session or in future sessions.

Month, year and age when pain started?

This tells the therapist how long the woman has been living and trying to cope with the pain and gives an idea of age and time of onset. The woman may also outline what investigations and treatments they have tried to date.

Description of the pain?

Ratings of pain out of ten are asked for, including duration of pain, for example, a dull ache with some sharp stabbing pains. The psychologist can establish if there are set patterns with the menstrual cycle or whether the pain seems to occur randomly. Finding out if it is worse in the morning, afternoon and/or evening will help with future management and helping women assess what factors may trigger the pain and how to pace their activities.

What makes the pain worse?

This helps the psychologist to establish what factors exacerbate the pain, to help determine effective interventions later in therapy. For example, with pelvic congestion, a vascular condition, we have established that the following factors influence pain:

1.   Gravity, which allows the blood to pool in the veins; therefore, standing and sitting for any length of time, can bring the pain on.

2.   Exercise, sexual arousal and intercourse also exacerbate the pain. It is proposed that these activities cause an increase in bloodflow but the veins are unable to clear the blood effectively, which results in pain. Again, giving information about the condition can help to give the woman a model, which in turn helps to alter her beliefs, assumptions and understanding of the condition and pain, which can help reduce anxiety and fear, and therefore with the management and reduction of pain.

3.   Emotional and cognitive factors: it is known that emotions such as anxiety and depression can increase the experience of pain. Hence the psychologist will ask if the patient has noticed this effect. Some of the patients, having had the condition explained to them by the doctor, will have made this connection by the time of the psychological assessment, and this can be a significant realisation for the woman, helping to provide a model with which to understand her condition. Others will not have made the connection and some will be quite sceptical about this. It is important that the woman is allowed to air her views freely, so that the psychologist can make a thorough assessment about her understanding and thinking about her condition.

What have they found reduces the pain, if anything?
How do they cope with the pain?

This line of questioning helps to establish what 'coping mechanisms' they use if any. In my experience, most women will say 'nothing really helps'. A number have found that lying down can ease the pain and so can a hot water bottle. Other than these strategies they feel quite helpless at managing their pain. The psychologist will ask specifically about the following three areas:

Relaxation skills

Research shows that relaxation can be helpful for managing chronic pain.[19] Hence, the psychologist will ask if they are able to relax or if they have found this helpful. In our experience, many of the women referred with CPP reply 'I never relax', 'I can't relax', 'I am always on the go'.

Future management will involve teaching specific relaxation exercises. Relaxation is an integrated physiological response that is characterised by generalised decreases in the sympathetic nervous system and metabolic activity.[43,44] Standardised instructions[45] or meditative techniques[43,46] are typically used to elicit the 'relaxation response'. This is often combined with teaching diaphragmatic breathing. Women are also taught that relaxation can release the body's natural pain-killers, 'endorphins', which will help them to manage their pain far more effectively. Relaxation is a characteristic part of most psychological interventions for pain.[47] We will recommend a tape that has a selection of exercises for the woman to use on a daily basis at home.[48]

It must be noted that many of the women we see at the clinic find it difficult to relax, so it is important that the psychologist asks the woman about their relaxation practice at each session, and also whether they are starting to use the relaxation exercises when they experience pain. It is also important to note that emotional issues, psychological factors and personality type may be hindering effective relaxation; hence, teaching relaxation exercises on their own is not sufficient with this client group. They may not be able to fully relax until other psychological and emotional factors are addressed first.

Cognitions (thoughts, beliefs, perceptions, meaning, assumptions, coping mechanisms etc.)

If the psychologist continues with this line of questioning, for example, 'When you are in pain, or when you do lie down due to the pain, what thoughts or images go through your mind?' The woman will often reply 'This pain is awful, why me? When will this pain stop? It is ruining my life. I am a useless mother and wife. What if my partner leaves me? What if I lose my job? Everyone thinks I am making this up, as they can't find anything wrong with me. The doctors make me feel it is all in my head, but it's not it is very real. No one understands. What if it is due to something like cancer and they haven't found it yet?' This type of anxiety-provoking thinking, also known as 'catastrophising', increases anxiety and depression, which can exacerbate the experience of pain. This is useful information to the psychologist when planning the continuing treatment strategy.

- *Cognitive coping strategies* The first part involves helping the woman to become more aware of her thoughts. Once the woman can start to monitor her thoughts she will often begin to see that if they are anxious, fearful, or depressing thoughts, then this will result in a feeling of anxiety, fear and depression, which we know can increase the experience of muscular tension and pain. She is then helped to devise more calming, reassuring thoughts when in pain, for example; 'I now recognise what brought this pain on, for example, overdoing the gardening, getting into an argument. The pain does not last forever. I will do some muscular relaxation, diaphragmatic breathing, think calming, reassuring thoughts. I will learn from this'.

• *Distraction and visualisation* Distraction is known to be effective in reducing the experience of pain, so the women are helped to find effective forms of distraction for them when in pain, such as doing a crossword or looking at a magazine. Visualisation and imagery skills, are helpful for pain management as they help to induce a feeling of calm and relaxation and are a form of distraction. The therapist will guide them through a variety of visualisations so they can find one they particularly like. For example, imagining lying on a warm, tropical beach, listening to the sound of the waves lapping against the shore, imagining the smell of the sun lotion and feeling her body getting warmer under the sun and relaxing. It can be helpful to use each of the five senses in the visualisation, what do they see, smell, hear, taste and touch.

Behavioural activities, both physical and mental

Both overdoing and underdoing activities can exacerbate the experience of pain. Hence, it is useful to assess the amount of activity being carried out to determine future therapy. As previously mentioned, many of the women when questioned say that they are 'always on the go, with so much to do'; 'can't stop and relax' or 'my mind is always on the go'. If the partner is in the assessment, he will often say, 'I am always telling her to stop and put her feet up, but even if she does stop you can see her thinking of all the things she should be doing or that need doing'. People with chronic pain conditions can be drawn into a cycle of not doing activities when in pain, then as the pain reduces they increase their activities, but can overdo activities, to try and 'catch up', which in turn can bring the pain on, so they have to stop and do nothing until the pain reduces, when they start again. This is not a helpful pattern to be in when trying to manage chronic pain.

• *Pacing skills* Continuing therapy will involve teaching the value of pacing their activities, both physical and mental. This may need the psychologist to ask about their daily schedule in detail, from waking to going to bed at night. Together with this they may need to learn how to prioritise their tasks, set realistic goals and learn assertion and communication skills to be able to say for example, 'no' to extra demands at work or home and to be able to ask for help when they need it. It will be helpful for the woman to learn the value of both 'pacing down' and 'pacing up' activities for pain management. For example, if she has a flare-up of pain, then it can help to 'pace down' activities for a while. Then when the pain has reduced and is more manageable, she can start to gradually 'pace up' her activities again, but still within a manageable range.

Women who are perfectionists tend to put excessive demands on themselves and others, and find it difficult to set healthy limits of activity. Likewise, a number of women we see have obsessive–compulsive disorder, involving excessive cleaning and tidying, which again puts excessive demands on their time and activities. This is also an anxiety disorder in itself, increasing the level of anxiety experienced by the women, which will exacerbate the experience of pain.

Emotional factors and current life events

To continue the assessment and gain further information, the psychologist will explain that certain emotions can increase the experience of pain and so will ask what are the woman's current issues causing, for example, anxiety, distress or conflict. These will often include the pain itself; the worry about what it is due to; all the doctors' appointments and investigations; the effect on her life, including relationships, work and social life. Together with this, there may be continuing life events causing emotional, cognitive and physical stress, for example, stress from continuing conflicts with their relationship with their partner, including their sexual relationship, relationships with family, friends or work colleagues, extra demands at work which are continuing, leading to the woman feeling pressurised or overwhelmed, buying and selling a house, with numerous problems along the way, a new baby in the house, especially with children already, leading to extra physical and emotional demands, conflicting with other established activities.

Psychological coping mechanisms

The psychologist will often assess and ask how they usually cope with emotions and life issues. A number of women may admit that they tend to 'bottle their emotions up', or try to ignore them or suppress them. Some people may not have a close friend to confide in and talk things over with. Continuing therapy will be about helping the woman to: (i) identify issues and conflicts, that may be contributing to making the pain worse; (ii) acknowledge them; and (iii) learn to use the therapy sessions to talk more openly about them and find ways to resolve, change or manage these issues more effectively. If there are particular relationship problems then specific couples therapy may be organised, either with the therapist in the clinic, or by referral to 'Relate'.

Personality type

Research has failed to identify a typical personality profile in patients with chronic pain and therefore studies are now more likely to investigate psychological profiles of subgroups of pain patients than to search for a typical pain patient profile.[7] Having said that, a number of the women that we see at the pelvic pain clinic, have an obsessive–compulsive personality (DSMIV – Axis II).[49] They may either show traits of this personality type or have a full personality disorder. They tend to be perfectionists and orderly, with particularly high expectations of themselves and others. A number also have obsessive–compulsive disorder (OCD) (DSMIV – Axis I), particularly to do with excessive cleaning and tidying. This is an anxiety disorder (Axis I) in itself, and the women often report feeling uncomfortable and anxious if their environment is not clean and tidy. This puts undue demands on their time and activities, making it particularly difficult for these woman to relax physically or mentally and they tend to overdo activities. Continuing therapy will be about working with the woman to help minimise the impact of the condition or personality on the pain condition.

Emotional factors and life events prior to onset?

As mentioned, the majority of cases that come to our pelvic pain clinic with CPP for which no cause has been established are found to have pelvic congestion. As it is believed that this is a functional condition, our experience has shown that stress is a significant factor in the onset and development of the condition. Stress is an umbrella word, which includes external stressors, such as life events, which interact with internal coping mechanisms, which are learnt, which interact with biological predisposition, genetic factors, or personality type.[50,51] Due to this, the psychologist will ask what was occurring in the woman's life six months to one year prior to onset. The stressors prior to onset fall into two broad categories: (i) life events as mentioned above, more often it is not necessarily one event but a number of events over an extended period of time and (ii) stress-prone personality type, for example the obsessive–compulsive personality, driven, or perfectionist type, with limited coping skills.

Continuing stress can lead to physical symptoms and then the development of disorders due to the action of the stress hormones adrenaline, noradrenaline and cortisol being released over an extended period of time. Many of the women we see with pelvic congestion, when we explain that it is thought to be a stress-related disorder, will say 'no wonder, of course, it all falls into place now, I had a very difficult, demanding or pressurised six months to a year prior to onset'. This information seems invaluable for some women and helps give them an explanation and model, which helps to put their condition in perspective and gives them much more of an idea of how to manage it.

Childhood

As part of the assessment, it is helpful to find out about the woman's childhood, including her relationship with parents and siblings. It can be helpful to ask about her parents' personalities, as unhealthy behaviour patterns can be learnt, for example if one parent was a 'workaholic' or had obsessive cleaning and tidying behaviour. It is helpful to ask if there was any history of abuse including emotional, physical or sexual abuse, each of which can result in emotional and psychological difficulties, which in turn hinder people's ability to manage emotions, relationships, stress and pain. The early literature suggesting that CPP is caused by unresolved psychic conflict being somehow 'somatised' has now been largely discredited.[52] However, it may still be true that for some women with pelvic pain somatisation remains an issue, and the association continues to be explored. Overall, however, assessing their childhood gives further helpful information about emotional and psychological coping skills and mechanisms they have learnt, as already mentioned. It highlights cognitive schemas learnt in childhood,[25] for example, messages they learnt about themselves and others which may still be having an effect on how they manage their life and relationships currently. It highlights life-management skills they may not have learnt, and need to learn, in order to manage lifestyle stress and pain more effectively.

Continuing pain-management therapy sessions

From the assessment the psychologist is able to build up a profile of the woman and see where the problem areas exist currently. If there are continuing life events causing

Table 7.1. Factors and skills that increase or reduce pain

Factors that increase pain	Factors/skills that reduce pain
Physical	**Physical**
Muscular tension; activated autonomic nervous system	Muscular relaxation skills; diaphragmatic breathing; release of endorphins
Behavioural	**Behavioural**
Overactivity; underactivity (physical and mental)	Pacing; prioritising; goal setting skills; assertion skills, saying 'no'; asking for help
Cognitive	**Cognitive**
Faulty assumptions; meaning; limited understanding of pain; anxiety-provoking thoughts focusing on pain	Education: condition and pain; cognitive coping strategies; calming, reassuring thoughts; distraction; visualisation
Emotional	**Emotional**
Anxious, upset, angry, unsupported; life issues/conflicts; bottled-up/ignored/suppressed emotions	Calm, relaxed, in control, supported; identifying issues, resolve, change; talking in safe, trusting relationship; counselling for couples

emotional conflict, it is important to identify these and acknowledge them as significant factors. It is important to identify their personality type, to assess how this is impacting on their pain condition. Together with this it is important to identify the coping skills they are lacking for managing life issues and chronic pain. This information will help the psychologist to determine the most suitable treatment strategies for the continuing sessions. Table 7.1 gives a summary of areas assessed and what future management hopes to achieve.

The areas covered in further sessions and the order and the amount of time spent on different aspects will obviously depend on the issues identified in the assessment phase, together with additional information that reveals itself in further sessions. The goal is to help the woman gain control over her pain and in effect reverse the vicious cycle of pain (Figure 7.1). The areas covered are often interrelated and overlap in therapy. The therapy is combined with a variety of counselling skills, including building a therapeutic relationship, being nonjudgemental, using empathy and having sensitivity around the timing of particular interventions, all of which are important therapist skills.

Alongside the pain and stress management sessions, we recommend relaxation tapes as mentioned,[48] together with a selection of books, if the patient is interested in further reading.[51-56]

Research

The model carried out at the pelvic pain clinic has helped women reduce their pain significantly, learn how to manage their pain far more effectively and improve their quality of life significantly.[39,57-60] Farquhar and colleagues[59] carried out a randomised controlled trial of ovarian downregulation with medroxyprogesterone acetate (MPA;

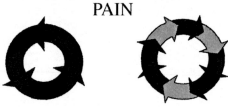

Reversing the vicious circle of
PAIN

- Pain – Tension – Anxiety – Fear – Increase pain
- Pain – Relax – Coping thoughts – Pacing –
  Realistic goals – Identify stress issues – Assertion
  skills – Reduce pain – Increase self-confidence

Figure 7.1.   Reversing the vicious cycle of pain

Provera) for 4 months at the Clinic, with and without cognitive–behavioural therapy for the treatment of pelvic congestion. The four groups were placebo, placebo and psychotherapy, MPA, MPA and psychotherapy. Pain scores were taken at four months and ten months using a visual analogue scale. The most effective group at ten months after start of treatment was the MPA and psychotherapy.

Peters and colleagues[61] carried out a randomised controlled trial and has shown that a 'biopsychosocial' model was significantly more effective with CPP than a 'traditional' management group where organic screening for pelvic pathology was ruled out by diagnostic laparoscopy. Similar multidisciplinary approaches, which emphasise management within a biopsychosocial model, have been shown to be effective in other pain syndromes such as chronic low back pain.[62]

The clinical effectiveness of the cognitive–behavioural approach to pain management has been demonstrated in well over a 100 studies,[30] with a wide range of pain syndromes, including headaches,[63] rheumatoid arthritis,[64] temporomandibular pain disorders,[65] debridement of burns,[66] low-back pain,[67] atypical chest pain,[68] cumulative trauma injury[69] and heterogeneous samples of chronic pain syndromes.[70-72] A number of these studies have reported follow-up data ranging from six months to two years, indicating that the improvements have been maintained.[30]

The Department of Health has just published a 62-page report on *Treatment choice in psychological therapies and counselling – evidence based clinical practice guidelines.*[73] Under somatic complaints they list 'chronic pain' and state: 'Cognitive and behavioural therapies, including biofeedback, show evidence of being effective in the treatment of chronic pain. This was based on three eight-rated reviews of psychological treatments for chronic pain'.[74-76]

Following on from chronic pain comes: Gynaecology: 'No high quality review evidence was identified'. As mentioned, this could be more due to the fact that there are still few specialist pelvic pain clinics, so there are still relatively few people doing research. However, they did include supplementary evidence: 'There is growing evidence from recent randomised control trials (RCTs) that psychological approaches have utility. Pelvic pain benefited from a cognitive–behavioural approach'.[57,61]

Therapist and patient variables

Assuming a good standard of therapist training, as a counsellor and a member of the British Association of Counsellors and Psychotherapists (BACP),[42] a psychotherapist and a member of the United Kingdom Council for Psychotherapists (UKCP),[41] or a psychologist and a member of the British Psychological Society (BPS),[40] then along with treatment variables, it is important to recognise that therapist and patient variables[77-80] and the quality of the relationship[81,82] also influence outcome. Research indicates that therapist qualities linked to good outcome include the personality of the therapist, help in understanding the problems, encouragement to face up to difficult issues gradually and coming across as an understanding person who the patient feels comfortable talking to.[83]

Pain clinics

There are a number of specialist pain clinics in the UK and the 'Pain Society' and 'Pain Concern' can provide a list of them. These clinics are for people suffering chronic pain due to a variety of conditions and are multidisciplinary, usually including psychologists, physiotherapists and doctors. The psychological approach to pain management usually follows a cognitive–behavioural approach. As gynaecologists refer relatively few women for pain management, these clinics do not often treat a large number of patients with CPP. However, if gynaecologists did begin to refer more women, then their experience and expertise would develop. It needs to be decided if women with CPP, both with and without pathology, should be treated in a multidisciplinary team at their local hospital, or be referred to a specialist pelvic pain clinic of which there are very few or, referred to a general pain clinic.

Conclusion

Pain conditions are multi-causal and pain itself is a multidimensional phenomenon that needs a multi-theoretical treatment approach incorporating sensory, affective, cognitive and behavioural factors. The cognitive–behavioural approach to pain management, carried out in an integrated multidisciplinary team, has been found to be effective at helping women with chronic pain due to a variety of conditions, including CPP, to reduce their pain and manage it far more effectively. Hence, the IASP[38] recommends that chronic pain should involve both medically trained and psychologically trained health professionals.

There have been a number of research studies now into the effectiveness of the cognitive–behavioural approach and the management of pain for a wide variety of conditions as already mentioned, however, there is still little research for CPP. This is probably because the field of gynaecology has yet to realise the benefits of psychological interventions, and so there are relatively few psychologists working in this area to carry out research. When gynaecology does realise the benefit, as other disciplines now have, it is hoped that more clinics will be set up and more funding will be made available for specific research into exactly what treatment variables are the most effective for this client group.

References

1. Gillibrand PN. The investigation of pelvic pain. Presented at the scientific meeting on 'Chronic pelvic pain: a gynaecological headache', Royal College of Obstetricians and Gynaecologists, London: RCOG; 1981.

2. Steege JF, Stout AL. Resolution of chronic pelvic pain after laparoscopic lysis of adhesions. *Am J Obstet Gynecol* 1991;**165**:278–83.

3. Fedele L, Parazzini F, Bianchi S, Arcaini L, Candiani GB. Stage and localization of pelvic endometriosis and pain. *Fertil Steril* 1990;**53**:155–8.

4. Vercellini P, Trespidi L, De Giorgi O, Cortesi I, Parazzini F, Crosignani PG. Endometriosis and pelvic pain: relation to disease stage and localization. *Fertil Steril* 1996;**65**:299–304.

5. Stout AL, Steege JF, Dodson WC, Hughes CL. Relationship of laparoscopic findings to self-report of pelvic pain. *Am J Obstet Gynecol* 1991;**164**:73–9.

6. Gamsa A. Clinical Reviews. The role of psychological factors in chronic pain. I. A half century of study. *Pain* 1994;**57**:5–15.

7. Gamsa A. The role of psychological factors in chronic pain. II. A critical appraisal. *Pain* 1994;**57**:17–29.

8. Stengel E. Pain and the psychiatrist. *Br J Psychiatry* 1965;**111**:795–802.

9. Stengel E. Pain and the psychiatrist (reply to open letter written by E Slater). *Br J Psychiatry* 1966;**112**:329–31.

10. Fry RPW, Crisp AH, Beard RW. Sociopsychological factors in chronic pelvic pain: A review. *J Psychosom Res* 1997;**42**:1–15.

11. Beecher HK. Pain in men wounded in battle. *Ann Surg* 1946;**123**:95–105.

12. Beecher HK. Relationship of significance of wound to the pain experienced. *JAMA* 1956;**161**:1609–13.

13. Melzack R, Wall PD. Pain mechanisms: a new theory. *Science* 1965;**150**:971–9.

14. Weisenberg M. Cognitive aspects of pain. In: Wall PD, Melzack R, editors. *Textbook of Pain.* Edinburgh: Churchill Livingstone, 1994. p. 275–89.

15. Craig K. Emotional aspects of pain. In: Wall PD, Melzack R, editors. *Textbook of Pain.* Edinburgh: Churchill Livingstone; 1994. p. 261–74.

16. Keefe FJ, Lefebvre JC. Behaviour therapy. In: Wall PD, Melzack R, editors. *Textbook of Pain.* Edinburgh: Churchill Livingstone; 1994. p. 1367–80.

17. Williams C. Dysfunctional illness behaviour. *Br J Health Psychol* 1997;**2**:153–65.

18. Flor H, Turk DC. Psychophysiology of chronic pain: do chronic pain patients exhibit symptom-specific psychophysiological responses? *Psychol Bull* 1989;**105**:215–59.

19. Jessup BA, Gallegos X. Relaxation and biofeedback. In: Wall PD, Melzack R, editors. *Textbook of Pain.* Edinburgh: Churchill Livingstone; 1994. p. 1321–36.

20. Melzack, R. Pain theory: exceptions to the rule. *Behav Brain Sci* 1980;**3**:313.

21. Ellis A. *Reason and Emotion in Psychotherapy.* New York: Lyle Stuart; 1962.

22. Beck AT, Rush AJ, Shaw BF, Emory G. *Cognitive Therapy of Depression.* New York: Guilford Press; 1979.

23. Beck AT, Emory G, Greenberg RL. *Anxiety Disorders and Phobia.* New York: Basic Books; 1985.

24. Beck AT, Freeman A., Pretzer J, Davis DD, Fleming B, Ottaviani R, *et al. Cognitive Therapy of Personality Disorders.* New York: Guilford Press; 1990.

25. Young JE. *Cognitive Therapy for Personality Disorders: A Schema-Focussed Approach.* Sarasota, FL: Professional Resource Press; 1999.

26. Turk DC, Meichenbaum D, Genest M. *Pain and Behavioural Medicine: A Cognitive-Behavioural Perspective.* New York: Guilford Press; 1983.

27. Turk DC, Holzman AD, Kerns RD. Chronic pain. In: Holroyd KA, Creer TL, editors. *Self-Management of Chronic Disease.* New York: Academic Press; 1986.

28. Holzman AD, Turk DC, Kerns RD. The cognitive-behavioural approach in treating chronic pain. In: Holzman AD, Turk DC, editors. *Pain Management: A Handbook of Psychological Treatment Approaches.* New York: Pergamon Press; 1986.

29. Turk DC, Rudy TE. An integrated approach to pain treatment: beyond the scalpel and syringe. In: Tollison CD, editor. *Handbook of Chronic Pain Management,* 2nd edn. Baltimore: Williams & Wilkins; 1993.

30. Turk DC, Meichenbaum DH. A cognitive-behavioural approach to pain management. In: Wall PD, Melzack R, editors. *Textbook of Pain.* Edinburgh: Churchill Livingstone; 1994, p. 1001–9.

31. Fordyce WE, Fowler R, Lehmann J, DeLateur B, Sand P, Trieschmann R. Operant conditioning in the

treatment of chronic pain. *Arch Physical Med Rehab* 1973;**54**:399–408.

32. Fordyce WE. *Behavioural Methods for Chronic Pain and Illness.* St Louis: CV Mosby; 1976.
33. Grace VM. Problems women patients experience in the medical encounter for chronic pelvic pain: a New Zealand study. *Health Care Women Int* 1995;**16**:509–19.
34. Grace VM. Problems of communication, diagnosis and treatment experienced by women using the New Zealand health services for chronic pelvic pain: a quantitative analysis. *Health Care Women Int* 1995;**16**:521–35.
35. Selfe S, Matthews Z, Stones RW. Factors influencing outcome in consultations for chronic pelvic pain. *J Women's Health* 1998;**7**:1041–8.
36. Elcombe S, Gath D, Day A. The psychological effects of laparoscopy on women with chronic pelvic pain. *Psychol Med* 1997;**27**:1041–50.
37. Price JR, Blake F. Chronic Pelvic Pain: the assessment as therapy. *J Psychosom Res* 1999;**46**:7–14.
38. Fields HL. *Core Curriculum for Professional Education in Pain.* Seattle, WA: IASP Press; 1991.
39. Audit of the Pelvic Pain Clinic, Northwick Park Hospital. Unpublished. 1998.
40. British Psychological Society (BPS). St Andrews House, 48 Princess Road East, Leicester, LE1 7DR, UK.
41. United Kingdom Council for Psychotherapists (UKCP). 167–169 Great Portland Street, London, W1W 5PF, UK.
42. British Association for Counselling and Psychotherapy. (BACP). 1 Regent Place, Rugby, Warwickshire, CV21 2PJ, UK.
43. Benson H. *The Relaxation Response.* New York: Morrow; 1975.
44. Benson H, Pomeranz B, Cutz I. The relaxation response and pain. In: Wall P, Melzack R, editors. *Textbook of Pain*, 1st edn. Edinburgh: Churchill Livingstone; 1984, p. 817–22.
45. Jacobson E. *Progressive Relaxation.* Chicago: University of Chicago Press; 1938.
46. Kabat-Zinn J. An outpatient program in behavioural medicine for chronic pain based on the practice of mindfulness meditation: theoretical considerations and preliminary results. *Gen Hosp Psychiatr* 1982;**4**:33–48.
47. Turner JA, Chapman CR. Psychological interventions for chronic pain: a critical review. I. Relaxation training and biofeedback. *Pain* 1982;**12**:1–21.
48. Talking Life, PO Box 1, Wirral, L47 7DD, UK. 'Coping with Pain' audio tape and 'The Relaxation Kit' audio tape.
49. American Psychiatric Association. *Diagnostic and Statistical Manual of Mental Disorders*, DSM-IV, 4th edn. Washington DC: American Psychiatric Association; 1994.
50. Powell TJ, Enright SJ. *Anxiety and Stress Management.* London and New York: Routledge; 1990.
51. Jones H. *I'm Too Busy To Be Stressed.* London: Hodder & Stoughton; 1997.
52. Savidge CJ, Slade P. Psychological aspects of chronic pelvic pain. *J Psychosom Res* 1997;**42**:433–44.
53. Catalano EM, Hardin KN. *The Chronic Pain Control Workbook*, 2nd edn. Oakland, CA: New Harbinger Publications, Inc.; 1996.
54. Davis M, Eshelman ER, McKay M. *The Relaxation and Stress Reduction Workbook*, 5th edn. Oakland, CA: New Harbinger Publications, Inc.; 2000.
55. Wells C, Nown G. In Pain. *A Self-help Guide for Chronic Pain Sufferers.* London: Optima; 1993.
56. Shone N. *Coping Successfully with Pain.* London: Sheldon Press Publications; 1995.
57. Pearce S, Knight C, Beard RW. Pelvic pain, a common gynaecological problem. *J Psychosom Obstet Gynaecol* 1982;**1**:12–17.
58. Pearce S. A psychological investigation of chronic pelvic pain in women. PhD Thesis, University of London. 1986.
59. Farquhar CM, Rogers V, Franks S, Pearce S, Wadsworth J, Beard RW. A randomised controlled trial of medroxyprogesterone acetate and psychotherapy for the treatment of pelvic congestion. *Br J Obstet Gynaecol* 1989;**96**:1153–62.
60. Beard RW, Gangar K, Pearce S. Chronic gynaecological pain. In: Wall PD, Melzack R, editors. *Textbook of Pain.* Edinburgh: Churchill Livingstone; 1994. p. 597–614.
61. Peters AA, van Dorst E, Jellis B, van Zuuren E, Hermans J, Trimbos JB. A randomized clinical trial to compare two different approaches in women with chronic pelvic pain. *Obstet Gynecol* 1991;**77**:740–44.
62. Bendix AF, Bendix T, Lund C, Kirkbak S, Ostenfeld S. Comparison of three intensive programs for chronic low back pain patients: a prospective, randomized, observer-blinded study with one-year follow-up. *Scand J Rehabil Med* 1997;**29**:81–9.
63. Newton CR, Barbaree HE. Cognitive changes accompanying headache treatment: the use of a thought-sampling procedure. *Cogn Ther Res* 1987;**11**:635–52.
64. O'Leary A, Shoor S, Lorig K, Holman HR. A cognitive-behavioural treatment for rheumatoid

arthritis. *Health Psychol* 1988;**7**:527–44.

65. Olson RE, Malow RM. Effects of biofeedback and psychotherapy on patients with myofascial pain dysfunction who are non-responsive to conventional treatments. *Rehab Psychol* 1987;**32**:195–205.

66. Wernick R, Jaremko ME, Taylor PW. Pain management in severely burned patients: a test of stress-inoculation training. *J Behav Med* 1981;**4**:103–9.

67. Linssen ACG, Zitman FG. Patient evaluation of a cognitive behavioural group program for patients with low back pain. *Soc Sci Med* 1984;**19**:1361–7.

68. Klimes I, Mayou RA, Pearce MJ, Fagg JR. Psychological treatment for atypical non-cardiac chest pain: a controlled evaluation. *Psychol Med* 1990;**20**:605–11.

69. Spence SH. Cognitive behaviour therapy in the management of chronic occupational pain of the upper limbs. *Behav Res Ther* 1989;**27**:435–46.

70. Kerns RD, Turk DC, Holzman AD, Rudy TE. Efficacy of a cognitive-behavioural group approach for the treatment of chronic pain. *Clin J Pain* 1986;**2**:195–203.

71. Thorn BE, Williams DA, Johnson PR. Individualized cognitive behavioural treatment of chronic pain. *Behav Psychother* 1986;**14**:210–25.

72. Nicholas MK, Wilson PH, Goyen J. Comparison of cognitive-behavioural group treatment and an alternative non-psychological treatment for chronic low back pain. *Pain* 1992;**48**:339–47.

73. Department of Health. Treatment choice in psychological therapies and counselling. Evidence-based clinical practice guidelines. London: Department of Health; 2001.

74. Compas BE, Haaga DAF, Keefe FJ, Leitenberg H, Williams DA. Sampling of empirically supported psychological treatments from health psychology: smoking, chronic pain, cancer and bulimia nervosa. *J Consult Clin Psychol* 1998;**66**:89–112.

75. Morley S, Eccleston C, Williams A. Systematic review and meta-analysis of randomised controlled trials of cognitive behaviour therapy for chronic pain in adults, excluding headache. *Pain* 1999;**80**:1–13.

76. Scheer SJ, Watanabe TK, Radack KL. Randomized controlled trials in industrial low back pain. Part 3. Subacute/chronic pain interventions. *Arch Physic Med Rehab* 1997;**78**:414–23.

77. Bergin AE, Lambert MJ. The evaluation of therapeutic outcomes. In: Garfield SL, Bergin AE, editors. *Handbook of Psychotherapy and Behaviour Change*, 2nd edn. New York: Wiley; 1978. p. 139–89.

78. Orlinsky DE, Howard KI. Process and outcome in psychotherapy. In Garfield SL, Bergin AE, editors. *Handbook of Psychotherapy and Behaviour Change*, 3rd edn. New York: Wiley; 1986, p. 311–84.

79. Lambert MJ. Psychotherapy outcome research: implications for integrative and eclectic therapists. In: Norcross JC, Goldfried MR, editors. *Handbook of Psychotherapy Integration*. New York: Basic Books; 1992. p. 94–129.

80. Lambert MJ Shapiro DA, Bergin AE. The effectiveness of psychotherapy. In: Garfield SL, Bergin AE, editors. *Handbook of Psychotherapy and Behaviour Change*, 3rd edn. New York: Wiley; 1986, p. 157–212.

81. Gelso CJ, Carter JA. The relationship in counselling and psychotherapy: components, consequences and theoretical antecedents. *The Counselling Psychologist* 1985;**13**:155–243.

82. Clarkson P. *The Therapeutic Relationship*. London: Whurr Publishers Ltd.; 1995.

83. Sloane RB, Staples RF, Cristol AH, Yorkston NH, Whipple K. *Psychotherapy Versus Behaviour Therapy*. Cambridge, MA: Harvard University Press; 1975.

Chapter 8

Pain and pain relief

Discussion

Discussion following Professor Li Wan Po's paper

Collett: There has been some recent work that has looked at the use of morphine in rats and compared the difference on tail flick test and abdominal constriction between female rats and male rats. It showed that, in the female rats, morphine was not so efficacious as in the male rats. There has also been a clinical study by Gear,[1] who looked at the use of butorphanol and nalbuphine after third molar extraction, which showed that these κ-agonists were efficacious in women but were not particularly efficacious in men. My question is: do you think that by using new agonists we are using the wrong type of analgesic in women?

Li Wan Po: I really don't know at the moment because the clinical trials that have been conducted are not sufficiently fine-tuned to be able to separate those things. In any case, when we talk about pieces of selectivity and receptors of types we do not actually sample the patient population that we are looking at. We are starting to get information from the genomic world in relation to quite a number of drugs and we know that there are different distributions and that some of them are bimodal. Therefore, perhaps what we should do is not even to treat on the basis of gender but to individualise treatment. That would make sense anyway, given the complexity of the management of pain, because everyone has different inputs there.

Steege: My contacts in the drug industry tell me that, currently, one outgrowth of the Human Genome Project is to consider typing individuals specifically for their reactions to drugs and receptiveness to drugs. It would cost US$10,000 a piece to do that, so it is not going to happen any time soon, but the expectation is that in the next five or ten years the per-patient cost will come down and we will see designer approaches to drugs that we cannot even dream of now.

Li Wan Po: Perhaps I am a little more sceptical than you on this, simply because when we do the genotyping it is on the basis of genes that we know have an influence on the response. The problem is that most of the responses are not monogenic; they are polygenic, with many interactions. Therefore, typing for one gene would not predict a response when there are multi-genes involved.

Thornton: You mentioned that the opioid receptors were G-protein linked. I did not understand about the signal transduction mechanism. Could you briefly describe that? Secondly, with a number of G-protein-coupled receptors, constitutive activity has been described. I wonder whether you feel that constitutive activity – in other words, receptor activity in the absence of an agonist – is important for the mechanism of action of opioid receptors?

Li Wan Po: You are quite right. I don't know whether you have more information than I have in that sense because I am not sure whether the downstream events are all that well defined or that we have the sensitivity to pick out the differences to which you are alluding. The problem is, it is fairly generic and average behaviour and what we need is to be able to count the number of receptors. Unfortunately, these populations are so heterogeneous and so widely dispersed that the noise itself does not enable us to identify what are the downstream events and whether there are other differences.

Berkley: I want to add to the comment about genetic specificity. It is not only the interactions but how the gene expression changes over time as a result of experience, so that a person at one moment is a different person than he or she was before. Is not that part of the problem? There are certain absolutes. Certain people are missing enzymes and, in that case, a drug that is not going to be metabolised will not work if the liver enzymes are not there. Most of the other cases would end up being more complex and go back to this whole issue of developmental history. Would you agree with that?

Li Wan Po: In some cases it is actually absolute. For example, I am a lousy drinker because my alcohol dehydrogenase is not very good. Therefore, you will see me drink one glass of wine only. That is clear and it is quite common among people of Chinese descent. We also know that in the African sub-population they have genetic differences. For example, in the metabolism of some of the anti-tuberculous drugs, isoniazid being one of them, and also some of the anti-malarial drugs, there is no doubt at all that the dosing schedule should be different. But on the whole, when people come into the surgery, aside from the very clear examples, being able to genotype is very difficult. There have been many experiments about phenotyping – looking at population differences. For example, if you look at the Malaysian population, you have an Indian sub-population, a Chinese sub-population and a Malay sub-population (which is a mix of the two way back in history), and you can actually see the polymorphism. If you do that and you then genotype, there is no correlation with response, because response rates may be due to diet, and I am sure that culture has an effect, and how to dissociate those very different components is difficult. The genes tell you one thing but the test results do not correlate. The culture does and the phenotype – how they look correlates to the responses – but we cannot relate it to the genotype.

There are three explanations for this. The first is that what we think is monogenic is not really monogenic. The second is that what we thought was an important gene is really not important in the fullness of things. The third is that there are a lot of other interactions affecting the response, and I suspect that that one is probably the most important.

Sutton: I am going to lower the tone a little and ask you about the chilli powder cream you use when you castrate your people back home. We had a patient recently who, four weeks after hysterectomy, had the most appalling abdominal pain – you could not touch her abdomen. We could find no cause for this and the neurologists were unhelpful, but we rang Chris Glynn in Oxford and he had heard of this syndrome – he sees it once or twice a year, particularly after hernia operations but occasionally after hysterectomy. He suggested the use of chilli cream and it worked instantly and miraculously. Can you tell me why that is?

Li Wan Po: The current theory is that it depletes the nerve cells of substance P, so you get to a state where there is no response any more. Initially it is very painful. From experience, we know that when we start eating chillies they start hot but then we get accustomed to them. One intriguing thought that has crossed my mind is how do people who eat a lot of chillies day in, day out, have responses to pain – for example, from the abdomen? I am not sure. I suppose the pain sensitivity threshold would be much higher than in those who are not used to taking chillies – the plasticity that Professor Berkley mentioned.

Berkley: There are data available. A group in Mexico has been doing this work and vaginal sensitivity decreases with people who eat a lot of chilli peppers. May I ask Professor Sutton – where did the women apply it?

Sutton: I don't know.

Berkley: If they had applied it to their forehead, do you think it would have worked?

Li Wan Po: There are two modes of delivery. I have not mentioned delivery systems. With many of the new drugs we need to have parenteral delivery. Therefore, for many patients, just keeping that will be very painful. In terms of capsaicin, the chilli drug, I wonder, with topical applications for post-herpetic neuralgia, where it is sure to be effective, whether we need systemic delivery for some of the internal organs. Rubbing it might have an effect as a counter-irritant activity – rubbing fibres and then having the second pathway coming into effect – but I suspect that with internal organs we probably need to have oral delivery.

Berkley: Dr Clare Fowler is the neurologist with whom I am working at Queen Square. She invented intracervical treatments with capsaicin for hyperactivity and it works quite well in selected patients. So there are data.

Li Wan Po: Except that trials are extremely difficult to conduct because capsaicin is actually quite hot and therefore it is difficult to have a placebo control. What you find is that you do not know whether it is psychological or biochemical in terms of activity. There are some new derivatives now that are non-pungent. Those are being trialled and it will be interesting to see whether they work just as well, so that we can dissociate the psychological component from the pharmacological biochemical component.

Crowhurst: Professor Li Wan Po has just said that he did not mention drug delivery systems and pharmacokinetics. Most of you will know that, in obstetrics, certainly in the acute pain area, the story of epidurals and administering drugs as close to the site of spinal receptors as we can get it has been a great success and it has now spread into other areas of analgesic therapy. We are on the threshold of an era where we can administer some of these drugs in minute doses, getting them very close to the drug receptors.

I should like to ask Dr Smith about pelvic pain. I wonder how much of pelvic pain goes back to poor experiences of childbirth with either failed analgesia or a fixed attitude to somebody who comes into labour with a birth plan set in stone – no gas, no pethidine, no epidural, no nothing. Then it finishes up with a labour with a bad outcome or one where they have to have all of those things. Is that a common aetiological factor in pelvic pain?

Smith: If I am looking at factors prior to onset for women with pelvic congestion, sometimes it will start around the birth. If they have had a particularly bad experience it can do, but I would say that is rare. It is not something that I get coming up recurrently.

Thornton: I have a question for Professor Li Wan Po. I completely accept the tissue distribution and the constitutive and inducible forms of the cyclo-oxygenase (COX) enzymes. I was under the impression that COX-1 and COX-2 both acted on exactly the same substrate with exactly the same products, but one of your slides demonstrated that the products of COX-1 and COX-2 were different. Could you clarify that for me, please?

Li Wan Po: Do you mean in terms of drugs? We have very selective agents now that will only act on the COX-2 isoform. For example, celecoxib, rofecoxib and nabumetone are selective COX inhibitors. Ibuprofen, naproxen and aspirin would be non-selective: they actually attack both.

Thornton: I was thinking more of the enzymes themselves than their selective inhibitors.

Li Wan Po: In terms of distribution?

Thornton: In terms of the products formed by those enzymes, whether the products from the arachidonic acid effects of COX-1 and COX-2 are identical or whether different products are formed from both of those enzymes.

Li Wan Po: The prostaglandins are obviously different. For example COX-1 and COX-2 inhibition leads to differential effects on the kidney.

Discussion following Dr Newton-John's and Miss Smith's papers

Stones: I should like to address a question to both of the psychologists. We have heard a bit about some of the models and clearly you use psychological models in your work. We have also heard this afternoon that in a way the models that some of us have become used to, such as the gate control theory, are superseded in current thinking. Is that a problem? Should we be trying to treat patients with the very latest post-modern neuroscience/culturally informed model? Or does it not matter? Is it just useful to have a model that is an operational construct which will be a useful vehicle for a discussion? Is that really what is happening? Or is the nature of the model important?

Smith: Just keep it quite simple. If you speak to people who work with chronic pain in groups, the more complex the explanations become, the more likely you are to fall out of treatment. I will use that gate control theory because it is quite a straightforward, simple model that women can take on board and I find that it is the most effective. I am aware that there are more complex models about where pain pathways go in the brain and the cortex and thinking processes, but I do not feel that they really need to know that. If they are very inquisitive, then yes, I may explain more about the science of pain, but I do not feel it is really necessary. So keep it simple.

Stones: Is it the case that for a patient to accept a model or to plug into a model is part of the treatment? And if they cannot do that, is it a problem for them?

Smith: Some people take the model on board very quickly and it can be a significant intervention for them. With other people it can take a while, so it is just having the sensitivity to work with them, to work with their understanding and perceptions over time and gradually help them to come around to that way of thinking. I may be contradicted on the cultural issues, but that is what I have found to be most effective. It can take five minutes or it can take five sessions – it depends.

Newton-John: In terms of models I agree. Most of us do not have a great deal of time to go through the detail. I also believe that patients on the whole do not take away a great deal of detail. What they do take away is the physician's attitude towards them, the degree to which the doctor asks questions and listens to answers, and the judgmental approach. If patients go away feeling not blamed for their condition if there is no obvious aetiology for it, but understood and listened to and supported by the doctor, and it is a collaborative approach, that is really what it is about – not sophisticated understanding of gate control versus biopsychosocial or whatever.

Berkley: Can I back that up? I would get very upset if I heard you saying this is the mechanism for pain, or there are much better ones – like the things I showed in my talk. I agree that it really does not matter as long as people come to understand that their pain is a multidisciplinary kind of event and how one's nervous system creates it is a multidisciplinary event. Whenever I give talks to audiences, one of the biggest things that is gone over and I get the most requests for is the table I showed you, in a format so that they can bring it to the clinician and they can have an exchange over that table. I hear that from the people who have listened to me who could not give a hoot about my carrying on about this mechanism or that mechanism but what they love is the opportunity to have a look at this optimism – 'I've something to talk about now.' I have given it out and told them to add to it. Despite my carrying on about mechanisms, I would back that up.

MacLean: Can I follow Mr Stones' point and perhaps question whether clinicians should ever pursue these areas? I know that clinicians become involved more and more, but there is surely a boundary beyond which clinicians should not venture. One of Miss Smith's recommendations was that in managing chronic pain gynaecologists should have access to psychology and psychotherapy. Do we really put that as a recommendation, or should we be saying that unless you are working in a special clinic situation, when you get to a particular stage those patients should be referred either to a special clinic such as you have at Northwick Park or to the local pain clinic? Rather than each of us having our own psychologist who comes to the gynaecology clinic, it might be better to recognise those patients who would benefit more by going to a specialised pain clinic. Any thoughts?

Smith: I understand the restrictions of having a psychologist on board with your team. I suppose that is being quite idealistic. So yes, when you find these patients you definitely need to do something with them that involves a psychologist and that may mean referring them to a specialist clinic or pain clinic, or making links with your clinical psychology department and then having set times every month, say, for a ward round on particular patients. That might be another way – so that you start to make more links with the clinical psychology department that is usually in each hospital.

Newton-John: I slightly disagree, as a clinical psychologist. There is a slight danger in partitioning off the approach to managing chronic pain to different disciplines. Certainly at the extremes of the normal curve there are people who need specialist input, but my feeling is that we should be very aware that in every interaction with every health professional there is a psychological process occurring and that every professional needs to be very aware of how to maximise that inter-reaction at every point. Any clinician who is open and honest and is working collaboratively in this way, talking about the treatment options with the patient and getting them to elicit the patient's anxieties about this one versus another one and planning this through carefully – it does not need a clinical psychologist to do that. Certainly to have access to specialist input where that is required is important, but there is a slight danger in thinking that we do the biomedical stuff and the other people do the psychology. It is incumbent upon us to understand the biomedical as best we can, but it also up to everybody to understand the psychosocial nature of these problems.

In relation to who to refer and when to refer, there are numerous pain measures and reviews of the measures and updates on the reviews, and it does not take a great deal of time for anybody to be distributing a brief battery to the patients coming through, to score that quickly and to get what is a pretty rough rule of thumb but it is better than nothing from standardised questionnaires to get an idea of who is exhibiting significant levels of distress and may therefore need referral out. You do not need to do a full psychiatric interview to be able to detect where the problems are.

Collett: I should like to endorse a good deal of what you have said. In our pelvic pain clinic we spend quite a lot of time going back through the notes with the patient and explaining what diagnoses they have had in the past and why certain diagnoses may not be true. One thing that I would like to know from either of you is this. Do you think that these patients are best managed in a group or on an individual basis? That may help answer some of the questions that have been raised.

Newton-John: The group has potentially a very powerful effect. Patients coming together and realising that they are not alone in their condition, certainly not alone in their experience of the condition, is extremely powerful. On group treatment for chronic pain the evidence is equivocal. A group is very much dependent upon the screening and selection that goes into that, and you could have too many disparate individuals within a group that breaks down. There are good formats for running groups but it is very important not to see a group as a kind of dumping ground for anybody who vaguely comes under the heading of chronic pain. If you are able to select carefully and put people together who have similar kinds of experiences, the group can be tremendously powerful as an ongoing support after the treatment is finished.

Collett: Not for the treatment itself?

Newton-John: For the treatment as well, but the treatment may be eight or 12 sessions. Their pain problem does not end there; it is an ongoing thing. Often in the programme where I work patients stay in touch and act as their own support group, which again is pretty useful.

Stones: I would like to comment on the access to psychology services that there may or may not be in different parts of the country. I work in a trust where there is no psychology service. You can only have psychology input if it is to do with child sexual abuse or alcohol. My colleagues in pain management have managed to get some resources for psychology through some of the primary-care trust routes, but the trust itself does not fund any psychology, so the question of whether it should be in one setting or the other is academic. It is a serious issue for this Study Group in terms of recommendations. We are probably an extreme, but in other parts of the country there may be similar difficulties in having any access to any sort of psychology, and I would want that to be very much on the agenda of recommendations from this Study Group.

Overton: I would echo those sentiments, working in a place where we do not get that degree of psychological support. I have one concern, however. A striking feature to me this afternoon was that despite a wealth of scientific evidence about the various models of pain and various ways of tackling the pain, there seems to be a dearth of good, scientific, controlled studies about the benefits of pain management in the gynaecological setting. It seems to be a glaring deficit in the information that we have at the moment and I would have thought that before we can make specific recommendations about how we are to manage such patients, a recommendation that we would need to make strongly before we go along that pathway is for the overwhelming need to have good scientific studies upon which to base such recommendations – especially when we may well be making recommendations which in the present set-up in this country would be impossible to achieve in a large majority of units that come into contact with such problems.

Beard: If you read the literature you will find that those studies do exist. The psychological literature is filled with first-class studies on the benefits of managing pain with the sort of psychotherapy that we have been hearing about. The gynaecological studies I suppose are not that many, but we did a good treatment trial on ovarian downregulation that was referred to – the Farquhar study[2] – which was a randomised control trial. At some time or other you have to make a decision as to whether there is enough evidence to make a formal representation, and I believe that if you look hard enough it is there.

It is absolutely vital that gynaecologists understand about the psychological issues because they are unconvincing to their patients if they do not. This is a further reason for gynaecologists and psychologists working side by side in the pain clinic to understand one another's objectives and combine to create a satisfactory cohesion of care. I believe that we should be going for these things now.

MacLean: I disagree with Tim Overton. I know this is Professor Foster's area, but there are drugs like amitriptyline that are used for dysaesthetic vulvodynia, based on very limited experience by Marilynne McKay in Atlanta. Some of us are now using gabapentin, and although that perhaps has some advantages in neuropathic pain, no one has really shown that it has clear advantages over amitriptyline in the management of vulvodynia except that many of our vulvodynia patients do not like the thought of taking amitriptyline because they do not think you believe them. There probably is a need to try to identify certain areas. No individual clinic can accrue sufficient patients to be able to do studies and get information, but collectively there probably are groups and it may be that one of the results of this will be to identify some of the agents that Professor Li Wan Po has already indicated are drugs that have use and then to identify areas and people who could work in a much more collaborative way.

Foster: Just a comment on the research on vulvodynia. We have had a couple of problems that might be peculiar to vulvodynia; they may not be. One is the fact that we do not have good prevalence data. In order to go to drug companies in the States and ask to start a randomised trial, the first thing they ask is what is the prevalence of the disease, because they want to know the bottom line. The other problem is that the National Institutes of Health in the USA has also been fairly reticent to break its habit of paying for basic science work and randomised clinical trials. I believe that they are changing to a degree, but we really have not had the funding available for large-scale multi-institutional clinical trials for a number of our pelvic pain and vulval pain problems.

Lees: This is rather going away from this topic, but I would like to ask Dr Newton-John about a statement he made. You said that the female of the species has a lower pain threshold. I wondered what evidence you had for that.

Newton-John: There was a large review published in 1996 in the journal *Pain* on gender differences in pain, experimental as well as clinical, and one of the conclusions was that within experimental settings women reported a lower pain threshold than men. But the whole issue and the difficulty in teasing the things apart is that that report does not necessarily mean experience; it means report. As I mentioned, the gender of the experimenter can have a significant influence on pain report. It may be simply that the women are more willing to report a stimulus as being painful than are men in these essentially first-year undergraduate laboratory psychology department settings. It does not necessarily mean that women who experience pain have a lower pain threshold in terms of their underlying experience of their pain, but they are simply more willing to report it at an earlier point in the intensity increase than are men – in general.

Lees: Thank you very much. I asked the question in no barbed way. It was because the only conclusion I have drawn from my clinical life is that I have an undying admiration for women who have had to withstand the most ghastly pain that I could see. Second, from the records of war, women withstand pain and deal with it incredibly well. If you look at the Special Operations Executive and the individuals who won George Crosses, proportionally women were very much ahead of men.

Whorwell: Just to give a gastroenterological perspective, it is impractical to have psychologists in a team for the reasons that have been described. What I would suggest is that all trainees go through a specialised unit. That is what we do. A lot of our trainees do not give a toss about irritable bowel syndrome but at least they will go through our unit and see how we deal with it so that they then at least recognise the problem and possibly refer people on. There is also the first encounter. If they are sympathetic to it – they may not like the condition but if they just show some sympathy with it and then say 'Look, I know a man who can', they will send it on, rather than this terrible negative first impact. That first consultation, that first negative, shaking-head consultation, is so important.

Newton-John: I would like to echo that from the perspective of somebody who gets the referral in the end. A lot of bad work can be created at that first consultation. Equally, a lot of the distress and uncertainty and unpredictability can be resolved at that consultation. Perhaps there is more work that can be done, but we are all psychologists when interacting with patients and it is important to try to maximise that where we can.

Berkley: I want to speak on the issue of sex/gender differences in pain. There is going to be a report from the National Academy of Sciences in the form of a book – I was on the committee and we have just finished our work – on understanding the biology of sex and gender differences. That was the remit we were given, so you can imagine what went on at these meetings. On the issue of sex and gender differences in pain, you will probably agree that it is not just a simple matter of women being more or less tolerant. You can drive any study on assessing responses to noxious stimuli in any direction you want by manipulating history, by manipulating the presence of other illness, by manipulating the experimenter – and it is not always the sex of the experimenter, it is also the attitude of the experimenter. So you can drive the situation in whatever way you want and get any result that you want. That is one of the issues that comes up in, for example, things like whether we give women different drugs from men. It is the individual more than it is the woman.

This sits in the context of culture and someone's developmental sociology. For most women, if you think about the developmental history of assessing – how the brain is learning to assess a situation and whether to call it pain or not, whether the brain is going to make a decision 'Is this something worrisome, should I do something about it or not?', pain is an outcome. 'Should I think this is threatening or not?'

Most of women's, as opposed to men's, sociocultural – whatever you want to call it – background and upbringing encourages them to nurture, to pay attention, to care. Therefore something is more likely in a generalised way to be threatening to a woman, either to threaten her child or her family or someone near her or herself, than it would be for a man. This is very general background. Therefore one could say that women do not have lower thresholds for pain: they are more attuned to the possibly damaging consequences of certain stimulus conditions. We do not respond to pain unless we have it and are giving ourselves drugs; we respond to stimulus circumstances, and the perception of pain comes out of what the nervous system puts on it.

In a sense, this issue of gender differences is an example of what we have been talking about all day, about how the body handles information from itself to give us disabling sorts of pain or pain that is useful. If a woman says OK, this is painful, and you say she has a lower threshold to pain, or she can endure it – it all has to do with the meaning – again, what we have been talking about – meaning in past history of the stimulus circumstances. I am sorry, I am passionate on this issue and I had to respond to what was being said.

Newton-John: It is an obscuring of sex difference versus gender difference a lot of the time. What people are trying to say is that there is a sex difference. In fact, it is much broader – it is the meaning, the context of a whole lot of other variables that are affecting the report of pain as opposed to anything else.

Grace: This is a question for Dr Newton-John or Miss Smith. Dr Newton-John, in your talk you were making the point – I believe in the context of referring to the problem of the mind–body dualism – that where there is organically identified pathology there tends not to be a focus at all on the psychological. Do you think that we need to focus on the psychological dimensions when there is identified pathology? Do you in your practices actually do that? I am wondering whether the approaches that you take to dealing with that with clients, patients, is different. Do you find that it needs to be different in that circumstance?

Newton-John: I would say 'yes' to all of those points. It strikes me as being incredible that from the base at Queen's Square there are no psychological services for multiple sclerosis. That seems to be a fairly striking example of how that is an identified organic problem and therefore psychology is less relevant, whereas within the Pain Society chronic pain mandate to call a pain clinic a pain management clinic it has to have a psychologist involved. There seems to be an ongoing lack of recognition of the psychology involved in recognised – or medically sanctioned – pathologies.

In terms of differentiating individuals who have a label versus ones who do not, a lot of the setting-up of the model and the engaging in treatment is often for those without the validating label, helping them to develop this broader contextualisation of their problem rather trying to resolve the conflict of 'Well, if it isn't real, what is it?' and so on. It does not necessarily make the work easier with individuals who have a label but there is that whole dimension that is taken care of when people have that label. It is a chicken-and-egg thing in some ways because as the fibromyalgia term has become more widely acknowledged, there are people who are very aware of the validity of their label, who are joining support groups and are very involved in identifying strongly with it as a label to explain their pain – almost so as to be unhelpful in the other direction. It is no easy balance.

Smith: It goes back to the recommendation that in terms of training for doctors, doctors deal with pain but they need to be taught about the whole aspect of pain including the psychology of it because, as Dr Newton-John pointed out, we are all psychologists in a sense, dealing with the patient. Doctors are making interactions with patients that are very significant and can have quite a profound effect. Mr Stones and his team have been doing some research on doctor–patient consultations (see chapter 14) showing that the quality of the communication between the doctor and patient influences the outcome in pain. The more that can be brought into doctors' education the better. We may end up getting fewer people needing to be referred on if they are managed more appropriately and effectively at their first port of call.

Steege: A note on some of Dr Newton-John's reflections. It is well to remember that some of the literature of the 1970s arose out of pelvic pain clinics and the entry criterion for some of those clinics was a negative laparoscopy, which suggests that a person who does have endometriosis is not capable of developing chronic pain syndrome in a psychobehavioural sense, and obviously they are. We have come a long way from that. One of the difficulties we face in the USA in terms of the mental health world is also in terms of the physiotherapy, in that they are somewhat incomplete in their training as well. Many are still back with the mind–body split. I have had many mental health therapists tell me 'When she's cleared gynaecologically I can work with her'. I say that is not what I had in mind. The physical therapists are the same – they are beginning to learn about chronic pain as well, but some of them are still not there. Having a resource is wonderful, but it has to be the right kind of resource.

Coldron: I would like to respond to that, having been a lecturer in physiotherapy for the last ten years in various physiotherapy schools and I am now a lecturer to medical students as well as physiotherapy students. Certainly, all the physiotherapy schools that I know have massive psychosocial input into their syllabus: like a lot of the allied health professionals, the patient is the centre of their learning whereas in the medical schools I have to say it is still the diagnosis and the medicine that seem to be at the centre of the doctors' learning. There is a difference. We find the same problems in clinics as the psychologists may find. We do not just pay lip service to the psychosocial aspects of the patients; it is an integral part of our relationship with the patient and we cannot possibly examine and treat a patient without taking that into account. From what I have seen in my medical school – and perhaps it is unfair to take just one – I do not think that the medical schools are anywhere near that at the moment. I am teaching clinical skills to medical students at the moment and I find the big barrier, let alone the actual content, is the fact that they cannot communicate at third-year level with the person in front of them to say 'Good morning, my name is – I would like you to do this' – at that level, let alone anything that we have discussed today.

Tookman: This dialogue demonstrates one of the big issues about medical training.

We are taught to work as groups rather than teams, so if a recommendation is to be made I would suggest teamwork is probably a good recommendation, and learning how to work as an effective team, appreciating one another's skills and using them when appropriate.

Beard: I would like to ask Professor Sutton what he feels about the need for a psychologist. You deal with a great deal of so-called pathology-causing pelvic pain, particularly endometriosis and adhesions. Do you feel the need in some of those patients to have a psychologist there?

Sutton: We have one at the University of Surrey.

Collett: If we are talking about who should be in the clinic, we should also ask whether we need a women's health physiotherapist. If we are having that debate we need to include that.

MacLean: This has been an excellent discussion. Miss Smith had some recommendations in relation to training for obstetricians and gynaecologists in the teamwork, bearing in mind some of the points made by Dr Tookman, and the issues of funding which are clearly important and beyond the reach perhaps of some services and appropriate in others. I wonder whether you and Dr Newton-John want to have separate recommendations or whether you will do something together to cover those aspects.

I want to ask Professor Li Wan Po if he could put something relating to some of the newer pharmacological drugs appropriate for obstetricians and gynaecologists in this area.

One thing that will come out of this is if we can identify areas that need to be researched. WellBeing do not necessarily read these recommendations, but if we identify areas where funding should be made available and areas where research should be promoted, that is a good start. If we can identify some of the newer agents where multi-centre collaborative projects should be developed to look at these issues, there is something positive for that.

Some of the things that Professor Berkley said about understanding pain models are points that it behoves all of us to keep up to date with. Again, to identify that the last word in understanding pain is still far from written and that more research and more money should be put into looking at models of pain and, in particular, those that relate to gynaecological and obstetric pain.

Some of the things that Dr Grace was saying are very relevant to our education as post-graduates but also in terms of what undergraduates need to take into their medical education because that is an area where in health education we should be saying that people need to have a much broader understanding of some of these issues.

Berkley: This is a mechanistic question. Who is the audience for this? Where are these recommendations going to be put to use?

MacLean: The recommendations go into the book that is produced from the Study Group. They go at the back of the book, probably four or five pages. The audience is essentially Fellows and Members of the College, but sometimes the remit is much wider than that.

There is a series of things that will be disseminated to Fellows and Members with some guidance as to what people should know and where we should be heading.

One of the important benefits of a Study Group is to identify areas for study for young, enthusiastic researchers out there who are saying this is an area I am interested in and I would like to take this forward, and also for those people who hold the funds – and WellBeing is one of them. I would like to think that some of these would go through to the Department of Health and in areas of Women's Health people will say these are the areas that have been identified by the Study Group at the Royal College of Obstetricians and Gynaecologists and these are the areas where further funding is required. When I look at some of the 'research and development' targeted areas I wonder how on earth any of them were ever included on the list. There are many areas in Women's Health that we can identify and we should target, and research and development should be taking some of them forward. By all means, yes, they should go to WellBeing, but also further than that.

Berkley: One of the best recommendations this morning would come from Dr Lees' talk. We should all label the pictures of ourselves so that the future generations will know who we are! Wasn't Simpson's picture in question?

MacLean: I suspect that if you are a boy professor you probably do not have your portrait painted at that time. It is only when you become old and they are trying to capture you before you die that it happens.

References

1.   Gear RW, Miaskowski C, Gordon NC, Paul SM, Heller PH, Levine JD Kappa-opioids produce significantly greater analgesia in women than in men. *Nat Med* 1996;**2**:1248–50.
2.   Farquhar CM, Rogers V, Franks S. A randomised controlled trial of medroxyprogesterone acetate and psychotherapy for the treatment of pelvic congestion. *Br J Obstet Gynaecol* 1989;**96**:1153–62.

SECTION 3

PELVIC PAIN I

Chapter 9

Pelvic pain: an American perspective

John F. Steege and Anne Shortliffe

The physiology of acute pain and its management in the case of labour and acute gynaecological problems is complex enough. Chronic pelvic pain adds further layers of complexity due to multiple factors probably including but not limited to:

1.   Dimensions of personality influenced by both positive and adverse life experiences

2.   Prior and concomitant presence of other pain disorders

3.   Intrinsic variation in the degree of neurophysiological resilience in the face of continued nociceptive stimuli.

Pain theories have evolved to include ever more plasticity in the nervous system's handling of pain signals. While the theory of neuroplasticity has been devised to explain the development of chronic and intransigent pain states, the optimist in us must look forward to demonstration of the positive side of neuroplasticity: the ability of the nervous system to 'recover' from such undesirable circumstances.

Clinicians dealing with chronic pelvic pain seem to have widely varying views on the predominant aetiology of this common disorder. While most give at least nodding assent to the possible involvement of complex spinal cord mechanisms, the most common treatments still seem to spring from dearly held beliefs about the importance of either physiological or structural change in peripheral organ systems. Indeed, the aetiology of chronic pelvic pain seems to be in the eye of the beholder. For some, myofascial pain and trigger points lead the pack of potential causes while others focus on vascular changes, such as pelvic congestion, and still others believe that pharmacologically obliterating the reproductive tract with gonadotrophin-releasing hormone (GnRH) agonists is sufficient response to the complexity of these disorders.

Proponents of these various theories of aetiology see predominantly the disorder that they believe in most, and are left shaking their head in confusion or disbelief when the experience of others does not coincide with theirs. For many years, a number of us in this field have felt that the personal theoretic biases that most clinicians carry with them into this field rapidly become a source of bias in the referral of patients they see. Continued experience with patients selectively referred and continued interpretation of their problems in the light of the pre-existing bias reinforces their personal favourite theories. This is probably clinically appropriate, as we are often most effective in treating the disorders we like to treat most.

After many years of discussions in this vein with my colleagues in the USA, we decided for the purpose of today's presentation to collect some data concerning the power of referral bias. Rather than use further generalities the rest of the time will be spent discussing the results of the survey we performed of American members of the International Pelvic Pain Society.

The survey consisted of two parts. First, a retrospective description of each physician's practice, in which they listed their years in practice and described the source of their pelvic pain patients and, second, prospective collection of data concerning each new pelvic pain patient they saw over the ensuing month.

Slightly more than half of the 54 physicians circulated returned their retrospective surveys. They represented a mixture of physicians in private practice and those with primary or secondary academic affiliations. Of the 29 respondents, 12 were in private practice, ten in academic positions, and seven were in private practice with an academic affiliation. Over half reported regularly referring pelvic pain patients for physiotherapy, while smaller percentages referred their clients for mental health care, gastroenterological evaluation and urological studies. Less than 10% routinely recommended acupuncture.

For the prospective portion of the survey, questionnaire data were returned for 146 patients. They had an average age of 35 years and a mean parity of one. Taken as a group, approximately 50% were referred by gynaecologists to the physicians responding to the survey. In this group, 13% were referred for surgery and 74% for evaluation of chronic pelvic pain.

Table 9.1.   Presenting diagnoses in 146 women referred for evaluation and treatment of chronic pelvic pain

Diagnosis	% of referrals
Endometriosis	46.6
Adhesions	28.7
Vulval vestibulitis	15.1
Levator spasm	2.7
Vulvodynia	2.7
Interstitial cystitis	4.1
Myofascial pain	4.8

Table 9.2.   Prior treatments of 146 women referred for evaluation and treatment of chronic pelvic pain

Prior treatments	% of referrals
Any surgery	76
Prior laparoscopies	62
Prior laparotomies	29
Organs removed	
Hysterectomy	23
USO, BSO	22
GnRH agonist	20
NSAIDS	47
Narcotics	37
Psychotropics	29
Antiepileptics	5

USO, unilateral salpingo-oophorectomy; BSO, bilateral salpingo-oophorectomy; GnRH, gonadotrophin-releasing hormone; NSAIDs, nonsteroidal anti-inflammatory drugs

The average duration of pain was 5.44 years, with a range of 1–12 years. Their presenting diagnoses upon referral are listed in Table 9.1. Prior treatments are listed in Table 9.2. As a whole this group had incurred a high incidence of surgery, although removal of all pelvic organs was less common.

Modest numbers of women had been treated with GnRH agonists, narcotics or psychotropic drugs. The proportion who had prior psychiatric diagnoses was 22.6%, although this varied greatly from one practitioner's practice to another. A history of physical and/or sexual abuse was present in 26.4% of all subjects reported. This is similar to the prevalence found in population surveys, but less than the levels reported in some papers emerging from tertiary-care clinics.

Following evaluation by this group of physicians, the average number of diagnoses made was 2.51, with frequencies described in Table 9.3. Compared with the diagnoses rendered by referring physicians, the consultants more often diagnosed vulval vestibulitis, levator spasm, myofascial pain, neuropathic pain, interstitial cystitis and hernias. Treatment plans involved predominantly medical management (61.6%), with diagnostic or therapeutic surgery as a common part of the package (34.9%). Physical therapy was recommended in 32.2% of cases, distinctly lower than the retrospective estimate of 53%.

For the next and final section, the variation in some of these patterns found in different practices will be described. This variation might help to explain some of the therapeutic biases held by different specialists in this field. Although we had replies from 15 physicians, for the purpose of this chapter the three demonstrating the greatest extremes among the practices will be selected. In Table 9.4 we see that the percentage of patients referred by gynaecologists was relatively similar among physicians A, B and C. However, the reason for referral was surgery in as many as 40% of patients for physician C, but was not the reason for referral in any case in physicians A or B. Conversely, the proportion of patients referred for chronic pelvic pain evaluation only was somewhat reciprocal. The duration of pain endured by the patients in each practice was somewhat similar.

The entering diagnoses and surgical histories in patients referred to these individuals are seen in Table 9.4. The patients referred for surgery had a history of a greater number of prior surgeries. The proportion of patients having been previously treated with narcotics or psychotropics also varied widely among different patient groups.

The consultants' estimates of illness burden in their patients also varied widely, as measured by their assessed prevalence of other pain syndromes. Although the mean number of psychiatric diagnoses per patient was similar in the three practices, the history of prior abuse ranged from 17% to 26%.

Taken as a whole, despite the differences and the reasons for their referral, there seem to be many common denominators among the patients seen by physicians A, B and C. The differences emerge during examination of the diagnoses rendered and the treatment plans proposed.

Table 9.5 lists the diagnoses most commonly made by the three physicians profiled and compares their diagnostic patterns to the group taken as a whole. It is apparent that while most physicians dealing with pelvic pain recognise it as a multifactorial disorder, some specialists have a predilection towards rendering substantially more diagnoses than others. That is, they are 'splitters' rather than 'lumpers'. A rough examination of the clustering of these diagnoses would seem to imply a tendency to group together the diagnoses of interstitial cystitis, vulval vestibulitis, levator spasm and endometriosis all in the same patients.

Table 9.3. Diagnoses[a] made by 15 consulting physicians on 146 women referred for evaluation of chronic pelvic pain

Diagnosis	% of referrals
Specific diagnoses	
Vulval vestibulitis	32.9
Endometriosis	30.8
Levator spasm	28.1
Myofascial pain	27.4
Neuropathic pain	15.8
Interstitial cystitis	15.1
Adhesions	11.0
Hernia	10.3
Pelvic congestion	5.5
Irritable bowel syndrome	5.5
Vulvodynia	4.8
Visceral hyperalgesia	4.8

[a] Mean number of diagnoses, 2.51

Table 9.4. Characteristics of 146 women referred to 15 consultants for evaluation and treatment of chronic pelvic pain and for physicians A, B, and C

	Physician			
	A	B	C	All
n	18	21	23	146
Referred by gynaecologist (%)	55	67	78	50
Referred for surgery (%)	0	0	39	13
Referred for CPP evaluation (%)	100	71	56	74
Duration of pain (years)	5.8	5.0	4.1	5.4
Prior diagnoses:				
Endometriosis (%)	50	38	43	47
Adhesions (%)	11	19	43	29
Levator spasm (%)	11	0	0	3
Vulvodynia (%)	0	10	0	3
Vulval vestibulitis (%)	22	4	4	16
Interstitial cystitis (%)	11	0	0	4
Myofascial pain (%)	22	0	0	5
Prior surgeries:				
Any surgery (%)	67	67	91	76
Prior laparoscopy (%)	50	62	90	62
Prior laparotomy (%)	11	33	57	29
Hysterectomy (%)	28	24	17	23
USO, BSO (%)	22	10	22	22
Prior treatments:				
GnRH agonist (%)	22	14	26	20
NSAIDS (%)	44	14	26	47
Narcotics (%)	33	19	43	37
Psychotropics (%)	61	19	17	29

CPP, chronic pelvic pain; USO, unilateral salpingo-oophorectomy; BSO, bilateral salpingo-oophorectomy; GnRH, gonadotrophin-releasing hormone; NSAIDs, nonsteroidal anti-inflammatory drugs

Greater degrees of variance are also seen in the treatment plans recommended by the individual physicians. Physician C, who has a surgically biased practice, in fact operated on an even higher percentage of patients than those who were referred for

Table 9.5. Diagnoses rendered and treatments offered to 146 women evaluated by 15 consultant physicians for chronic pelvic pain and for physicians A, B, and C

	Physician			
	A	B	C	All
n	18	21	23	146
Mean number of diagnoses made	4.3	1.7	1.8	2.5
Adenomyosis (%)	0	0	4	3
Endometriosis (%)	22	19	39	31
Hernia (%)	33	0	4	10
Interstitial cystitis (%)	56	10	4	4
Myofascial pain (%)	50	14	17	27
Neuropathy (%)	33	29	0	16
Pelvic congestion (%)	28	0	0	6
Uterine retroversion (%)	6	0	0	3
Vulvodynia (%)	0	14	0	5
Visceral hyperalgesia (%)	0	0	0	5
Adhesions (%)	0	0	39	11
Irritable bowel syndrome (%)	6	5	0	5
Treatments offered				
Surgery (%)	44	10	65	35
Medical management (%)	94	86	35	62
Physical therapy (%)	50	10	13	32
Mental health (%)	10	0	4	10

surgery specifically. Medical management was, of course, employed by most but largely to the exclusion of surgery in the cases of physician B. In all cases, a smaller fraction of patients were referred for physical therapy or mental health care than was reported in the retrospective survey of these same physicians.

While these data describe the varying perspectives of American physicians, it is strongly suspected that similar variations exist among practitioners in this field in in Europe. Certainly the differences in the estimated prevalence of the various disorders may be influenced by referral mechanisms and prevailing notions of aetiology as well as by the intrinsic forces within the structures of the healthcare systems in each country that may influence referral patterns.

A few conclusions may be drawn from the data presented. As most of the disorders listed in this discussion do not have any definitive laboratory tests that describe them, we retreat to the traditional stance that diagnoses are made by history and physical examination. As these are both subject to investigator bias and to the personal interpretation of subjective variables, such as tenderness during examination, it is easy to see how entering biases can be continually reinforced by 'experience'. Personal professional experience has shown that patients tend to be referred by physicians whose beliefs are concordant with those of the consultant. For example, in a recent telephone call from an internal medicine colleague, he wanted to know what our diagnostic and treatment plan would be before we saw the patient, as he did not refer patients for 'invasive procedures'. If we talked about laparoscopy as a possibility, he clearly was not going to allow her to attend our clinic.

Perhaps more important than an understanding that equally well-intentioned and intelligent clinicians may hold differing views is the obvious conclusion that the most common painful disorders that we treat in gynaecology are woefully lacking in clear-cut diagnostic criteria and agreed-upon standards for diagnosis, much less treatment. Perhaps the time will arrive when at meetings such as this attempts can be made to standardise our diagnostic criteria and our clinical assessment.

Chapter 10

The epidemiology of chronic pelvic pain in the UK

Krina T. Zondervan and Stephen H. Kennedy

Introduction

Epidemiological studies aim to provide information on the distribution of conditions in different populations in terms of prevalence and incidence. They also aim to identify risk factors associated with the condition, to try to elucidate potential causes. This information is required for healthcare planning and resource allocation; it can also complement other lines of research, such as experimental, qualitative and health economic studies.

Until 1999, little was known about the epidemiology of chronic pelvic pain (CPP). Studies focused mainly on laparoscopic observations of pelvic pathology as an explanation for CPP,[1,2] and on attempts to explain the symptoms when no such pathology was found.[3-8] We published a review of the epidemiology of CPP in the general population.[9] The information retrieved was limited to a single community-based study that investigated the prevalence of CPP in the USA,[10] and one conducted in UK primary care.[11] In this chapter, we revisit the findings of our previous review and extend it with information that has become available since its publication in 2000.

Epidemiological concepts

The prevalence rate of a condition in a population is the proportion of the population that has the condition at a specific point in time (point prevalence) or at some point in a time period (period prevalence). The incidence rate is the number of new cases arising in a given period as a proportion of the 'person-time' at risk (i.e. the aggregated time that the members of the population spend in that population over the period, before the onset of the condition). The investigation of prevalence and incidence requires different study designs. Prevalence is assessed in cross-sectional studies, in which information on disease status and other information from a population are collected at one time-point. In contrast, incidence can only be determined through prospective study of a group.

Different types of epidemiological studies can be used to investigate risk factors. These can be prospective (cohort studies), retrospective (case–control studies), or cross-sectional. In cohort studies, two or more groups who are free of disease but who differ with regard to levels of exposure to the risk factor are followed prospectively to investigate who develops the disease. Cohort studies are seen as the standard for risk-factor analysis, because they allow the collection of unbiased risk-factor information. Disadvantages include cost and feasibility if the disease is rare or requires long-term follow-up.

When a condition is rare, case–control studies are an alternative. Their design, however, generally requires careful consideration, since the appropriate selection of cases and controls is crucial for an unbiased and meaningful outcome. In a case–control study, a group of incident cases with the disease is identified, their risk-factor information pre-dating the onset of disease is collected, and this information is compared with that provided by a carefully selected control group that is free of disease. A disadvantage of this design is that retrospectively collected risk-factor information may be incomplete (if it relies on previously recorded data) or biased (if it relies on recall).

Prevalent cases obtained through cross-sectional studies are also used in case–control studies, sometimes out of necessity, but more often because of the relative ease of data collection. This design introduces additional problems. First, it is more difficult to collect unbiased exposure data pre-dating the onset of disease. Second, there is potential for selecting a disproportionate number of cases with long duration of disease (who could well have a different risk-factor profile compared with incident cases). This means in general that, even when detailed historical risk-factor information is collected, causal relationships can never be inferred.

Essential ingredients in the design of all epidemiological studies are (i) the need for an unambiguous definition of the condition; (ii) an appropriate study population; and (iii) calculation of a sample size that is adequate for answering the questions under study. A clear disease definition is essential, not only for the accurate ascertainment of cases (and controls), but also to allow comparison of results between studies. The choice of the study population determines to what extent the results from the study sample can be generalised to the wider population. An adequate sample size is required to reduce the potential for 'chance' findings, as well as to increase the power of the study (the probability of finding a significant effect when there truly is one). These concepts are discussed in detail in many epidemiological textbooks.[12]

Unfortunately, no internationally agreed consensus yet exists on the definition of CPP. The one most commonly used only considers the location and duration of the pain: recurrent or constant pain in the lower abdominal region that has lasted for at least six months.[13] Women with pelvic pain related to pregnancy or malignancy are usually excluded, as are those who only experience dysmenorrhoea or dyspareunia.

Other definitions used have carried more subjective anatomic or affective–behavioural assumptions. The International Association for the Study of Pain[14] provided a specific definition for 'CPP without obvious pathology': chronic or recurrent pelvic pain that cannot be sufficiently explained by an apparent physical cause (also referred to as 'the pelvic pain syndrome' or 'pelvalgia'). However, this definition uses simple theories of pain perception: it assumes there is always a direct link between pain and tissue damage or pathology, and that causes of pain can be divided simply into 'organic' and 'non-organic'. Furthermore, it assumes that all possible pathology underlying pelvic pain is known and well established, that it can always be reliably detected through laparoscopy, and that all surgeons would interpret pelvic findings in the same way. It has become clear from the diverse literature on CPP causation that these assumptions cannot be met.

Some definitions of CPP have included a need for pain to be accompanied by 'significantly altered' physical activity or disturbance of mood, or 'significant' use of analgesics.[15,16] Although perhaps of value in more qualitative studies, these types of definition are clearly subjective and can never ensure reproducible findings in large-scale epidemiological studies.

Prevalence and incidence of CPP

In 1995, we conducted a systematic review into the prevalence and incidence of CPP in the UK general population.[17] The only study that had investigated the epidemiology of CPP in any setting was a hospital-based study of 559 pathology-free women who had undergone a laparoscopy for sterilisation or investigation of infertility.[1] The prevalence of CPP, defined as 'recurrent pelvic pain unrelated to menstruation or coitus' was 39%; this high rate was likely to be influenced by the inclusion of infertile women in the study.

Worldwide, the only truly community-based prevalence figure for CPP was that reported by Mathias and colleagues in the USA.[10] They conducted a telephone survey of 5263 women aged 18–50 years randomly selected from the general US population. The prevalence of CPP, defined as pelvic pain of at least six months' duration and with pain having occurred in the past three months, was 14.7% (95% confidence interval: 12.7–16.7%). In another US study by Jamieson and Steege,[18] the prevalence of pelvic pain was assessed in 581 patients and their female companions aged 18–45 years in waiting rooms of gynaecology and family medicine practices. Since the results of patients were pooled with those of companions, the results were unsuitable for generalisation to the population; 39% of women reported having some degree of pelvic pain, while 20% reported pelvic pain of more than a year's duration.

The lack of epidemiological data on CPP in the UK outside a hospital setting led us first to investigate its prevalence and incidence in primary care.[11] For this purpose, the MediPlus UK Primary Care Database (UKPCD) was used, which contains anonymised clinical and prescribing data from 1991 onwards on approximately 1 700 000 patients. The most common definition of CPP was used: 'constant or recurrent pain in the lower abdominal region lasting for at least six months, excluding pain related to pregnancy or malignancy, or pain that occurs only with menstruation or intercourse'. CPP cases were identified from a denominator of 278 509 women, on the basis of contacts for pelvic pain with the practices contributing information to the database between 1991 and 1995. The annual prevalence of CPP in women aged 15–73 years was 38 per 1000. This figure was higher than that reported elsewhere for migraine (21 per 1000), but comparable to figures for asthma (37 per 1000) and back pain (41 per 1000).[19] The annual prevalence for women aged 18–50 years was similar, at 37 per 1000. CPP prevalence was found to vary with age, from 18 per 1000 in 15–20-year-olds to 28 per 1000 in women older than 60 years. Regional variations were also found, with prevalence lowest in Scotland (16 per 1000) and highest in Wales (29 per 1000). Underlying differences in community-based rates as well as differences in healthcare-seeking behaviour could explain these variations.

The prevalence of a condition is approximated by the product of its incidence and mean duration. The monthly incidence of CPP on MediPlus UKPCD was relatively low, at 1.6 per 1000. Therefore, one explanation for the high prevalence was long symptom duration. In a second study using MediPlusUKPCD, we investigated CPP duration (defined as the time between the first and last contacts for pelvic pain), as well as patterns of diagnosis and referral.[20] A cohort of 5051 incident cases was followed for three to four years from their first contact for pelvic pain with primary care. Women with CPP had a median symptom duration of 15 months on the database, with a third of women having persistent symptoms after two years. These results were likely to have been influenced not only by the actual duration of symptoms, but also by healthcare-seeking behaviour. In turn, healthcare-seeking behaviour could have been influenced by many unknown factors, such as patient–doctor interaction and patient satisfaction with the care offered.

The study also revealed that a quarter of incident CPP cases received no diagnostic label during the three- to four-year follow-up and only 40% had evidence of referral to a hospital specialist. The majority of women received one diagnosis only, the most common being irritable bowel syndrome (IBS) and cystitis in all age groups. In addition, pelvic inflammatory disease (PID) was common in women aged up to 40, and other gastrointestinal diagnoses in women above 50 years. The likelihood of receiving a diagnosis varied with age: women under 20 years and older than 60 years were less likely than others to receive a diagnosis. The referral rate varied similarly with age: women in the 31–40 year age group were twice as likely to have been referred as the youngest or oldest women in the cohort.

The prevalence figures from MediPlus UKPCD must have underestimated general population rates, since they only provided information on women with CPP seeking health care. To investigate the true community prevalence, we conducted the Oxfordshire Women's Health Study.[9,21] This was a postal questionnaire survey among 4000 women, randomly selected from 141 400 women aged 18–49 years on the Oxfordshire Health Authority (OHA) register. It aimed to investigate (i) the prevalence of CPP in the community, (ii) its effect on women's lives in terms of pain severity, use of health care, and quality of life, (iii) symptom overlap between CPP, IBS, genitourinary symptoms, dysmenorrhoea and dyspareunia, and (iv) associated investigations and diagnoses reported by the women. A semi-quantitative questionnaire was developed for the purpose of the study, collecting information on a wide range of issues related to women's health (http://www.medicine.ox.ac.uk/ndog/cppr/frame.html). As in the MediPlus UKPCD study, CPP was defined as recurrent or constant pelvic pain of at least six months' duration, unrelated to periods, intercourse or pregnancy. Pain severity and quality of life were assessed using well-validated outcome measures. Of the 3206 questionnaire receivers, 2304 (74%) returned a complete questionnaire. Responders were similar to all women aged 18–50 years in Oxfordshire in terms of social class and ethnic distributions. The study group consisted of 2016 women, after exclusion of those who had been pregnant in the last 12 months.

CPP in the last three months was reported by 24.0% of the women (95% confidence interval: 22.1–25.8). This prevalence estimate was higher than the 14.7% reported by Mathias and colleagues in the USA. However, their study excluded women with ovulation-related pain, which our study did not, since many women were unable to say whether their pelvic pain occurred at mid-cycle. Exclusion of those able to report ovulation-related pain would have reduced our estimate to a similar figure of 16.9%.

We found that the prevalence of CPP varied slightly with age ($P = 0.02$); the lowest rate (20%) was found in the age groups 18–25 years and 31–35 years, and the highest (28%) in 36–40-year-olds. Non-Caucasian women had a much lower prevalence (10%) than Caucasian women (25%; $P = 0.003$); a risk ratio (RR) of 0.4 (95% CI: 0.2–0.8). Adjustment for age and social class did not affect this result. Prevalence did not vary with social class, marital status, or employment status. A third of women with CPP reported that their pain had started more than five years earlier.

General health status, assessed using the Short-Form 36 Health Survey (SF-36),[22] was compared between women with CPP and those with dysmenorrhoea only. Mean SF-36 physical and mental component summary scores and frequency of sleep problems – were significantly worse in women with CPP than in the comparison group. However, women with CPP who had consulted for pelvic pain in the year prior to the study (32% of the 483 cases) were most affected by their symptoms. Nearly 70% reported moderate or severe pain; 58% reported that the pain restricted their activities, and one-third had taken at least one day off work in the preceding 12 months due to the pain. Compared with other women with CPP, their general health status was appreciably reduced in terms of SF-36 summary scores and sleep quality, differences that could not be explained by a higher frequency of coexisting illnesses.

Women with CPP who had consulted for their symptoms more than 12 months previously (27% of cases) appeared slightly less affected by their symptoms than more recent consulters. However, a substantial number (43%) reported that the pain restricted their activities. The reasons why these women discontinued seeking medical advice despite continuing symptoms were unclear, and this warrants further investigation. Some women may have been controlling their pain after medical advice or treatment. It is also possible, however, that some may have been dissatisfied with their medical care. This is clearly a possibility, as a survey of 144 women in New Zealand who sought health care for CPP reported that 45% felt their GP had not adequately explained the diagnosis, that there had been occasions when they felt their pain was not taken seriously, or that they felt 'less and less in control' after numerous trips to a doctor.[23]

Women with CPP who had never consulted for pelvic pain (41% of cases) were similar in terms of general health, pain severity, use of health care, and measures of pain-related functioning to women with dysmenorrhoea alone. However, the reported effect of dysmenorrhoea on women's lives when they had the pain was not negligible: three-quarters used medication for symptom relief and one-third reported that the pain restricted their activities. Thus, non-consulting women with CPP appear to perceive their symptoms as no greater burden than having painful periods.

An important observation in our study was that one-third of women with CPP reported that they were anxious about their pain, particularly its cause. This symptom-related anxiety was common in non-consulters as well as consulters. A qualitative study of women with CPP interviewed 12–18 months after a negative laparoscopy reported similar findings:[24] most women stated that their pain negatively affected many aspects of their lives, that they were worried about the pain (mainly about its cause and possible long-term effects) and that this anxiety affected their mood, sleep and weight.

In summary, the Oxfordshire Women's Health Study showed a high prevalence of CPP in women of reproductive age in the community, many of whom were not seen by a GP for their symptoms. This could partly be explained by variation in the severity of the condition and its impact on daily life as perceived by the women. However, the large number of women – including non-consulters – reporting anxiety about the cause of their symptoms clearly emphasises the need for further research into potential causes. Furthermore, the high proportion of past consulters among women with CPP warrants research into possible reasons why women discontinue seeking medical advice despite continuing symptoms. In addition, more widespread awareness that the condition is highly prevalent is likely to benefit all women with CPP, including those who have so far not sought medical advice.

Symptom complexity and diagnoses

CPP is difficult to diagnose and treat, mainly due to the wide range of possible causes with overlapping symptomatology,[25] e.g. endometriosis, chronic PID, adhesions, irritable bowel syndrome (IBS), interstitial cystitis and the urethral syndrome. In gynaecology clinics, high IBS prevalence rates (50–79%) have been reported in women referred for CPP.[26] Similarly, high prevalence rates of dyspareunia (42%) and urinary symptoms (61%) have been reported in IBS patients.[27] Community-based data on the overlap between CPP and other abdominal symptoms are, however, limited. In the second part of the Oxfordshire Women's Health Study, we investigated the symptom overlap between CPP, IBS, genitourinary symptoms, dysmenorrhoea and dyspareunia in the community, and associated investigations and diagnoses.[28] The diagnoses were based only on the woman's recall and were not validated using information from GPs or hospitals. However, these results were important since they represented women's perceptions of the diagnoses given to them.

A substantial overlap was found between CPP, genitourinary symptoms and IBS. Approximately half of the 483 women with CPP had at least one additional symptom; 39% had IBS and 24% had genitourinary symptoms. Prevalence rates of dysmenorrhoea and dyspareunia were much higher among women with CPP (81% and 41% respectively) than among those without CPP (58% and 14%). These rates were high in all subgroups of CPP, irrespective of the presence of additional genitourinary symptoms or IBS. The results demonstrated the complexity of the diagnostic problems presented by a CPP patient. Moreover, the study found that women with CPP and additional genitourinary symptoms and IBS in particular were most affected in terms of pain severity and episode duration. This group also reported having received the widest range of diagnoses.

Consistent with the MediPlus UKPCD analysis,[20] IBS was the most common diagnosis received. However, the second most common diagnosis was stress. In clinical settings, high frequencies of stress, depression and anxiety observed in women with CPP have often been interpreted as providing a direct explanation for the pain (especially in those women for whom no 'obvious' pathological explanation is found). This dualistic approach is increasingly being recognised as unhelpful.[29] A meta-analysis showed that these psychological characteristics are linked to chronic pain states in general rather than specifically to CPP.[30] The overlap between CPP and other abdominal symptoms, the wide range of possible diagnoses, and the complexity of associated psychosocial issues provide further support for the requirement of multidisciplinary settings for effective assessment and management of CPP.

Risk factors for CPP

As detailed in our earlier review,[9] the investigation of risk factors for CPP provides a major challenge to the epidemiologist. Gradually emerging knowledge indicates that a host of somatic, psychological and socio-environmental factors may act and interact in its causation, together forming a multidimensional 'biopsychosocial' model of disease aetiology.[25] Women with CPP may suffer from various underlying somatic conditions, which may all have different or even conflicting risk factors. Furthermore, psychological factors (e.g. traumatic events, depression, illness beliefs) and socio-environmental factors (e.g. the role of 'significant others') may play a role in pain aetiology or maintenance. Risk of CPP may be influenced by a variety of these factors, some of which can be difficult to measure. Furthermore, different populations are likely to exhibit different frequencies of underlying somatic and psychosocial conditions, thus limiting comparability of results from one country to another.

The situation may be even more complex when CPP cases are identified from primary-care instead of secondary or tertiary care settings. Associations between CPP and risk factors in these settings may be different, because of differences in healthcare-seeking behaviour and referral patterns. For instance, if pelvic pain were common in young women but if they were less inclined to seek medical advice than older women, they would be less likely to be identified as CPP cases and risk of CPP in this group would be seen as low. Differences in referral patterns from primary to secondary or tertiary care between certain demographic groups may result in an even further distorted picture of CPP risk. Therefore, risk-factor analysis of CPP is at present only of some value using cases identified at community level and interpretation of the results remains complicated due to its multicausality.

There are no population-based cohort or case–control studies investigating risk factors for CPP. The information from cross-sectional studies is limited. The community survey in the USA by Mathias and colleagues[10] and the semi-community study of women and their companions in primary-care clinics by Jamieson and Steege[18] described the association between certain demographic factors and CPP. In a logistic regression model adjusted for age, ethnicity, education and marital status, Mathias and his associates[10] found a slightly decreased risk of CPP in women older than 35 years compared with younger women (OR: 0.7, 95% CI: 0.6–0.8). Jamieson and Steege[18] reported unadjusted results for the association between pelvic pain (defined as any current pain not associated with menstruation or intercourse) and age, with rates varying significantly from 49% in 26–30-year-olds to 22% in 36–40-year-olds. Mathias and colleagues[10] found a reduced risk in women of African American origin compared with Caucasian women (OR: 0.7, 95% CI: 0.5–0.95), whereas Jamieson and Steege[18] found an increased risk (53% vs. 35%, respectively). An increased risk was found in separated/widowed/divorced women compared with single women (OR: 1.5, 95% CI: 1.1–2.0) by Mathias and colleagues,[10] but not by Jamieson and Steege.[18] Neither study found associations with educational status, income or parity.

Despite its limitations, we conducted a risk-factor analysis in the cross-sectional Oxfordshire Women's Health Study for hypothesis-generating purposes (unpublished results). As outlined in the first section, using prevalent cases from a cross-sectional study is problematic if the intention is to identify predisposing factors that may explain the onset of disease. In our analyses, we therefore distinguished two categories of risk factors: 'exposure variables' (or proxies of unknown exposures), which could not have resulted from CPP or were unlikely to have done so. These included age, social class, ethnicity, height, use of intrauterine device, use of diaphragm, sterilisation and termination of pregnancy. The other category was termed 'associative' variables, which could contribute to or modify the risk of CPP but could also be the result of CPP or an underlying condition. This category included marital and employment status, smoking, alcohol consumption, oral contraceptive use, weight, body mass index, regularity of menstrual cycle, length of bleeding, age at first pregnancy, parity, miscarriage, ectopic pregnancy and subfertility. Unadjusted risk-ratios were first computed for each factor. For those borderline significantly associated with CPP ($P < 0.1$), a logistic regression model was built in which risk was adjusted for age, social class, ethnicity, height, contraceptive use, sterilisation and hormone replacement therapy use.

After adjustment, significant differences in risk were found only with age, ethnicity, height, condom use, length of bleeding and subfertility. Compared with women aged 18–25 years, odds ratios (ORs) of other age categories varied from 0.72 (95% CI: 0.44–1.18) for 46–49-year-olds to 1.30 (95% CI: 0.88–1.90) for 26–30-year-olds. Non-Caucasian women had a much lower risk of CPP compared with Caucasian women (OR 0.35, 95% CI: 0.16–0.78). Although this result was consistent with the findings of Mathias and colleagues,[10] it was based on only 80 non-Caucasian women participating in the study (an accurate reflection of the percentage of non-Caucasian women in the Oxfordshire population). The applicability to the general population may therefore be compromised.

Surprisingly, tallness (≥ 1.70 m) appeared to have an increased risk of CPP even after adjustment for possible confounding factors such as social class or ethnicity (OR = 1.37, 95% CI: 1.00–1.88). Cramer and colleagues have previously associated tallness with increased risk of endometriosis,[31] but were similarly unable to explain their result other than by suggesting residual confounding by other factors. Another unexpected result was the association of condom use (but not the diaphragm) with increased risk of CPP, but this effect was limited to use more than 12 months earlier only (OR 1.55, 95% confidence interval 1.17–2.05). A tentative explanation for this elevated risk could be that condom users may not have used this method consistently, and that they were less likely to be long-term users of oral contraceptives.

Longer bleeding periods (7+ days) were associated with an increased risk of CPP (OR 1.34, 95% CI: 1.00–1.80). Various studies have previously associated prolonged menstrual flow with increased risk of endometriosis.[32] Subfertility was also found to be positively associated with CPP (OR 1.50, 95% CI: 1.08–2.07). Since both pelvic pain and infertility are common in women with endometriosis, this association was also not surprising.

Conclusions

Emerging evidence from population-based studies in the UK has shown that CPP is a common condition and that women may suffer from their symptoms in varying degrees. However, many do not seek, or they stop seeking, medical advice despite the considerable impact the condition has on their lives and despite anxiety about its cause. Those who do see a doctor may receive multiple treatments and diagnoses before symptoms resolve or are reduced; for a large number of women no such solution is achieved. Thus, further research into the needs of women with CPP at various stages of the healthcare system is warranted, as is research exploring possible causation mechanisms. As outlined in the last section, the multidimensional pathway of CPP causation severely limits the potential for aetiological research. Development of non-invasive diagnostic tools for underlying conditions such as endometriosis or chronic PID will be an important step in allowing better investigation of the relative importance of these conditions in CPP patients. In addition, a large-scale prospective study that collects information on various lifestyle, somatic, social and psychological risk factors before the onset of CPP would provide a significant step towards unravelling its causation.

Acknowledgement

The work described in this review was supported by the BUPA Foundation, registered charity no. 277598.

References

1. Mahmood TA, Templeton AA, Thomson L, Fraser C. Menstrual symptoms in women with pelvic endometriosis. *Br J Obstet Gynaecol* 1991;**98**: 558–63.
2. Liu DTY, Hitchcock A. Endometriosis: its association with retrograde menstruation, dysmenorrhoea and tubal pathology. *Br J Obstet Gynaecol* 1986;**93**: 859–62.
3. Beard RW, Highman JH, Pearce S, Reginald PW. Diagnosis of pelvic varicosities in women with chronic pelvic pain. *Lancet* 1984;**2**: 946–9.
4. Hogston P. Irritable bowel syndrome as a cause of chronic pain in women attending a gynaecology clinic. *BMJ* 1987;**294**: 934–5.
5. Fry RP, Crisp AH, Beard RW, McGuigan S. Psychosocial aspects of chronic pelvic pain, with special reference to sexual abuse. A study of 164 women. *Postgrad Med J* 1993;**69**: 566–74.
6. Low WY, Edelmann RJ, Sutton CS. A psychological profile of endometriosis patients in comparison to patients with pelvic pain of other origins. *J Psychosom Res* 1993;**37**: 111–16.
7. Hodgkiss AD, Sufraz R, Watson JP. Psychiatric morbidity and illness behaviour in women with chronic pelvic pain. *J Psychosom Res* 1994;**38**:3–9.
8. Waller KG, Shaw RW. Endometriosis, pelvic pain, and psychological functioning. *Fertil Steril* 1995;**63**:796–800.
9. Zondervan KT, Barlow DH. Epidemiology of chronic pelvic pain. *Baillière's Clin Obstet Gynaecol* 2000;**14**:403–14.
10. Mathias SD, Kuppermann M, Liberman RF, Lipschutz RC, Steege JF. Chronic pelvic pain: prevalence, health-related quality of life, and economic correlates. *Obstet Gynecol* 1996;**87**:321–7.
11. Zondervan KT, Yudkin PL, Vessey MP, Dawes MG, Barlow DH, Kennedy SH. Prevalence and incidence in primary care of chronic pelvic pain in women: evidence from a national general practice database. *Br J Obstet Gynaecol* 1999;**106**:1149–55.
12. Rothman KJ, Greenland S. *Modern Epidemiology*, 2nd edn. Philadelphia: Lippincott-Raven; 1998.
13. Campbell F, Collett BJ. Chronic pelvic pain. *Br J Anaesth* 1994;**73**:571–3.
14. International Association for the Study of Pain. Classification of chronic pain. Definitions of chronic pain syndromes and definition of pain terms. *Pain* 1986; Suppl: S1–S221.
15. Steege JF, Stout AL, Somkuti SG. Chronic pelvic pain in women: toward an integrative model. *Obstet Gynecol Surv* 1993;**48**:95–110.
16. Howard FM. The role of laparoscopy in chronic pelvic pain: promise and pitfalls. *Obstet Gynecol Surv* 1993;**48**:357–87.
17. Zondervan KT, Yudkin PL, Vessey MP, Dawes MG, Barlow DH, Kennedy SH. The prevalence of chronic pelvic pain in women in the UK – a systematic review. *Br J Obstet Gynaecol* 1998;**105**:93–99.
18. Jamieson DJ, Steege JF. The prevalence of dysmenorrhea, dyspareunia, pelvic pain, and irritable bowel syndrome in primary care practices. *Obstet Gynecol* 1996;**1**:55–9.
19. McCormick A, Fleming D, Charlton J, editors. *OPCS. Morbidity Statistics from General Practice. Fourth national study 1991–1992.* London: HMSO; 1995.
20. Zondervan KT, Yudkin PL, Vessey MP, Dawes MG, Barlow DH, Kennedy SH. Patterns of diagnosis and referral in women consulting for chronic pelvic pain in UK primary care. *Br J Obstet Gynaecol* 1999;**106**:1156–61.
21. Zondervan KT, Yudkin PL, Vessey MP, Jenkinson CP, Dawes MG, Barlow DH, Kennedy SH. The

community prevalence of chronic pelvic pain in women and associated illness behaviour. *Br J Gen Pract* 2001;**51**:541–7.

22. Brazier JE, Harper R, Jones NMB, O'Cathain A, Thomas KJ, Usherwood T, *et al*. Validating the SF-36 Health Survey Questionnaire: new outcome measure for primary care. *BMJ* 1992;**305**:160–64.

23. Grace VM. Problems of communication, diagnosis, and treatment experienced by women using the New Zealand health services for chronic pelvic pain: a quantitative analysis. *Health Care Women Int* 1995;**16**:521–35.

24. Savidge CJ, Stewart P, Li TC. Women's perspectives on their experiences of chronic pelvic pain and medical care. *J Health Psychol* 1999;**3**:103–16.

25. Moore J, Kennedy SH. Causes of chronic pelvic pain. *Baillière's Clin Obstet Gynaecol* 2000;**14**:389–402.

26. Prior A, Wilson K, Whorwell PJ, Faragher EB. Irritable bowel syndrome in the gynecological clinic. Survey of 798 new referrals. *Dig Dis Sci* 1989;**34**:1820–24.

27. Whorwell PJ, McCallum M, Creed FH, Roberts CT. Non-colonic features of irritable bowel syndrome. *Gut* 1986;**27**:37–40.

28. Zondervan KT, Yudkin PL, Vessey MP, Jenkinson CP, Dawes MG, Barlow DH, Kennedy SH. Chronic pelvic pain in the community: symptomatology, investigations and diagnoses. *Am J Obstet Gynecol* 2001;**184**:1149–55.

29. Grace VM. Mind/body dualism in medicine: the case of chronic pelvic pain without organic pathology. A critical review of the literature. *Int J Health Serv* 1998;**28**:127–51.

30. McGowan LPA, Clark-Carter DD, Pitts MK. Chronic pelvic pain: a meta-analytic review. *Psychol Health* 1998;**13**:937–51.

31. Cramer DW, Wilson E, Stillman RJ, Berger MJ, Belisle S, Schiff I, *et al*. The relation of endometriosis to menstrual characteristics, smoking, and exercise. *JAMA* 1986;**255**:1904–8.

32. Mangtani P, Booth M. Epidemiology of endometriosis. *J Epidemiol Community Health* 1993;**47**:84–8.

Chapter 11

Pelvic congestion: a functional disorder of the menstrual cycle?

Richard W. Beard

Introduction

Chronic pelvic pain (CPP) among young women, who are otherwise healthy in every way and who should be at the peak of their effectiveness in daily life, obstinately remains a problem of management. Considerable doubt exists about the aetiology of CPP, with psychologists and psychiatrists, gastroenterologists, gynaecologists, rectal surgeons and urologists all claiming some ownership of the symptom. It seems that a likely reason for this doubt is that, for gynaecologists, working in a specialty which is still predominantly surgical, there are few surgical solutions in the largest group of women, which contains those with CPP with no obvious pathology to account for their pain. There is now general agreement that for at least 65% of all women who suffer from disabling pelvic pain between the ages of 18 years and 50 years,[1] no surgical solution can be easily found because of their age. Within some specialties, there is an increasing recognition that the explanation may lie with the'functional disorders', which include such disabling conditions as irritable bowel syndrome and constipation. The purpose of this chapter is to explore the possibility that pelvic congestion is a gynaecological functional disorder of the menstrual cycle which has both psychological and somatic components and for which effective treatment can be found.

The hypothesis

It is proposed that: (i) pelvic pain is caused by pelvic congestion, and (ii) pelvic congestion is a functional disorder of the menstrual cycle with stress mediated through the hypothalamo–pituitary–ovarian system inducing ovarian dysfunction. This hypothesis is expressed diagrammatically in Figure 11.1.

In order to explore this hypothesis, our knowledge of the clinical presentation of pelvic congestion, its physiology, endocrinology and the psychology of chronic pain caused by congestion are summarised and referenced in the six boxes within the text.

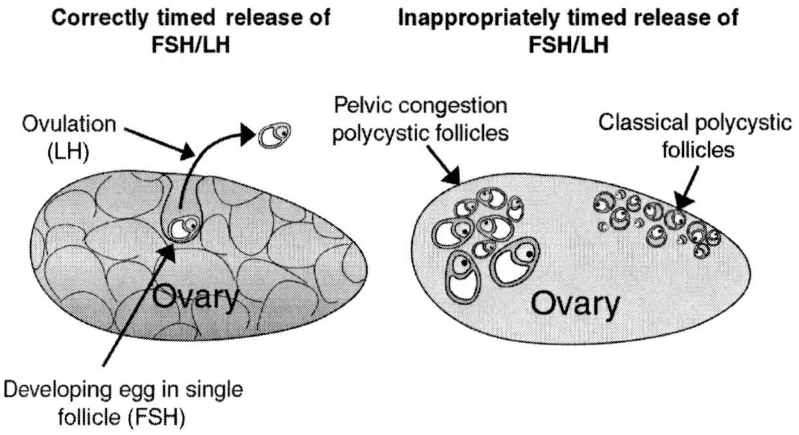

Correctly timed release of FSH/LH   **Inappropriately timed release of FSH/LH**

Ovulation (LH)   Pelvic congestion polycystic follicles   Classical polycystic follicles

Ovary   Ovary

Developing egg in single follicle (FSH)

Figure 11.1. Diagram illustrating the proposed mechanism for the genesis of pelvic congestion

Clinical presentation of CPP and pelvic congestion (Box A)

What is pelvic congestion?

Physiologically, vascular congestion is an accumulation of blood in the peripheral circulation of the affected tissue, associated in time with tissue oedema and often accompanied by reduced venous return from the affected area. Pain in the congested tissues is of variable intensity and time of onset. This occurs in response to poor vascular perfusion leading to a disturbance of local homeostatic mechanisms, leading to the disorganisation of metabolic processes and the accumulation of pain-producing substances. The epidemiology, presenting symptoms and physical signs of pelvic congestion are shown in Box A.

The link between congestion and pelvic pain

A good example of transient congestion occurs in runners who develop cramp. The leg muscles go into spasm at a critical point when their metabolic needs are no longer met by perfusion and only relax when the demands on them (exercise) diminish, and an adequate circulation is re-established. Interestingly, women with pelvic congestion often describe their background pelvic pain as being like cramp. They also complain that the pain is brought on or made worse by standing, when gravity impedes venous return with the resultant development of congestion.

Box A. Clinical features of women with pelvic congestion	References
Epidemiology	5,18,44
Confined to women of reproductive age	
Parity normally distributed	
Major cause of CPP in the 65% of women with no obvious pelvic pathology	
Population-based study required to determine prevalence	37, 45
Condition more pronounced in luteal phase (congestive dysmenorrhea)	
Symptoms and pain characteristics	
Dull, 'crampy' ache interspersed with acute episodes	6,18,44–46
More commonly on one side, but always occasionally the other	
Exacerbated by exercise, standing, rise in intra-abdominal	
pressure, menstrual cycle, sexual excitement (deep	
dyspareunia, postcoital ache), defaecation, stress	
Relieved by lying down, local heat, suppression of ovarian activity	
Menstrual dysfunction – menorrhagia (days 1 and 2)	6,18,38,45
or congestive dysmenorrhoea	
Poor quality of life – domestic, social, sexual, sleep and work	
Physical signs	
Anxious appearance +/– hostile manner	
'Ovarian point' tenderness on deep palpation	
Abdominal bloating	
Vaginal examination – vaginal 'blueing', excess discharge	
Bimanual – ovary(ies) always tender on compression	
– uterus sometimes tender	

The possibility that pelvic congestion is flow-dependent was investigated in a formal single-blind crossover study by Reginald and colleagues,[2] in which women with pelvic congestion were given intravenously either the specific venoconstrictor, dihydroergotamine tartrate, or saline during an acute attack of pelvic pain. Dihydroergotamine is known to increase venous flow velocity[3] and to reduce the diameter of congested veins by 23%.[4] A consistent and significant reduction in the pain scores of the women who were given the dihydroergotamine was reported, whereas the same women given saline showed only a transient, probably placebo, response. These findings reveal a close association between pelvic venous flow and the severity of pelvic pain due to congestion.

The demonstration of pelvic congestion in women with CPP without obvious pathology

Until recently, most of the information available on pelvic vascular function in women with congestion, had come from venographic studies. In one of these,[5] 85% of women with CPP with a median duration of 3.5 years for which no obvious cause could be found on laparoscopy were found to have significantly reduced venous clearance as compared with women who had no pain. This ranged from delay to complete stasis, accompanied by dilatation of many of the pelvic veins, in particular the ovarian vein. These findings give rise to the reintroduction of the concept of pelvic congestion, originally described by Taylor in the USA in 1949[6] but subsequently discredited because of his inability to find a surgical solution to the condition. With the re-establishment of pelvic congestion as a demonstrable cause of CPP has come the need to characterise it as a clinical condition and to determine its cause.

The anatomy, function and pathology of pelvic veins (Box B)

The pelvic circulation is part of the larger visceral circulation. It is unique in that it forms an all-embracing plexus with arteriovenous communications creating links between the ovarian, uterine, vesical, mesenteric and rectal circulations. Pelvic veins have few valves as compared with veins in the legs, so that modulation of venous pressure (and of flow) by some other mechanism is necessary. Anatomical studies of the ovarian vein[7] have shown that it is a thick-walled vessel with both longitudinal and circular muscle coats, with nerves and nerve endings situated in the outer longitudinal layer of muscle. This layer also contains many vasoactive endothelial substances or their precursors, such as substance P, bradykinin and nitric oxide synthetase, which contribute to the autoregulation of the ovarian circulation.[8-10] It has been shown by venography that the pelvic veins can be dilated up to a diameter of 13 mm.[5] The ovarian vein is also capable of considerable spontaneous activity and on surgical removal may go into spasm lasting up to half an hour (personal observation). It is these properties that enable veins in an autoregulated circulation to control venous pressure and bloodflow without the assistance of valves, unless the control system is in some way compromised, as will be described shortly.

The role of nitric oxide

Many studies have shown the importance of nitric oxide as a smooth muscle relaxant, capable of regulating bloodflow and in particular the adaptation of the maternal circulation in pregnancy.[11] Oestrogen is known to stimulate its formation through the enzyme nitric oxide synthase.[12] Kingden-Milles and Arndt[13] have drawn attention to a lesser known action of nitric oxide in modulating central and peripheral neuronal function. They cite the study of Haley and colleagues,[14] which revealed that in the periphery, nitric oxide, in addition to relaxing smooth muscle, is involved in the transmission of sensory signals to the brain. Kingden-Milles and Arndt showed that this latter function can be blocked by a nitric oxide synthetase inhibitor which led them to postulate, and then to demonstrate in human volunteers, that pain elicited by injecting bradykinin into a vein on the back of the hand can be blocked by pre-injecting

Box B. Physiology of pelvic congestion	References
• Dilatation of peripheral circulation involving whole genital tract or individual pelvic organs	5,47
• Delayed venous return	
– in supine but particularly in erect position	5,47
– clinically evident in the erect position with an increasing tendency to syncope, and exacerbation of CPP (analogous to 'runner's cramp')	15,48
• Attenuation of peripheral vascular reactivity in response to a rise in venous pressure	
• Evidence that oestrogen may be responsible for the circulatory dysfunction of pelvic congestion:	15,17,49
– it stimulates release of nitric oxide	12
– it interferes with autoregulation of the pelvic circulation	8,9
– it interferes with control of the circulation by the autonomic nervous system	8,50

that vein with the nitric oxide inhibitor, N-mono-methyl-L-arginine. This is evidence that nitric oxide is likely to be a major contributor to the genesis of the pain of pelvic congestion.

The possibility that pelvic congestion is not confined to the pelvis alone, but may involve the whole circulation, was investigated.[15] The reactivity of the peripheral circulation was studied in the skin of the foot by measuring changes in laser Doppler flux in response to head-up tilt. A group of women with pelvic congestion and a matched control group of no-pain women were studied in the supine position followed by 45° head-up tilt. In the control group during the follicular phase of the menstrual cycle, there was a constant reduction in flux in response to tipping, providing presumptive evidence of peripheral vasoconstriction, whereas in the luteal phase 30% of the same women had an increase in flux. These findings strongly suggest a cyclical influence of ovarian steroids on peripheral vascular reactivity. When the same study was carried out in women with pelvic congestion, there was a variable response, with reduced flux (constriction) and increased flux (dilatation) in both phases of the cycle, similar to that seen in the control group of women. Treatment of the pelvic congestion women by suppression of ovarian activity to alleviate their pain[16] resulted in a return of their peripheral vascular response to tilting to the follicular phase type of response exhibited by the control group. These findings can be interpreted as strong evidence in support of the role of ovarian hormone(s) in the genesis of pelvic congestion. The return of the peripheral circulation to physiological responsiveness is illustrated by the finding that before treatment, with prolonged standing, 40% of women with pelvic congestion developed symptoms of syncope compared with 7% in the no-pain control group. After treatment, only one woman in the pelvic congestion group (5%) complained of syncope with standing.

In order to compare the relative peripheral vascular responsiveness of the skin of the foot with that of the vagina and rectum in a similar group of women without pain, the same study design was use.[17] An identical pattern of change in peripheral flux in response to head-up tilt and relative to the stage of the menstrual cycle was observed, with the exception that the magnitude of the change in flux was much greater in the vagina as compared with the rectal mucosa or skin.

These findings are evidence that the peripheral, and probably the whole circulation of the pelvis, normally responds according to the phase of the menstrual cycle. In the case of women with pelvic congestion, there is a considerable variability of peripheral vascular responsiveness throughout the cycle. This is good evidence of the link between peripheral vascular responsiveness to ovarian activity, and suggests that ovarian dysfunction increases that variability. Whether or not this variability is the product of the local hyperoestrogenism still has to be determined. Finally, these findings offer a basis for the treatment of pelvic congestion by ovarian downregulation as described in Box F.

Ovarian dysfunction (Box Ci and Cii)

The above data have pointed to the likelihood that ovarian dysfunction is a major contributor to the genesis of pelvic congestion. Pelvic congestion is a condition confined to women who have functioning ovaries. Typically, 65% of them complain of menstrual dysfunction[18] and on closer questioning most admit to passing clots on the

---

**Box Ci.   Evidence of endocrine dysfunction in women
with pelvic congestion**   **References**

Clinical features
- Pelvic congestion is confined to women with ovarian function   22,45
- Chronic pelvic pain is cyclical in its onset and severity   18,45
- Menstrual dysfunction is common, particularly menorrhagia   18,45
- The pain is relieved by suppression of ovarian activity   16,20

Investigative features
- Uterine volume and endometrial thickness are greater than normal   16,23,51,52
- Suppression of ovarian activity results in a change from peripheral
  vasodilatation to vasconstriction in response to a rise in venous
  pressure at the same time as relieving the chronic pelvic pain
  of congestion   15

**Box Cii.   Evidence of ovarian dysfunction in women
with pelvic congestion**   **References**

- An increased prevalence of abnormal ovarian morphology – 56%
  (polycystic and pelvic congestion cystic ovaries)   16,19,22,23
- Likely cause is inappropriately timed released of gonadotrophins   53
- Pelvic congestion cystic ovaries are different in morphology and function
  from classical polycystic ovaries   19
  i)   – an excess of large follicular cysts randomly arranged
       – ovarian stroma is reduced and spongy
       – ovarian cortex thickness is normal
  ii) response to gonadotrophin stimulation
       – granulosa cells – estradiol response to follicle-stimulating hormone
         stimulation is reduced for pelvic congestion cystitis with ovaries, while it is
         increased for classical polycystic ovaries
       – theca cells – androstenedione response to luteinising hormone stimulation is
         increased for both classical polycystic ovaries and pelvic congestion cystic ovaries

---

first two days of menstruation. In addition, the occurrence and severity of CPP associated with pelvic congestion is related to the menstrual cycle. It often starts as congestive dysmenorrhoea, with pain preceding menstruation, and then spreads into the remainder of the cycle. Women usually state that their pelvic pain is worse in the second part of the menstrual cycle and occasionally at midcycle.

Studies with ultrasound scanning, using the criteria described in Table 11.1 below, have shown that 50–60% of women with pelvic congestion have ovaries with multiple follicles,[16,18] either as classical polycystic ovaries (PCO) or with multiple follicular cysts irregularly arranged throughout the ovarian stroma, referred to as pelvic congestion cystic ovaries (PCCO).[19] These occur with equal prevalence in women undergoing bilateral oophorectomy and hysterectomy for pelvic congestion.[20]

Table 11.1.   Ultrasound criteria proposed for distinguishing between PCO and PCCO[23]

The classical polycystic ovary	The pelvic congestion cystic ovary
<>> 10 follicles, diameter 2–8 mm	Follicles (cysts) 7–11 mm diameter
Follicles peripherally distributed	Distribution of follicles random
Stroma increased in volume and density	Stroma 'spongy' and often reduced
Tunica thickened	Tunica normal
Ovarian volume <>> 9 ml	Ovarian volume usually normal

Reference has already been made to the effectiveness of downregulation of ovarian function or bilateral oophorectomy in suppressing pelvic pain due to congestion and of returning peripheral vascular responsiveness to normal.[15] From these general comments, it can be seen how the concept of ovarian dysfunction being responsible for pelvic congestion has arisen and this will now be considered in greater detail.

Ovarian dysfunction

It was Taylor[22] who first noted the association between women with CPP and cystic ovaries. Subsequently, Adams *et al.* (1990)[23] reported a prevalence of cystic ovaries in 56% of women with pelvic congestion and noted that the morphology of many of these ovaries was different from that of the 'classical' PCO. The morphological differences between these two of these two are described in Table 11.1 and are shown graphically in Figure 11.2.

Much of the work on ovarian dysfunction has concentrated on the PCO syndrome. Polson *et al.*[21] investigated the prevalence of PCO in the general population of young women between the ages of 18–36 years whose menstrual cycles were spontaneous, and who 'had not found it necessary to consult a doctor for menstrual disturbance, infertility or hirsutism'. Using their ultrasound diagnostic criteria, they found that 23% of these women had morphological evidence of PCO. However, while the majority of menstrual cycle defects and 'hirsutism' in their study population were in the PCO group, their biochemical markers were not so clear-cut in distinguishing between the ultrasound normal and PCO groups. No significant differences were present between the groups for basal luteinising hormome (LH), follicle-stimulating hormone (FSH) or

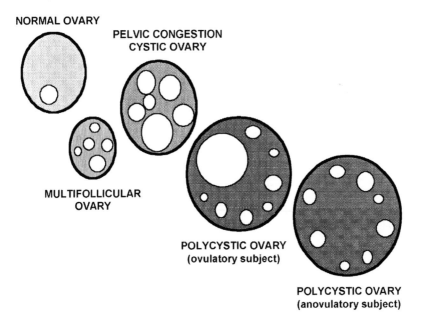

Figure 11.2. Diagram illustrating the variations in the morphological distribution of follicular cyosts relative to the clinical syndrome[19]

testosterone. In addition, the authors reported that 45% of the PCO group had an ovarian volume within the normal range. These findings raise the possibility that ultrasound scanning may not be such a good discriminant between PCO and normal ovaries, or with some ovaries with multiple follicular cysts (PCCO) not being PCO.

Further support for this view has recently been provided by Gilling-Smith et al.,[19] who reported on the follicular fluid content of ovarian steroids and the steroidogenesis of granulosa and theca cells in PCO, PCCO and normal ovaries. There are clear differences between the two types of ovaries, with an ovular PCO showing a significant increase in his oestradiol secretion in response to FSH stimulation of granulosa cells, while the granulosa cells from PCCO showed a reduced response. Theca cell secretion of androstenedione, both basal and LH-stimulated, was higher in the PCO and PCCO than normal ovaries. The conclusions of the authors were that, not only was the morphological appearance of PCCO different from those with PCO, but functionally, while the cysts of PCO ovaries are fully active, those of PCCO have a high proportion of atretic follicles than either normal or PCO ovaries.

Psychological dysfunction in women with CPP (Box D)

It has long been accepted that a range of psychological factors influences the relationship between physical damage to tissues and subjective pain intensity in all parts of the body.[24] This concept of the interaction between psychological (psyche) and physiological (soma) components of pain is a model that is central for the management of all painful conditions, whether due to functional or other causes. The history of the development of this concept of women with chronic pelvic pain has been reviewed by Pearce and Beard.[25] These authors propose a model of interaction between psychological and somatic factors shown in Figure 11.3.

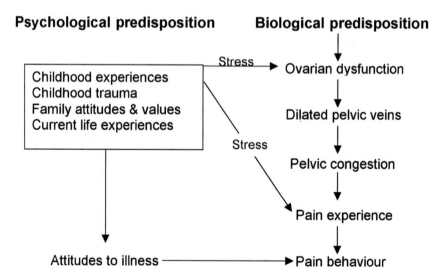

Figure 11.3.   Proposed model of interaction between psychological and biological factors responsible for the development of pelvic congestion (adapted from ref. 54)

Studies in women with CPP of unspecified origin

Most studies have characterised the psychological status of patients with CPP without addressing such issues as whether psychological dysfunction precedes CPP, with the implication that it might be seen as possibly responsible for the pain or, alternatively, that the psychological dysfunction is a product of the pain. It is unfortunate that, in the research on the subject, such a wide variety of questionnaires has been used to determine whether psychopathology is present or not that there is a lack of comparability which makes it difficult to summarise the findings in a convincing manner. Inevitably, most of the research has been carried out on women referred to hospital clinics, and this is likely to be reflected in a higher proportion being psychologically dysfunctional than among women with CPP in the general population. Bearing this in mind, there does seem to be general agreement that women with CPP do have certain psychological abnormalities, which are listed in Box D. As a group, there is an increased prevalence of anxiety, neuroticism, sexual dysfunction, hostility and a tendency to somatise their feelings.[24,26-28] There is some disagreement as to whether depression is significantly more common among this group, with authors being about equally divided for and against. There is, however, now general agreement that women with CPP, as a group, more commonly have a history of emotional trauma, and of physical and sexual abuse.[27-30] Prevalence rates for sexual abuse vary from 40% to 60% but, here again, there are methodological problems in defining what constitutes sexual abuse and how this information was obtained from subjects being interviewed.

The authors of the laparoscopic studies reviewed who have distinguished between the presence or absence of pelvic pathology,[30-33] have drawn the following conclusions:

1. The prevalence of psychological abnormalities is significantly higher in the CPP group as compared with the no-pain control group, regardless of whether pelvic pathology was present or not.

2. There is no significant difference in the prevalence of psychological abnormalities in women with and without pelvic pathology.

Box D. Psychological dysfunction

a) In all women with CPP   **References**
- Increased prevalence of anxiety, neuroticism, sexual dysfunction,
  hostility and somatisation: 24,27,28, 30,31,33,54
  - the increase is present in women with CPP as a group rather
    than being confined to those with pelvic congestion
  - when pelvic pathology (endometriosis, adhesions) is present,
    the prevalence of psychological dysfunction is no different
    from those without pathology   28,32,55–57
  - the severity of CPP is not related to the severity of the pathology
- There is an increased prevalence of a history in childhood or   24,29,30,32,60
  adult life of:
  a. sexual abuse
  b. physical abuse
  c. emotional abuse

b) In women with pelvic congestion   27, 29,30,32
In addition to the dysfunction above, women with pelvic congestion have:
- increased prevalence of disease conviction and of paternal
  overprotection in childhood   24,30,32
- major stressors, both emotional and physical, which contribute   29,31,36
  to a persistent state of chronic stress

3. The single study of treatment by Richter and colleagues[33] showed that, at postoperative follow-up, the prevalence rates for psychopathology and for persistence of pain were high and not significantly different between the laparoscopy-negative women (no specific treatment) and those who were laparoscopy positive (surgical treatment).

4. In several studies the prevalence of pelvic pathology between the pain and the control groups was not significantly different. In addition, Elcombe and colleagues,[34] in their laparoscopic study of women with CPP, concluded that only 10% of women with CPP had pelvic pathology likely to be a cause of their pain. These findings suggest that much of the pathology reported at laparoscopy for CPP is coincidental, particularly when it is limited to occasional deposits of endometriosis or a few fine adhesions. More objective studies are needed, such as those that use the laparoscopic pain mapping technique by laparoscopy described by Reginald and colleagues,[35] before this matter can be resolved.

The above results can be interpreted as showing that women with CPP have an increase in psychological dysfunction as a group, regardless of whether pelvic pathology is found at laparoscopy. Whether this dysfunction is a cause or a consequence of their CPP is uncertain, the undoubted increase in prevalence among these women of emotional trauma and physical and sexual abuse in childhood does suggest that as a group they are more stress-prone and likely to somatise with pelvic symptoms.

Studies of women with CPP due to pelvic congestion

Women with pelvic congestion do not appear to be markedly different from the general population of women with CPP, except in a few aspects.

1. There is an increased prevalence of paternal over-protection in childhood,[29] disease conviction and exposure to death and separation within the family in childhood.[31,36]

2. There is an increased prevalence of major stressors, both emotional and physical, which contribute to a persistent state of chronic stress.[28,36,37] However, it must be recognised that, by itself, pelvic pain soon becomes the major stressor, not only because of the disagreeable sensation, but often because of the continuing uncertainty as to the cause of that pain.

Conclusions

This review of recent publications on this important aspect of women with CPP illustrates how relevant it is for psychologists, psychiatrists and gynaecologists to be aware of each others' interests. There can be little doubt that women with CPP do suffer generally from being over-anxious and sensitive to all forms of stress. A combined psychological and biochemical study found that many of these women had features of post-traumatic stress disorder.[30,32] These findings emphasise the importance of obtaining a history of possible emotional antecedents and current stressors in the

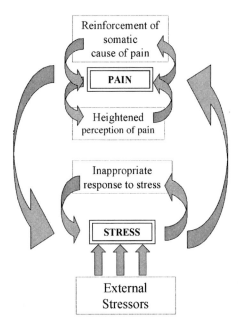

Figure 11.4.   Diagram illustrating the vicious circle of stress/pain/stress acting on women with CPP and the exogenous and endogenous factors which maintain the interaction

management of women with CPP, particularly as it is not usual for GPs or gynaecologists to do this when first presented with this type of problem. Equally, it is important for a psychologist or psychiatrist in the same position to have a good working knowledge of the somatic causes of CPP recognised by their gynaecological colleagues, because most women who have had CPP for years, believe deeply that there must be some pathology, as yet undetected, which is causing their pain.

Much more research into the important link between psyche and soma still needs to be done. However, the high placebo response of the condition and the significant improvement that results from a combination of medical and psychological treatment[16,38] is encouraging as evidence of the clinical reality of such a link. Figure 11.4, showing the interaction between pain and stress, is particularly useful in this respect because it describes a process a woman with CPP and her partner know only too well when an attack of pain starts. It also provides a basis for explaining the treatment programme proposed to them.

Treatment of women with pelvic congestion (Boxes E and F)

Treatment of the patient with CPP starts from the time when she and her partner first come into contact with the clinic. As Grace has described so graphically,[39] these women have often been emotionally traumatised by previous encounters with the medical profession, being labelled as 'neurotic' or 'a psychological problem', and they arrive at the clinic as dissatisfied sufferers.[40] There are many advantages in taking the services provided for women with CPP out of the general gynaecology outpatient clinic into a tertiary care setting[38] where women can meet receptive and knowledgeable carers who they feel have time to listen to them.

An important component of the above approach is to carry out standard investigations – a structured questionnaire to be completed by the patient, laparoscopy with photography, a detailed transvaginal ultrasound scan and, if necessary, pelvic venography, and a psychological assessment, the purpose and results of which are explained to the patient and her partner. In managing these patients, good communication (and this includes sending copies of letters to GPs to the patient) is, at all times, an essential component of effective treatment. Experience has shown that it is best to withhold the results of investigations from the patient until she meets the consultant for the first time at the assessment visit. With the results of these investigations in front of them, the consultant will be able to make a more balanced diagnosis than if these are revealed to the patient before a clear diagnostic picture has emerged. The use of photographs taken at laparoscopy, ultrasound scans, venograms and the diagrams shown in Figures 11.1 and 11.4 is helpful in this session.

It is essential that the patient and her partner understand the rationale for making a final diagnosis and, to aid this process, a leaflet containing a description of pelvic congestion and its management is provided. Possibly, the most important aspect of this visit is that the patient and her partner understand and accept the link between psyche and soma and the consequent need for psychotherapy (pain and stress management). Patients tend to feel threatened and are highly sceptical of any suggestion that there is a psychological component to CPP. If they are not persuaded of this link by the time they leave the session with the consultant, then it is unlikely they will attend the counselling sessions.

From the nature of the work, it is obviously important to have the counsellors working alongside the gynaecologists. It is also important for all gynaecologists seeing women with CPP, particularly the consultant gynaecologist, to have a working knowledge of the pain and stress management programme, and to meet regularly with the counsellor(s) for clinical discussions. Finally, patients should be encouraged from when they are first referred to the clinic but, in particular, when they are on treatment, to keep in contact with the clinic and this can be done with a 24-hour telephone 'help line' service, which has proved to be invaluable for this purpose.

Box E. Findings on investigation of women with CPP due to pelvic congestion	References
• *Laparoscopy:*	37,45
– visible peritoneal hyperaemia of variable distribution (uterus, broad ligament pelvis)	
– dilated pelvic veins > around hilum of ovary, ovarian vein, broad ligament	18
– +/– multiple cysts under cortex of ovary	16,23
– with or without pelvic pathology	
• *Pelvic ultrasound (TVA):*	4
– visible veins in the broad ligament and around cervix (2–6 mm)	
– reduced Doppler flow of dilated veins	
– +/– pelvic congestion cystic ovaries or classical polycystic ovaries	
• *Pelvic venogram:*	5
– dilated ovarian +/– myometrial veins	
– increased density and persistence of dye due to delayed clearance	

Treatment programmes – Box F

Medical

As pelvic congestion is confined to women of reproductive age, conservation of ovarian function is of paramount importance when planning treatment. The therapeutic philosophy adopted by the Northwick Park Pelvic Pain Service is of a combination of ovarian downregulation for six months, which provides pain relief that persuades the patient that a correct diagnosis has been made. At the same time, she will be expected to attend at least four of the planned six sessions of pain and stress management.

Specific therapy

Ovarian downregulation has been shown to significantly reduce pelvic pain due to congestion in 75% of women.[16] This was shown by using medroxyprogesterone acetate (MPA) at a dose of 50 mg a day but without addback hormone replacement therapy (HRT). Frequently, adverse effects, such as weight gain, flushes and sweats, were found to be worrying to women with CPP. For this reason, the gonadotrophin-releasing hormone analogues (GnRHa) drugs (leuprorelin acetate or goserelin acetate) were substituted, with the addition of addback HRT in the form of conjugated equine oestrogens 0.625 mg and MPA 5 mg daily during the period of downregulation.[37] The use of addback HRT has been shown to reduce the incidence of adverse effects but, the higher the dose of oestrogen, the greater the tendency for vaginal bleeding to develop and, in the experience of the author, for the pelvic pain to return or worsen. Increasing the duration of downregulation is sometimes necessary if the patient does not feel ready to cope with the pelvic pain that she is told will return when ovarian activity restarts. Irregular vaginal bleeding during downregulation has been reported in 25% of women using addback HRT and can usually be stopped by increasing the dose of the addback progestogen, which in the case of MPA, is to a maximum dose of 30 mg/day.

Psychotherapy

The benefits of adopting a combined medical and psychotherapeutic approach to achieve long-term improvement in the management of CPP from pelvic congestion have already been discussed. It is important that a patient entering the pain and stress management programme should understand the following. First, that stress management is demanding and she may have to make major changes to her lifestyle, such as changing her job, reducing her general level of daily activity, and reassessing her relationships (see chapter 7). Second, she should recognise that the pain management programme, consisting of a series of relaxation exercises on tape, has to be learnt, so that it can be implemented at any time as soon as an attack of pelvic pain starts. Understanding this is a part of the acceptance by the patient that, while she has functioning ovaries, stressful events may cause the pelvic pain to return but that relaxation can effectively prevent the spiral of anxiety–pain–more anxiety developing into a severe attack of pelvic pain. It also requires acknowledgement that the therapists are providing her with a 'self-help' programme rather than the more traditional cure that most people expect when going to see a doctor. Third, the relaxation tape provided

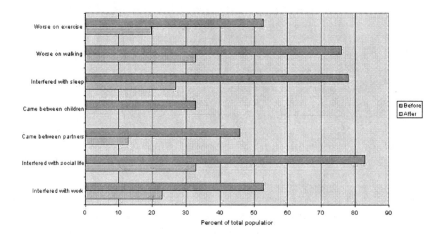

Figure 11.5. Outcome of combined therapy measured a year after completion of treatment, by quality of life indicators of 33 women with CPP due to pelvic congestion by ovarian downregulation and pain management; NWP Pelvic Pain Clinic 1997–98[38]

by the clinic may not suit her, and that alternative therapies such as yoga, reflexology or aromatherapy can achieve the same therapeutic aims as relaxation exercises, if they are acceptable.

Figure 11.5 shows the benefit of the combined approach to treatment in a group of 33 women, in terms of quality of life.[38] After periods of treatment, varying from three to 12 months, there was an improvement in the quality of life indicators that ranged from 61% to 100%.

Surgical treatment

From the outset of the treatment programme, it should be emphasised that the purpose of the treatment programme is to conserve ovarian function. Exceptions to this rule are women nearing the end of their reproductive life and those with trapped ovaries.[41] In addition, there is a small number of women who, despite having obtained relief from their CPP or no relief at all on ovarian downregulation, usually because of unresolved stress, require a surgical solution. This is relatively uncommon, and Beard and colleagues[20] reported that only 36 of 775 women (4.6%) referred to a pelvic pain clinic with CPP eventually needed to be treated by hysterectomy and bilateral salpingo-oophorectomy. A review from the same clinic for follow-up for five years of 84 women who had undergone the same operation for CPP due to congestion showed that 85% of them had remained pain-free.[42]

The removal of the ovaries of a woman of reproductive age with CPP due to congestion must be accompanied by advice on the importance of the use of HRT until at least the age of 50 years. The follow-up of such women for up to five years on HRT[42] has shown how effective this form of treatment is in allowing them to return to a normal life and preventing them from developing postmenopausal symptoms. The philosophy of the Pelvic Pain Service is that, if a patient and her partner have thought long and hard about the advantages and disadvantages of oophorectomy, particularly if

Box F. Treatment of women with CPP due to pelvic congestion	References
Medical (conservative) treatment	
• Treatment of women with CPP has a high 'placebo' response (approx. 40%)	16,34
• Ovarian downregulation with a progestogen or GnRH analogue in combination with 'addback' HRT is effective in alleviating CPP while on treatment; CPP returns with the onset of ovarian activity	16,58
• Psychotherapy is effective in the treatment of women with CPP, in particular, pain and stress management	31,34,40,59
• The first visit for assessing the psychological status of a woman with CPP may have some therapeutic effect	40
Combined treatment	38
• Ovarian downregulation, combined with psychotherapy is effective in the short- and long-term treatment of CPP	
Surgery	16
• Bilateral oophorectomy combined with hysterectomy relieves the pain of CPP due to pelvic congestion in 85% of 84 women followed up for 2–5 years postoperatively	20,42
• Bone mineral density remain unchanged following bilateral oophorectomy followed by HRT	42
• Embolisation of ovarian veins under radiological control has a 50–80% success, but a trial of treatment is required to verify this figure	43

they have tried more conservative management, and finally decide that bilateral oophorectomy and hysterectomy is the right way forward, then this course of action will be agreed.

Other more conservative surgical approaches to the treatment of CPP, such as hysterectomy with conservation of the ovaries, have all been tried without apparent success in the long term because it is the ovaries that are usually the cause and site of the CPP but, because of the high placebo rate that any surgical treatment of CPP carries, further experience is needed on this point. Surgical embolisation of the ovarian veins under radiographic control has been tried with a reported success rate varying from 50% to 80%.[43] However, as with all the treatments for CPP due to congestion referred to in this chapter, evaluation of them in a large enough population is needed, as is the development of new approaches as knowledge of the condition increases.

Conclusions

Figure 11.6 summarises, in a graphic form, the cycle leading from chronic stress to ovarian dysfunction to pelvic congestion to pelvic pain which, in turn, reinforces chronic stress. The probable adverse effects are shown of both endocrine dysfunction and stress on circulatory control by the autonomic system.

The proposed mechanism for the genesis of pelvic congestion shown above illustrates the interaction between psyche and soma and thus fulfils the requirements for a functional disorder involving the menstrual cycle, thereby supporting the hypothesis proposed in this chapter.

Pelvic congestion is a common cause of CPP when none of the traditional causes of

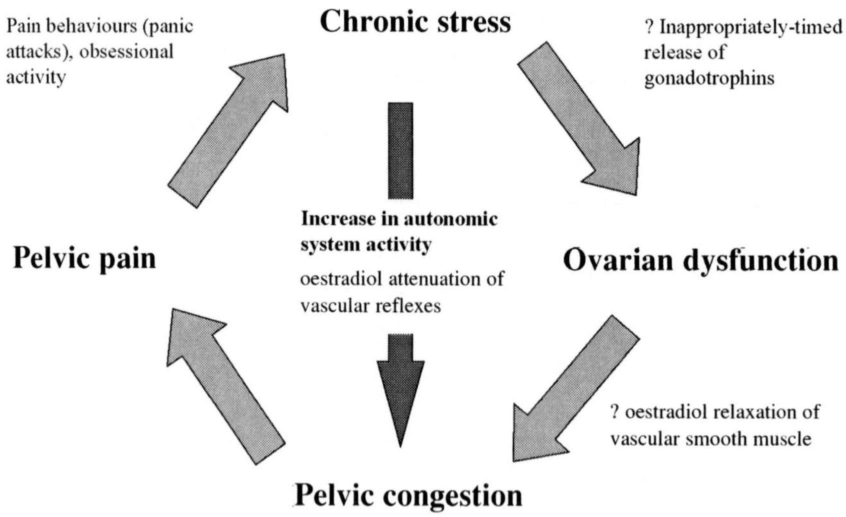

Pain behaviours (panic attacks), obsessional activity

Chronic stress

? Inappropriately-timed release of gonadotrophins

Pelvic pain

Increase in autonomic system activity

oestradiol attenuation of vascular reflexes

Ovarian dysfunction

? oestradiol relaxation of vascular smooth muscle

Pelvic congestion

Figure 11.6.   Summary of the conclusion that can be drawn from the data presented in support of the hypothesis

'pain-producing' pelvic pathology, such as endometriosis or adhesions, have been found. It is also likely that pelvic congestion is the cause of CPP in some cases when such pelvic pathology is present, but further study is required to investigate this.

Pelvic pain due to congestion is a treatable condition using the combined approach of medical (or occasionally surgical) management combined with stress and pain management counselling.

Acceptance and understanding, by health professionals, of the interaction between psyche and soma is an essential requirement for the effective treatment of women with CPP due to pelvic congestion.

Acknowledgements

I am grateful to all those colleagues who have helped me over the years in this work, and in particular to Cynthia Knight, Amanda Smith and Elaine MacWilliams for advising on, and reading, the early versions of this chapter.

References

1.   Mathias SD, Kupperman M, Liberman RF, Lipschutz RC, Steege JF. Chronic pelvic pain: pain prevalence, health quality and economic correlates. *Obstet Gynecol* 1996;**87**:321–7.
2.   Reginald PW, Beard RW, Kooner JS, Mathias CJ, Samarage SU, Sutherland IA, Wadsworth J. Intravenous dihydroergotamine to relieve pelvic congestion with pain in young women. *Lancet* 1987;**1**:351–3.

3. Muhe E, Burhardt KH, Kolb W, Stroberl G. Eine neue methode zur prophylaxie postoperativ venethrombosen. *Klinkartz* 1975;**4**:88–92.

4. Stones RW, Rae T, Rogers V. Pelvic congestion in women: evaluation with transvaginal ultrasound and observation of venous pharmacology. *Br J Radiol* 1990;**63**:710–11.

5. Beard RW, Highman JH, Pearce S, Reginald PW. Diagnosis of pelvic varicosities in women with chronic pelvic pain. *Lancet* 1984;**2**:946–9.

6. Taylor HC. Vascular congestion and hyperaemia. The clinical aspects of congestion fibrosis syndrome. *Am J Obstet Gynecol* 1949;**57**:637–53.

7. Stones RW, Turmaine M, Beard RW, Burnstock G. The fine structure of the human vein. *J Anat* 1994;**185**:285–94.

8. Stones RW. Local vascular control in the human ovarian circulation, MD Thesis. London: University of London; 1994.

9. Stones RW, Loesch A, Beard RW, Burnstock G, Substana P. Endothelial localisation and pharmacology in human ovarian vein. *Obstet Gynecol* 1995;**85**:273–8.

10. Cockell AP, Poston L. Effects of 17-beta-oestradiol on flow-induced vasodilatation of small arteries in female rats. *Am J Obstet Gynecol* 1997;**77**:1–7.

11. Poston L, McCarthy AL, Ritter JM. Control of vascular resistance in the maternal and fetoplacential arterial beds. *Pharmac Ther* 1995;**65**:150–59.

12. Van Buren GA, Yong D, Clarke KE. Oestrogen-induced vasodilatation is antagonised by L-nitroarginine methyl ester, an inhibitor of nitric oxide synthesis. *Am J Obstet Gynecol* 1992;**167**:828–33.

13. Kingden-Milles D, Arndt JO. Nitric oxide as a chemical link in the generation of pain from veins in humans. *Pain* 1996;**64**:139–42.

14. Haley JE, Dickenson AH, Shacter M. Electrophysiological evidence for the role of nitric oxide in prolonged chemical nociception in the rat. *Neuropharmacology* 1992;**31**:251–8.

15. Foong LC, Gamble J, Sutherland LA, Beard RW. Altered peripheral vascular response of women with and without pelvic pain due to congestion. *Br J Obstet Gynaecol* 2000;**107**:157–64.

16. Farquhar CM, Rogers V, Franks S. A randomised controlled trial of medroxyprogesterone acetate and psychotherapy for the treatment of pelvic congestion. *Br J Obstet Gynaecol* 1989;**96**:1153–62.

17. Emmanuel AV, Kamm MA, Beard RW. Reproducible assessment of vaginal and rectal mucosal and skin blood flow: laser doppler fluximetry of the pelvic microcirculation. *Clin Sci* 2000;**95**:201–7.

18. Beard RW, Reginald PW, Wadsworth J. Clinical features of women with chronic lower abdominal pain and pelvic congestion. *Br J Obstet Gynaecol* 1988;**95**:153–61.

19. Gilling-Smith C, Mason H, Willis D. In-vitro ovarian steroidogenesis in women with pelvic congestion. *Hum Reprod* 2000;**15**:2570–76.

20. Beard RW, Kennedy RG, Gangar KF. Bilateral oophorectomy and hysterectomy in the treatment of intractable pelvic pain associated with pelvic congestion. *Br J Obstet Gynaecol* 1991;**98**:988–92.

21. Polson D, Adams J, Franks S. Polycystic ovaries – a common finding in normal women. *Lancet* 1988;**1**:870–72.

22. Taylor HC. Vascular congestion and hyperaemia: their effect on the structure and function of the female reproductive system. *Am J Obstet Gynecol* 1949;**57**:211–30

23. Adams J, Reginald PW, Franks S, Wadsworth J, Beard RW. Uterine size and endometrial thickness and the significance of cystic ovaries in women with pelvic pain due to congestion. *Br J Obstet Gynaecol* 1990;**97**:583–7

24. Walker GA, Katon WJ, Hansom J, Harrop Griffiths J, Holm L, Jones ML, *et al.* Psychiatric diagnoses and sexual victimisation in women with chronic pelvic pain. *Psychosomatics* 1995;**36**:531–40.

25. Pearce S, Beard RW. Chronic pelvic pain in women. In: Bass C, editor. *Somatization: Physical Symptoms and Psychological Illness.* London: Blackwell Scientific Publications; 1990. p. 259–75.

26. Melzack R. *The Challenge of Pain.* London: Penguin Books; 1999.

27. Collett BJ, Cordel CJ, Stewart CR, Jogger C. A comparative study of women with chronic pelvic pain, chronic non-pelvic pain and those with no history of pain attending general practitioners. *Br J Obstet Gynaecol* 1998;**105**:87–92.

28. Pearce S. The concept of psychogenic pain: a psychological investigation of women with pelvic pain. *Curr Psychol Res Rev* 1987;**6**:219–28.

29. Fry RPW, Beard RW, Crisp AH, McGuigan S. Sociopsychological factors in women with chronic pelvic pain with and without pelvic venous congestion. *J Psychosom Res* 1997;**42**:1–15.

30. Ehlert U, Heim C, Helhammer DH. Chronic pelvic pain as a somatoform disorder. *Psychother Psychosom* 1999;**68**:87–94.

31. Pearce S. Chronic pelvic pain: a psychological approach, PhD Thesis. London: University of London; 1986.

32. Heim C, Ehlert U, Hanker JP, Hellhammer DH. Abuse-related posttraumatic stress disorder and alterations of the hypothalamic-pituitary adrenal axis in women with chronic pelvic pain. *Psychosom Med* 1998;**6**:309–18.

33. Richter HE, Halley RL, Chandraiah S, Varner RE. Laparoscopic and psychological evaluation of women with chronic pelvic pain. *Int J Psychiatr Med* 1998;**28**:243–53.

34. Elcombe S, Gath D, Day A. The psychological effects of laparoscopy on women with chronic pelvic pain. *Psychol Med* 1997;**27**:1041–50.

35. Reginald PW, Iyer L, Fell R. Conscious pain mapping: pain evaluation at laparoscopy under local anaesthesia in women with chronic pelvic pain. In: Gomez FG and Palacios S, editors. *Perspectives in Gynaecology and Obstetrics: Selected Papers Presented at the XIV European Congress of Obstetricians and Gynaecologists, Granada, Spain, 1999*. London: Parthenon; 2000. p. 153–6.

36. Duncan CH, Taylor HC. A psychosomatic study of pelvic congestion. *Am J Obstet Gynecol* 1952;**64**:12.

37. Beard RW, Gangar K, Pearce S. Chronic gynaecological pain. In: Wall P, Melzack R, editors. *Textbook of Pain*, 3rd edn. London: Churchill Livingstone; 1991. p. 597–613.

38. Audit of Clinical Activity in the Pelvic Pain Clinic, Northwick Park Hospital 1997–98 (unpublished).

39. Grace VM. Problems women patients experience in the medical encounter for chronic pelvic pain: a New Zealand study. *Health Care for Women International* 1995;**16**:509–19.

40. Price JR, Blake F. Editorial – Chronic pelvic pain: the assessment as therapy. *J Psychosom Res* 1998;**46**:7–14.

41. Siddum-Allum J, Rae T, Rogers V, Witherow R, Flanagan A, Beard RW. Chronic pelvic pain caused by residual ovaries and ovarian remnants. *Br J Obstet Gynaecol* 1994;**101**:979–85.

42. Reid BA, Gangar KF, Rogers V. Longterm results of bilateral oophorectomy for the treatment of chronic pelvic pain: relief of pain and special hormone replacement therapy requirements. *J Obstet Gynaecol* 1996;**16**:538–43.

43. Venbrux AC, Lambert DL. Embolization of the ovarian veins as treatment for patients with chronic pelvic pain due to pelvic venous incompetence (pelvic congestion syndrome). *Curr Opin Obstet Gynaecol* 1999;**11**:395–9.

44. Steege JF, Stout AL, Somkuti SG. Chronic pelvic pain in women: towards an integrative model. *Obstet Gynecol Survey* 1993;**48**:95–110.

45. Beard RW, Reginald PW. Chronic pelvic pain in gynaecology. In: Shaw WP, Stanton SL, editors. *Textbook of Gynaecology*. London: Churchill Livingstone; 1992. p. 777–88.

46. Gooch R. *On Some of the Most Important Diseases Peculiar to Women. The Irritable Uterus.* Republished by the Sydenham Society, London; 1859. p. 299–331.

47. Thomas DC, McArdle FJ, Rogers VE, Beard RW, Brown BB. Local blood volume changes in women with pelvic congestion measured by applied potential tomography. *Clin Sci* 1991;**81**:401–4.

48. Reginald PW. Investigation of the pelvic congestion or a cause of chronic pelvic pain in women with no pathology, MD Thesis. London: University of London; 1989.

49. Henriksen O, Sejrsen P. Local reflex in microcirculation in human cutaneous tissue. *Acta Physiol Scand* 1976;**98**: 227–31.

50. Taylor HC. Pelvic pain based on a vascular and autonomic nervous system disorder. *Am J Obstet Gynecol* 1954;**67**:1177–96.

51. Saxton DW, Farquhar CM, Rae T, Beard RW, Anderson MC, Wadsworth J. Accuracy of ultrasound measurements of female pelvic organs. *Br J Obstet Gynaecol* 1990;**57**:211–30.

52. Polson DW, Franks S, Adams J. The distribution of oestradiol in plasma in relation to uterine cross-sectional area in women with polycystic or multifollicular ovaries. *Clin Endocrinol* 1987;**26**:581–8.

53. Nadaraja R, Hansel W. Hormonal changes associated with experimentally produced cystic ovaries in cows. *J Reprod Fertil* 1976;**47**:203–8.

54. Pearce S, Knight C, Beard RW. Pelvic pain: a common gynaecological problem. *J Psychosom Obstet Gynaecol* 1982;**1**:12–17.

55. Fedele L, Parrazini F, Bianchi S, Areaini L, Candiani GB. Stage and localisation of pelvic endometriosis and pain. *Fertil Steril* 1990;**53**:155–8.

56. Vercellini P, Trespidi L, DeGiorgio O, Cortesi I, Parrazini F, Crouignani PG. Endometriosis and pelvic pain: relation to disease stage and of localisation. *Fertil Steril* 1996;**65**:299–304.

57. Stout AL, Steege JF, Dodson WC, Hughes CL. Relationship of laparoscopic findings to self-report of pelvic pain. *Am J Obstet Gynecol* 1991;**154**:73–9.

58. Gilling-Smith C, Rogers V, Wright M, Beard RW. GnRH analogue and medroxyprogesterone acetate for the treatment of pelvic congestion – a pilot comparative study. *Br J Obstet Gynaecol* 2001; submitted for publication.

59. Pearce S. A review of cognitive-behavioural methods for the treatment of chronic pelvic pain. *J Psychosom Res* 1983;**27**:421–40.
60. Walker GA, Katon WJ, Neraas K, Jemelka RP, Massoth D. Dissociation in women with chronic pelvic pain. *Am J Psychiatry* 1992;**149**:534–7.

Chapter 12

Pelvic pain I

Discussion

Discussion following the papers of Professor Steege, Mr Kennedy and Professor Beard

Stones: Professor Steege, what do you think about the different diagnoses that were being produced by the different doctors? Are we in the situation that it does not matter which model you are following as long as you have a model? Is that true for medical diagnosis?

Steege: What we do not know is whether the outcomes of treatment differed among these varying physicians. We have no data to address that. Perhaps interpretation of success is as biased as interpretation of ideology, I do not know.

Whorwell: As an outsider, may I suggest that you have a huge problem here with nomenclature. We used to call irritable bowel syndrome (IBS) mucus colitis, spastic colon, chronic constipation, painless diarrhoea. All those terms just served to confuse, and you almost need to step back and just call this chronic pain. It is a pity it has this slightly unfortunate term, and if you could come up with a new term it would be nice. But once you start attributing slightly suspect causes to your pain you have a problem. Concerning interstitial cystitis – I had never heard of vestibulitis, I thought you were talking about the ear to begin with.

Another problem you may have which we had in the irritable bowel world is where in the textbooks it said that IBS was a diagnosis of exclusion and you could not have Crohn's disease. That is entirely wrong because I see patients with Crohn's who have irritable bowel. They are being given steroids and made hugely Cushingoid for non-active Crohn's when their symptoms are IBS. I wonder whether you have the same problems here with endometriosis, that you are finding endometriosis and attributing their pain, and they have CPP – whatever that is. I believe that we will find the cause of all these conditions in the end, and then the psychology will fall into place. And I believe that the psychology is usually an effect rather than the cause of these conditions.

One very interesting paper in *The Lancet* looked at appendices that have been taken out for acute appendicitis – normal appendices.[1] They had all been classed as normal, nothing wrong with this appendix. They looked at them and found that they were stuffed full of substance P and therefore they must have an abnormality. We are just not good enough yet at detecting these abnormalities and perhaps the pelvic organs in all these people are stuffed full of substance P or something much more subtle than all the things that we are looking for today. In gastroenterology we do a colonoscopy, an ultrasound and perhaps a white cell scan, and say they are normal. But we are just scratching the surface.

Foster: I have a question for Professor Steege. It was disconcerting to see that physician C had a 74% rate of identifying sexual abuse, the highest surgical rate and one of the lowest referrals to mental health services of 4%. I wondered if you had any comments on that. Is that something that one would consider acceptable or is it just normal variation? To me it sounds as though surgery is another form of trauma to these.

Steege: I can speak with some authority because I happen to know physician C very well. It is me! Our referral pattern is unusual in that it is highly surgically biased. There is also an extraordinary institutional sensitivity to abuse in general. There is an extraordinary programme going on suggesting that every patient who walks through the door must be asked, and so forth. We also have a lower referral rate to mental health services because we handle a lot of that ourselves. I have a skilled nurse who works with me and manages much of that.

We have a lot of people referred in because the astute primary-care physician has detected a history of abuse, but it is relatively clear that it is not an active issue in the present. That is subject to the eye of the beholder for sure, but we do investigate pretty carefully whether it is an issue that is currently affecting their present way of thinking and ways of dealing with relationships and with life in general. That may explain some of that. It is artefactual.

To anticipate what Professor Berkley is going to say, she will start to look at the organ working interactions. Picking up what Mr Kennedy was saying in the epidemiological study, you have a significant proportion of people with overlap between their pelvic congestion, their bladder symptoms and their bowel symptoms. We have cross-talk between various organ systems that suggests that there is an undercurrent of visceral hyperalgesia that we are tapping into, depending on which speciality we happen to be looking from. One talks to the other.

Berkley: My question is a more mechanical one. Physician A with the multiple diagnoses and your situation with the predominantly surgical approach – to what extent do you think that finance has to do with this? In the USA that multiple diagnostic routine – if he/she is coding a number of different diseases those patients have freer access to pain beds because their insurance pays for it if they are coded that way, whereas your practice may not be so insurance based as other practices. So in the USA there may be an impact of our different HMO (Health Maintenance Organization) situations across the country. Do you believe that is part of the story?

Steege: To my knowledge, I do not think we get paid more if we make more diagnoses.

Berkley: I was not talking about you. I was talking about the patient. In some cases a physician in the USA will make a more extreme diagnosis for a patient than the physician actually believes the patient has in order for the patient to be eligible to get funding for his or her medication and treatment. I thought that multiple diagnoses might be an environment in which that is needed for the patient to get the financial support that the patient needs.

Steege: To the extent that in many HMOs a routine annual visit may not be reimbursed very well but a visit for a diagnosable illness would be, that may be a factor. But I am not sure whether the making of four diagnoses rather than one changes that reimbursement.

Beard: I should like to add to what Professor Steege said about functional diseases in the pelvis. If you look at the data from the various specialities, chronic constipation and pelvic congestion and interstitial cystitis are diseases uniquely in young women: more than 90% of the people who come to St Mark's Hospital, North London, for constipation are young women and the same for interstitial cystitis. So you have to ask what is affecting this, and it is my belief that it is ovarian function that is the key factor. But that is a long shot. I once asked a gastroenterologist what he thought the reason was. He pointed to his head and said, 'They're funny in the head.' They are not: they are very intelligent, normal women.

MacLean: Professor Steege, can I ask about access to health care? One of the interesting points that Mr Kennedy showed was that many patients only get as far as primary care. In this country there are implications for referral on to hospital and, certainly, once you are in hospital, there is no guarantee that you will have access to, for instance, diagnostic laparoscopy because of delays on waiting lists; no guarantee you will get referral to other consultants unless you go back to primary care and the GP agrees to facilitate referral elsewhere. In the USA, on the other hand, once you actually have your foot in the system, that can be facilitated and provided your insurance will pay the costs, you can get almost anything and go anywhere. But maybe I do not understand because I have not practised there.

Steege: That varies tremendously from one health plan to another. Five or six years ago the gatekeeper function was probably even more powerful than it is now. There has been a strong public protest against such constraints, so there is a little more freedom now than there used to be. But in many ways, five or six years ago the system was modelled much after the National Health Service in that you had to go back to your primary-care doctor in order to get referred – if you have seen the gynaecologist you have to go back to the primary-care doctor in order to get referred to a gastroenterologist and go back to be referred to a urologist and so forth. However, many plans have discovered that that is not necessarily cost-effective and so they have allowed more freedom. The public protested as well.

There is probably more consultation in the USA than the UK but I am struck by the similarities in the number of people who are left without a diagnosis in Mr Kennedy's epidemiological study and in the Matthias study,[2] for which I was on the tail end of the authorship, and I wonder if there are simply a certain number of women out there who experience pelvic pain at various levels but it is not top of their personal priority list; they have other problems on their plate and it goes undiagnosed because they simply do not pursue it far enough.

Kennedy: I did not show some data about the level of anxiety produced by having the pain. Remarkably, irrespective of how much pain they had, or whether they were consulting a GP or hospital doctor or not, women were still concerned about the nature of the pain.

I should like to expand on something that Professor MacLean said. What interests me, given the overlap in symptoms, is why some GPs will refer a woman to a gynaecologist, others to a gastroenterologist or a genitourinary medicine doctor. It is only once we begin to dissect patterns of referral and the reasons why woman are referred that we can come up with good guidelines for improving the interface between primary and secondary care.

MacLean: I will make just one comment. There is information that has to get through to general practice and the gatekeepers, as Professor Steege called them, and one of the recommendations that should come out of this morning's session is that GPs must be more aware of the diagnosis of chronic pelvic pain and the access to people who can help their patients. If that goes through as a health educational policy, it will perhaps have some impact for patients and for general practitioners.

Sutton: I have a question for Professor Beard. I can see that you are perhaps not obsessed but fairly certain in your own mind that there is an ovarian dysfunction behind this. If you just assume that it is purely a vascular dysfunction in much the same way as varicose veins in the legs or haemorrhoids, have you looked at the effect of, say, embolising those veins or doing a high ligation of the ovarian vessels as another way of trying to treat the disorder?

Beard: There have been studies done where people have surgically attempted to remove all the veins, but it is a *tour de force* surgically and with all the blood loss and so on people have tended to abandon that, particularly as results were not very good. I have included in the chapter the work that has been done by the people who have been embolising – it looks very encouraging. The problem with such studies is that no one has subjected it to the scientific rigour of a prospective study. They are individual cases.

Berkley: I have a recommendation. Given what has just been said and some of the occasions when I have had to write editorials in different medical speciality journals, one recommendation that might come out of this is some cross-talk between gastroenterologists, obstetricians, gynaecologists and urologists – I do not know how to phrase this but I would support some multidisciplinary sessions between different pelvic organ specialists. Seeing all these overlaps between the different classifications of illness, what might come out of that are some issues held in common that would lead to a different class of recommendations that cross pelvic organ boundaries.

Steege: May I correct one thing? For my notorious physician C the abuse percentage was 26%, not 74%. That may make you feel a little better.

Whorwell: A comment on the route for referral. In gastroenterology and, I suspect, in your area, these people are very polysymptomatic; they have a whole list of symptoms. I believe it is a lottery as to which one they mention first to their primary-care person; if it happens to be dyspareunia and they happen to have IBS, then they go the gynaecology route. I am sure it is almost as simple as that.

Tookman: Just to take that one step backwards, in the palliative care literature it has been well shown that the gatekeeping role of the primary-care physician is reliant on many issues. One of the major issues is social group. For example, socially disenfranchised people, low social class, get far less access to specialist palliative care services because of the GP gatekeeping role. I would guess that it is the same in accessing specialist advice about pelvic pain.

Thornton: I have three questions rolled into one because I had so many questions on Professor Beard's talk. It follows on from Professor Sutton's question. When you talked about the ergotamine–saline study you mentioned that that was single-blind. Is there a reason why it was single as opposed to double blind? Given the emotional overlay in this problem, I wondered whether you had evidence that the beneficial effects that you demonstrated were a direct effect on the pelvic vasculature.

Following along the same line, I wondered whether the medroxyprogesterone acetate (MPA) study was double-blind.

Thirdly, was it possible in your study of abdominal hysterectomy and bilateral salpingo-ovariectomy to look at the effect of unrelated surgery on an individual with chronic pelvic pain to see whether surgery *per se* had an effect rather than the abdominal hysterectomy and bilateral salpingo-oophorectomy.

Beard: Professor Sutton could probably reply to that last question. We have a problem of the ethics of doing a sham surgical procedure. Perhaps in the future a case can be made for it. However, I believe we were right to do a simple survey initially and say the results look encouraging.

The single-blind aspect of the DHE (dihydroergotamine) study was imposed on us by the ethics committee and the person who was blinded was the patient – she did not know which she was receiving. However, it was felt necessary with a drug like DHE that the operator should know whether he was giving the saline or the DHE. The MPA study was double-blind but it ran into the problem that when a subject is taking a placebo that has no side effects on her menstrual cycle she will suspect that she is not taking the MPA. However, there was no exchange between patients of their experiences as far as we could see. They all came from different areas at different times. But I accept that is a potential weakness of that study.

Steege: I have a few comments about the placebo phenomenon. I noticed, Professor Beard, that in your MPA study if you look at the placebo response at nine months versus four months, it is the same or even possibly a little greater at nine months, so our stereotype of a third of people responding for three months may not hold in many studies. Certainly in the old literature on placebo response and sham surgery, internal mammary arterial ligation studies[3,4] showed that the placebo response to sham surgery ranged between 55% and 100% at one year. So before we interpret surgical results for anything we have to look at the placebo response rather differently.

Beard: That is absolutely right. The group in Oxford with Elcombe, Gath and Day published a good study on a look at the effect of laparoscopy alone.[5] They showed that some 50% benefited from the laparoscopy and continued to benefit – and they took them to six months.

May I raise one interesting issue? When one has been working with this subject a long time you come to recognise that there are two major groups of patients – the copers and the non-copers. The copers are generally those who have life fairly sorted out and, when they are told that there is nothing in their pelvis, everything is fine, they tend to go away and say thanks very much, that is all I needed to know. The non-copers, on the other hand, are the ones who are alarmed that nothing has been found because they hoped that something would be found. There are a lot of new developments in this aspect of interaction between the psychologists and the gynaecologists that are important in this subject.

Steege: There is one other point in my data, which is not the world's most scientific study. People's incoming diagnoses were heavily weighted towards endometriosis and adhesions. Their outgoing diagnoses were much less so. So a lot of the people we see are those who have some sort of pathology identified, but they may be an innocent bystander, or they have not been effectively treated for that part of their problem. What they are left with are the musculoskeletal components of the other functional disorders that have been left undiagnosed and untreated. And that is what we do for a living.

Beard: I absolutely agree with that. In fact, in one of the psychological studies[6] where the gynaecological diagnoses were very well documented, they used women who were being sterilised as their control group and they found the prevalence of endometriosis and adhesions was the same in their control group as in their so-called chronic pelvic pain group. That suggests very much that a good deal of the pathology that has been documented is an innocent bystander and not the cause of the pain.

References

1.	Di Sebastiano P, Fink T, di Mola FF, Weihe E, Innocenti P, Friess H, *et al*. Neuroimmune appendicitis. *Lancet* 1999;**354**:461–6.
2.	Mathias DS, Kupperman M, Liberman RF, Lipschutz RC, Steege JF. Chronic pelvic pain:prevalence, health-related quality of life and economic correlates. *Obstet Gynecol* 1996;**87**:321–7.
3.	Cobb LA, Thomas GI, Dillard DH, Merendino KA, Bruce RA. An evaluation of internal mammary artery ligation by a double-blind technique. *N Engl J Med* 1959;**260**:1115–18.
4.	Dimond EG, Kittle CF, Crockett JE. Comparison of internal mammary artery ligation and sham operation for angina pectoris. *Am J Cardiol* 1960;**5**:483–6.
5.	Elcombe S, Gath D, Day A. The psychological effects of laparoscopy on women with chronic pelvic pain. *Psychol Med* 1997;**27**:1041–50.
6	Stout AL, Steege JF, Dodson WC, Hughes CL. Relationship of laparoscopic findings to self-report of pelvic pain. *Am J Obstet Gynecol* 1991;**154**:73–9.

SECTION 4

PELVIC PAIN II

Chapter 13

Endometriosis and pain

Angela Barnard

Introduction

I have a deep understanding of endometriosis and pain that has developed over many years of personal experience. I have also listened to a considerable number of women whose narratives have allowed me to explore and understand beyond the scope of my own experience and establish a reliable body of knowledge on this subject. This is common knowledge, but it is not commonly heard. It speaks of a level of human suffering that is not acknowledged and is therefore not addressed, despite the existence of both the knowledge and expertise that could do so. It is the cause of isolation and despair for those who endure it and of distress and impotence for those who witness it. It is shrouded in the stigma of dysfunctional female reproduction and is thereby denied the social recognition and support that it needs and deserves. This is strong language. The language of pain is strong and, although muted by forces beyond an individual woman's control, when given an outlet (such as those offered by the National Endometriosis Society) it is expressed unequivocally.

What follows does not speak for all women with endometriosis, but for that group of women for whom pain is a primary symptom of their disease.

What is normal?

From an early age we associate pain with injury or illness. Without realising it, we define for ourselves a 'norm' of physical existence that is free from pain. We will only tolerate pain that we can understand and endure, and seek to eliminate pain that persists and is intense. This may seem a simplification, but it becomes relevant when a young woman encounters her first 'period pain'.

Here, suddenly, is a pain that is 'normal'. There is no injury or illness. It can endure for minutes, hours, or days. Our peers and elders teach us to expect this pain and to accept it as normal. There is a whole language of pain that we quickly learn, whether or not we really know what it means. For example, I was over 30 before I experienced cramp in a leg muscle. I had talked about stomach cramps for decades, because that is part of the language of periods and pain. Yet they bore no resemblance whatsoever to the pain in my leg. What do we really mean when we talk about period pain? The expression eventually loses all meaning in the face of the variety of pains that women experience.

The most significant, yet unstated, function of this language about pain is that it serves to confirm our identity as women. This is part of being a woman. Periods are natural to women and they are naturally painful. Giving birth (the reason why we have periods) is also natural and also painful. We share this language of apparent mutual understanding without question, and veil detail in evasion. Graphic descriptions of periods or giving birth are virtually non-existent. Not surprisingly, it is difficult to find anyone who can define a 'normal period' but, more worryingly, few women seem able to define an abnormal period. This is not surprising, since the whole concept of 'normality' and the experience of period pain have achieved an unlikely marriage, which forms part of our experience of womanhood. Yet, in almost every other aspect of our experience, such pain would signal abnormality or injury and would not be tolerated.

From normal to symptomatic

Many women with painful endometriosis say that they have experienced that pain from the onset of periods or soon after. Not surprisingly, in the two surveys that the Endometriosis Society has carried out, over 50% of women thought that their symptoms of endometriosis (including pain) were normal. Of course they did – that is what they have learnt in the absence of any other knowledge, and it is a brave woman who complains about pain during periods. It is therefore hardly surprising that doing so to a doctor presents such a challenge.

The heart of that challenge is simple – a woman feels that by seeking medical help for her period pain she is putting herself outside the norm. She has decided that, even though other women probably experience more pain, she cannot bear hers and therefore must be weak. She also feels that her doctor may consider that she is wasting their time when there are other patients who are really ill. In fact, she is likely to conclude that she either has a very low pain threshold or that the severity of the pain is exaggerated in her mind. In doing this she has (unwittingly) assumed the mantle of a victim and accepted the terms of dependency that the victim culture implies.

Some or all of this is almost certain to be present, however subliminally, when a woman is describing her pain to a doctor. In fact, many of us admit to this between ourselves after a safe passage of time has elapsed. By going to a doctor a woman has admitted that there is not just something wrong with her periods, but, by inference, with herself as a woman. It is worth noting here that women will sometimes wait until their pain is so severe that they pass out before seeking help. This gives some indication of how tenacious the conviction of 'normal pain' is and the depth of the fear of being abnormal. Far from rational, this behaviour is the messy consequence of the erroneous folklore that surrounds female reproduction and, by inference, female identity.

Here are some messages recently posted on our web site that help to highlight some of the dynamics involved.

Request for help:
'Hi everyone, I am getting really nervous now waiting to see gynae, and would just like to ask if people can tell me when they get the pains and where they are. It's just that mine seem to be so on and off and change like the wind. One minute I have a horrendous period and can hardly move and then it fades only to come back days later in my back, bottom and bladder area. It feels like a knife is stuck inside me and when I move it presses into something. Then when I can take no more I have a mild month. I find this so confusing and wondered is it just me or what??? I do not want the gynae to give me the same treatment I had years ago – "take these pills and go home, it's your IBS that's causing the pain" – even though they found endo on ligaments and just left it alone and said it couldn't be causing pain. Sorry if I'm repeating myself and this is so long but I'm getting desperate now.'

Response 1:
'I don't have any advice for you on your situation, but I can sympathise completely. I am in a very similar situation. No one was in the least bit bothered about my painful periods (everyone gets it – some people just make more fuss about it – type of attitude) until my husband and I were unable to conceive.'

Response 2:
'First of all I would not say that you're being a fraud at all. I felt pretty much like that at first, but I think it's because you get used to the pain and then think that you are making a big deal about nothing. I can remember thinking I was going round the bend until they told me that something was actually wrong.'

The writer of the request for help expresses uncertainty about her judgement in the words, 'is it just me or what'? In other words, is there something different about me?

In the first response there is an acknowledgement of the norm in parenthesis – everyone gets it. So too, is the recognition of a prevailing attitude that dismisses complaint about pain – '…some people just make more fuss about it'.

In the second response there is an overt admission to the feeling of being a fraud and a good explanation of why this can happen. This is followed by another overt admission. The insidious worry that the pain is all in the mind is reinforced when no physical cause can be found.

I remember being told that successive tests proved negative and there was clearly an expectation that I would receive this as good news. As more and more possible causes were eliminated, I could only begin to conclude that the pain was all in my mind and that I was, indeed, 'going mad'.

To summarise, the step between accepting pain as normal and regarding it as abnormal is huge, and should not be underestimated. In fact, it may take a woman years to reach this point. Even then, it is likely that she is still experiencing strong self-doubt and is highly susceptible to the suggestion that there is nothing wrong. The next hurdle she faces is to convince a doctor that her pain is not 'normal'. For many this can take as long as, if not longer than, they took to convince themselves.

Communicating pain

I have vivid memories of sitting in front of doctors trying to explain the pain. I have already illustrated how inaccurate the descriptions of pain can be in the example of the cramp in my leg and so-called stomach cramps during periods. There were also always the doubts about whether or not I should be there in the first place. I was determined that the pain should not be mistaken for 'period pain' and tried to find different ways of describing it. Another problem lay in the fact that only one of us had any real understanding of the various organs in the female pelvis and how they work – and it certainly wasn't me!

Typically, doctors will suggest possible descriptions of pelvic pain. These will be words like sharp, dull, cramping, prolonged, heavy, etc. The most accurate and honest description is probably that it ******* hurts! But we remain polite and civil and try to negotiate bland descriptions that we hope mean the same thing to each other.

By contrast, the words used by women to describe endometriosis pain are quite precise, extremely evocative and various. They include: 'like a knife…when I move it presses into something'; 'like a grater – sometimes a nutmeg grater and sometimes a cheese grater'; 'like a girdle of pain, sometimes getting tighter'; 'barbed'; 'like a migraine'; 'pulling or catching'; 'not just stabbing but tearing'; 'as if something is going to fall out'; 'as if something is in the wrong place'; 'as if something is there that shouldn't be there'.

These pains, many of which can be present simultaneously, are mostly episodic and can vary greatly in intensity and duration. However, there is one pain that persists and which women refer to as 'endo pain'. It may be like a background hum, almost indistinguishable at times, but can rise in pitch until it becomes literally unbearable – the point of blackout. Such a pain does not easily fit on to linear scales from one to ten. It is more like the gradations of shade between white (no pain) and black (passing out). This use of shading captures the depth of pain more accurately than a line.

I have often been struck by the accuracy with which women describe the pain of endometriosis. It reflects the rigour of subjective expression over the passive quality of generalised study. In many ways, the language women use describes endometriosis itself – pulling, catching, tearing, in the wrong place. I have heard these words used so often that I cannot consider them coincidental. Before they are diagnosed, women are often describing their disease when they describe their pain. Indeed, as far as the woman is concerned, they are the same thing.

What seems to be the matter?

Like many women, when I went to my doctor I was asked what 'seems to be the matter?' I said that it was pain. It has often struck me since that, even in this simple exchange, we were not really talking about the same thing. I thought I was there to have the pain taken away. The doctor, however, was intent on discovering the cause of the pain. An apparently reasonable proposition, except that the pain itself was one of the measures being used to identify its source. 'If I push down, thus, does the pain carry on when I take my hands away?' It often felt as though it would carry on for eternity after such an examination. It frequently took days to revert to its usual level. Of course the pain carried on, and I am no longer surprised at the number of women who lost an appendix in the process of discovering endometriosis.

Another significant departure from my priorities took place when endometriosis was finally diagnosed. I had thought that pain was the reason I sought help. I was wrong. It was endometriosis. I realise that it was causing the pain but was dismayed that successive treatments did not relieve it. Like many women, I was never told what different treatments existed, what their effects might be and whether or not they were appropriate. There was no question of choice, I was simply told to take this or that and come back in six months. The only painkillers I was prescribed might just as well have been sweets. The focus of attention was not the pain I experienced but the invisible disease that I had never even heard of.

So the pain continued and was now accompanied by the various side effects of hormone treatments. I was fortunate. I was still able to get out of bed most days and hold down a job. However, I could no longer drive a car and walked only short distances at a snail's pace. When the pain was really bad, life went on hold. This scenario has been described to me so many times that I have become inured to it.

Beyond these physical effects, the effect of prolonged pain can be devastating. The fear of it, or of increasing it, becomes a preoccupation. The frustration that it is beyond control leads to grief, despair and anger. I have come across many women whose whole existence has become dominated by the pain of endometriosis. They are unable to lead normal lives and sustain close relationships. They are seldom, if ever, free from pain and will try almost anything to take the pain away. I have often heard (and felt) the wish that someone would cause another pain, just for the relief of feeling something different.

The most worrying version of this came to light recently. It was of a young woman who was relieved that her doctor did not 'tell her off' when he saw the burns on her abdomen and thighs. In order to gain some relief from the deep pain she was experiencing, she would put a scalding hot water bottle on her skin. It was frightening to realise that I knew exactly how she felt and to realise that she cannot be alone in doing this. I hope this example serves to illustrate two things. First, this is a very deep-seated pain. The only way she could escape it was to create another, superficial pain that would create an intense sensation. Most people would not consider scalding to be superficial pain. Compared with the pain of endometriosis, it is. In addition, it needs to be extremely intense pain in order to distract from the endometriosis pain. Second, it is very difficult to exaggerate the severity of endometriosis pain and, when prolonged, it can lead to desperate behaviour. The lesser forms of this, which are no less worrying, are excessive consumption of alcohol and or painkillers. I have heard many women admit to these.

What is so difficult about pain?

In the last months of his life my father was able to spend periods of time at home between sessions of chemotherapy. From the outset of his treatment, pain relief was a priority. As well as a regular dose, we were able to give him additional doses for breakthrough pain. My mother was frightened by the thought of giving him heroin and was unable to do so for a long time. I had no reservations. Whenever he asked, I gave him some. I knew what it was like to be physically and mentally overwhelmed by pain and I would not let an animal go through that, let alone my father. For his last few days, all the other medication stopped. Only intravenous pain relief was left.

This may seem an extreme example. I use it to illustrate the fact that it is possible to relieve pain but it is often reserved for those who are going to die. I have never really understood this. I know of one young woman with endometriosis who is occasionally referred to a hospice, just to get her out of the wheelchair and back on her feet for a few weeks or months. There is nothing else wrong with her, but her doctor recognises the expertise in pain control that exists in such places and is willing to send her there when necessary. I have heard from several women who regularly go to their local hospital for injections to control their pain.

Even using less aggressive measures, it is possible to gain greater relief by using painkillers differently. Simple and safe techniques exist but are not passed on to those who would benefit from them. For example, the fact that painkillers work better before or at the onset of pain is possibly one of the best-kept secrets there is! Mixing different types of painkiller at lower doses is another well-kept secret. It makes no sense that this kind of information is not routinely passed on to those who need it. The logical conclusion is that either this need is not recognised or that it is recognised and denied. The former is unlikely, since women report their pain, ask for pain relief, often from a variety of agencies, but still do not receive the help they need. Pain control is not an unreasonable expectation from a medical system that routinely administers it in other contexts.

Equally, it makes no sense that women who have been diagnosed with a condition that causes them such extreme pain are so often left without the resources to control that pain. It is one thing to treat the process called endometriosis but quite another thing to treat its symptoms as if they were the disease. As far as a woman is concerned, there really isn't any difference.

Conclusion and recommendations

The current mantra in health care is 'evidence-based' medicine. Those who work in the area of endometriosis admit that there is much that remains unknown. However, there have been trials and studies in many countries over the years that provide a base of evidence about treatments. Unfortunately, very few of these are grounded in anything other than the clinical model of the disease. Some seek to evaluate success based on the measurement of pain but, even among these, follow-up times are relatively short. It is important to recognise in such complex conditions that there are social and civil models that are of equal value to the clinical. Indeed, there is compelling evidence to suggest that, as a basis for understanding disease and developing appropriate treatments, the clinical model alone is inadequate.

As long as the clinical model persists in its search for the holy grail of a cure or a definitive treatment, the problems that women with endometriosis pain face will continue. By simply defining this disease as the biological process called endometriosis, the experience of having the disease is excluded. The proof of this is the fact that, despite advances in the clinical understanding of endometriosis, the experience of it, even among those who are being treated, remains unchanged – it still hurts. It hurts when I wake up, when I go to the toilet, when I make love, when I walk, when I go to bed and it stops me getting to sleep. For too many women, that is the reality of having endometriosis and it is that which needs to be addressed.

Treatments need to be individualised and regularly reviewed on the basis of each patient's needs and aspirations. This takes place in some centres, which need to be identified and signposted to all gynaecologists and to those in primary care. As well as offering the best available treatment for patients whose symptoms are proving difficult to manage, these would develop greater expertise in treatment and provide advanced training to the range of healthcare professionals involved in endometriosis care.

The variety, the intensity and the destructive effects of endometriosis pain need to be recognised. Treatment strategies that directly address this problem are urgently needed. These should be disseminated to clinicians and patients alike. Patients must be allowed to participate in the control of symptoms and not be relegated to the status of insentient recipients of prescriptions.

The continuing pain that endometriosis can produce is a strong indication of the need for a radical review of the current understanding and treatment of this disease. In order to develop treatments that are not exclusively based on the clinical model of medicine, patients need to be involved in the design and implementation of research projects as well as the design and delivery of patient care and clinical training, at every level. Without such reforms, we will undoubtedly be having the same conversations about the same problems ten years hence.

Chapter 14

Doctors, women and pain

R. William Stones and Susan A. Selfe

Summary and sources

Women report negative experiences from consulting doctors for the complaint of chronic pelvic pain (CPP). This chapter describes studies that have attempted to characterise medical attitudes in relation to pelvic pain and to identify the influence of the medical consultation on pain outcomes. The implications for medical education, service provision and research are discussed.

What do doctors think about women with pelvic pain?

Focus group discussions were conducted with groups of general practitioners, gynaecologists and patients.

Focus groups are interactive group discussions facilitated by one of the investigators, who aimed to prompt group members to expand on ideas or to clarify issues which might not have seemed of major importance to individual members of the group. In the context of a group discussion it is then possible to optimise participation and to help group members to develop and to verbalise insights that might not have been immediately apparent. Focus groups offer a means of tapping into a collective experience that specifically relies on group interaction. The aim of employing this methodology with both patients and doctors was to try and understand what each group thought and why they thought it and to determine if possible what had been responsible for forming their views.

It was anticipated that potential areas of relevance to medical attitudes would involve time constraints, communication and the demonstration of pathology. These issues were borne in mind to prepare 'prompts' for each group session. 'Prompts' are ideas based on broad issues that might be useful to provoke discussion. Separate focus groups were arranged for (i) practising gynaecologists from two nearby hospitals, (ii) general practitioners (GPs) attending a postgraduate course, and (iii) patients who had been referred for CPP within the previous six months but who had not taken part in any other pelvic pain studies. The groups each consisted of two to eight participants, in an informal setting. The sessions were tape recorded, transcribed and analysed for content with the aid of ethnographic software.

Themes common to all groups

There was an expression of the need to find a pathological cause for the pain, something which would provide a diagnosis. Issues relating to time were discussed by all groups and this was particularly related by hospital gynaecologists and GPs to aspects of communication. Both groups of doctors were aware of the possible stress-related and psychological influences of pain, although patients seemed to avoid direct discussion of psychological factors that may have been related to their pain.

Themes particular to GPs

GPs frequently mentioned diagnosis by exclusion, especially with respect to irritable bowel syndrome (IBS) and pelvic inflammatory disease (PID). They stated that the lack of a firm diagnosis meant that dealing with patients with CPP could be difficult, particularly in those patients who have experienced a 'negative' laparoscopy. If no visible pathology was seen at laparoscopy to account for the pain, GPs found it difficult to know how to proceed with persistent patients who 'keep coming back'. A provisional diagnosis, even if it was considered imprecise, could provide a label by which to justify the patient's symptoms. This applied especially to IBS and 'pelvic congestion'.

GPs recognised the value of effective communication, but acknowledged that a good rapport with a patient was unlikely to develop after one short visit. This was exemplified in the statement 'Often you've got this ten-minute slot or this seven-minute slot and you've got this thick record and they aren't compatible'. Repeat visits were likely to be necessary and indeed this was sometimes encouraged by GPs, particularly if they felt that at some point they would have to 'confront' a patient who had no obvious pathological cause for her pain. One GP felt that knowing the patient and her background was helpful, suggesting, 'it's quite a good investment of time though – if you deal with it and get to the root of the issue, you save yourself years of coming back and coming back and lots of pain relief'.

GPs also commented on the complexity of a complaint in which it was necessary to sort out 'the emotional components of the problem'. The psychological contributions to pain were frequently acknowledged, but some of the phrases used suggested negative connotations directed at both the patients and the hospital gynaecologists. For example, from one GP 'the chronic pelvic pain that's been around before and been seen a thousand times…the psychosomatic type or the psychosexual things'. In a similar vein when talking about referring patients to a hospital, 'you know there's definitely gynaecologists that make your patients feel particularly bad' and 'you just know that they're not interested in this kind of thing'.

Themes particular to hospital gynaecologists

Gynaecologists implied that identifying pathology would somehow validate the pain as 'real'. When visible pathology had been excluded by previous referrals to other specialties such as gastroenterology, comments included 'some patients are going to be afraid that you're going to think it's a psychological problem', and 'they [the patients] come in and they say I'm not mad you know'. There was a clear awareness that an anxious patient may make diagnosis difficult and that patients are alarmed by the suggestion of a psychological diagnosis, because they will be 'labelled'.

Many hospital gynaecologists felt that GPs expected them to focus on organic pathology and that this forced them to investigate specifically to exclude endometriosis and malignancy. Even when these conditions had been excluded, hospital gynaecologists acknowledged that counselling a patient without a diagnosis is difficult. Some also doubted the existence of certain diagnoses, for example pelvic congestion: 'I don't know if it really exists' and nerve entrapment syndromes, one individual having seen 'about four cases – allegedly'.

Hospital gynaecologists were acutely aware of the time sometimes necessary to deal effectively with patients suffering from CPP. Development of rapport was found to be 'difficult to establish in one outpatient session'. If needed, consultation time was extended, but doctors were concerned that 'you're filling up the waiting room', and there was anxiety that if, for example, a patient starts to divulge adverse psychosexual experiences, it may well become a lengthy consultation; the doctor thinks 'oh hell! I've got three patients in the waiting room'.

After a negative laparoscopy hospital gynaecologists felt the need to look for other causes, asking the question 'Have I missed something?' They recognised this as problematic as the patient is disheartened by not having a diagnosis, a 'label' by which to define her problem. One hospital gynaecologist felt that a patient would not be helped by what he considered 'collusion' between the patient and her GP that a continued search for visible pathology would yield results. One hospital gynaecologist thought that if no disease process was found, some patients would benefit from alternative therapies, which either influence the pain or help the patient to find ways of coping with it.

Themes particular to patients

Patients had expectations that making a diagnosis would demonstrate the cause of their pain and lead to curative treatment. One patient thought 'they'd sort it out instantly', another that she would 'tell them what the problem is and they'll fix it'. One patient said she had 'almost blind faith in the medical profession'. Not being able to locate a pathological cause left patients feeling 'disappointed' or in some cases 'fobbed off'. Such disappointment was given as a reason for not attending for a follow-up consultation after a negative laparoscopy and for requesting a second opinion.

Time is as valuable a commodity for patients as it is for doctors. They considered it 'time-wasting' to have to go back to their GP and wait for a further referral, rather than being referred on directly to another specialist by the gynaecologist. In a similar way having to explain the story to a succession of doctors over several visits was seen as 'wearing' and time-consuming. Patients did recognise that it was not always possible to see the same doctor, but because of the nature of the problem it would have been preferable.

One of the hospital gynaecologists acknowledged that patients needed time to talk, although not necessarily to doctors. The value of this statement became evident in one of the patient sessions when patients began to question each other, to offer each other explanations and to try and work out reasons for their pain, based on what they had been told at various times. They also attributed distinct incidents to the origins of their pain, for example as a result of childbirth, either natural or by caesarean section. There was an implicit suggestion that this may relate to a perception of body change following the birth of a baby. In the absence of a concrete diagnosis and the subsequent explanation from a doctor, patients visualise what might be happening inside their bodies. One patient imagined 'the process of healing' as incomplete; another imagined that after repeated infections her insides 'must be so yucky'.

Although patients did not explicitly discuss problems of a psychological nature, they clearly felt that finding a pathological, demonstrable cause would validate their pain. One patient would have preferred to find that a swab had been left in her pelvis after a caesarean section, rather than be told that there was no cause for the pain. If the pain was intermittent and the patient not in acute pain at the moment of seeing the doctor, she felt the problem was not taken seriously and that she had been made to feel silly. 'You feel a silly woman – you know – don't you? You feel silly'.

Can 'medical attitudes' to women with pelvic pain be characterised?

Attitudes and medical attitudes

An attitude can be defined as a learned disposition to respond to an object or person in a consistently favourable or unfavourable way.[1] Attitudes are influenced by group membership, for example, family, peers, school, employment and religious affiliation. In most cases subtle pressure is applied to force conformity to the group norm, rather than applying the weight of a specific argument.[2]

The acquisition of appropriate attitudes is now an explicit goal set for medical students during their training by the UK General Medical Council,[3] reflecting a view that attitudes, especially those desirable in a doctor, can be actively taught or inculcated rather than acquired through osmosis. The attitudinal objectives set out for undergraduate medical education include 'respect for patients and colleagues that encompasses, without prejudice, diversity of background and opportunity, language, culture and way of life', 'the recognition of patients' rights in all respects, and particularly in regard to confidentiality and informed consent', 'approaches to knowledge that are based on curiosity and the exploration of knowledge rather than on its passive acquisition, and that will be retained throughout professional life', 'ability to cope with uncertainty' and are summarised in a recommendation that 'attitudes of mind and behaviour that befit a doctor should be inculcated, and should imbue the new graduate with attributes appropriate to his/her future responsibilities to patients, colleagues and society in general'.[3]

Attitudes and behaviour

Many of the 'attitudinal' objectives set out for doctors in training are in fact behaviours. The assessment of attitudes is considerably more difficult than the assessment of behaviour, so that in medical education behaviour is often taken as a proxy for attitudes.

The theory of reasoned action[4] proposes that attitudes and subjective norms jointly determine intention, and that intention determines behaviour. This theory in itself is considered problematic because it relates to single acts, not complex, co-ordinated sequences and it excludes behaviour that requires skills, abilities and opportunities which may also demand the co-operation of other people.[5] This problem can be offset by identifying specific rather than general attitudes.

The theory of cognitive dissonance also links attitudes and behaviour, but suggests a reverse causality.[6] Behaving in a specific manner creates an unpleasant feeling as a result of inconsistency between one's thoughts and actions, producing the subjective experience of 'dissonance'. In an attempt to restore some balance and avoid the discomfort, the attitude is changed to suit the behaviour. This model may be particularly relevant to medical education in which the adoption of 'approved' attitudes brings the novitiate to full membership.[7]

Kelman[8] has emphasised the interplay between social and psychological factors in attitude formation. This model takes account of the structure of social settings and recognises stages in motivation to change and adapt, from compliance through identification to internalisation, and from superficiality to integration. In doing so, it takes into account the impact of significant relationships, highly relevant in the context of the acquisition of attitudes in medical education and practice from respected teachers.

The circumstances under which attitudes can exert a causal influence on behaviour are thus dependent on (i) psychological processes that determine behaviour, (ii) the influence of one's behaviour on attitudes, and (iii) the social context and relationships involved. A simple linear relationship would therefore be unlikely between an attitude rating scale and observed behaviour in a medical setting. However, identification of attitudes may help doctors to reflect on their responses to patients, and where further research reveals specific associations with behaviour and outcome for patients there will be implications for training.

Attitudes to patients with pain

The influence on the appropriateness of treatment of staff attitudes to patients has been recognised and used as a basis for training recommendations in the context of analgesia for cancer pain.[9] In non-cancer pain, physicians from different geographical areas and specialties had different opioid-prescribing habits and expressed differing treatment goals, with rheumatologists and GPs more likely than other specialists to emphasise symptom improvement as opposed to functional improvement.[10] Where doctors have identified a pathological process they may be more sympathetic and express recognition of the patient's suffering. Patients with rheumatoid arthritis were characterised as 'resilient', 'optimistic' and 'gallant sufferers',[11] language very different from that of the doctors and patients recorded in the present study of attitudes to women with chronic pelvic pain, who often do not have a clearly identifiable cause for their pain and whose pain impacts especially on their relationships and sexual function.

A questionnaire for gynaecologists about attitudes to women with pelvic pain

A sample of names from the register of Fellows and Members of the Royal College of Obstetricians and Gynaecologists was extracted and a 49-item questionnaire was sent to 300 individuals. The questionnaire development and sampling method is described in full in Selfe *et al.*;[12] 145 (48%) usable responses were received; 100 (69%) respondents were male, 124 (85.5%) Caucasian and the age distribution was 52 (35.9%) under 38 years of age, 36 (24.8%) were aged between 39 and 45 years, 40 (27.6%) were aged between 46 and 54 years and 17 (11.7%) were aged over 55 years. The number of years practising gynaecology ranged from 4 to 37 years, mean 16.9, SD 7.15.

Principal components analysis was used to identify groupings of variables that might indicate underlying attitudinal constructs. A solution with six factors accounted for just over one-third of the variance. It was possible to identify intuitively coherent constructs for five of the six factors identified by the principal components analysis. These were labelled as follows:

- **'Efficiency'** included the statement 'Repeated follow-up visits, even when there is no visible pathology, are a waste of everybody's time'.

- **'Complexity'** consisted of items relating to the emotional response provoked when treating women with CPP and included such statements as, 'During consultations with women with chronic pelvic pain, I experience a feeling of ambivalence'.

- **'Sociocultural liberalism'** consisted of questions relating to women's role in society in general, but also included items such as 'Alternative therapies such as acupuncture or herbal treatments are inappropriate in the treatment of chronic pelvic pain'.

- **'Pathology'** focused strongly on finding a pathological cause for the pain and included, for example, the statement 'The most important aspect of treating chronic pelvic pain is to exclude malignant conditions'.

- **'Communication'**, the final construct, included items such as the statement 'It is difficult to establish a rapport with patients with chronic pelvic pain'.

It was not possible to identify a single coherent or appropriate construct for the sixth factor from the questionnaire items included within it.

Factor scores were examined to identify any significant relationships with age, sex, ethnicity and the number of years practising gynaecology. This analysis showed that scores for 'sociocultural liberalism' were higher among gynaecologists in the younger age groups, women and those giving their ethnic origin as Caucasian (Tables 14.1–14.4).

What do the constructs mean?

'Efficiency'

Chronic painful conditions such as CPP are a significant burden on medical time and the economic impact of CPP has been emphasised. We have identified a corresponding attitude construct labelled 'efficiency'. The responses to the four items grouped within this factor suggest that there is a range of attitudes among gynaecologists, from those

Table 14.1.   Relationship of factor scores with age of gynaecologists questioned

Factor	<>>38 years (*n*=52)		<38 years (*n*=93)		*t*	*P*
	Mean	SD	Mean	SD		
'Efficiency'	12	2.5	12	2.8	−0.65	0.519
'Complexity'	19	3.7	19	4.2	−1.02	0.309
'Liberalism'	27	2.4	24	3.8	4.74	<0.001
'Pathology'	23	2.4	22	3.0	2.93	0.004
'Communication'	15	1.9	15	2.6	1.13	0.259

Table 14.2.   Relationship of factor scores with gender of gynaecologists questioned

Factor	Male (*n*=100)		Female (*n*=45)		*t*	*P*
	Mean	SD	Mean	SD		
'Efficiency'	11.9	2.6	11.7	2.8	−0.36	0.722
'Complexity'	19.5	4.2	18.2	3.4	−1.86	0.065
'Liberalism'	24.1	3.7	27.2	2.5	5.17	<0.001
'Pathology'	21.8	3.0	22.8	2.6	1.97	0.051
'Communication'	14.6	2.5	15.2	2.1	1.22	0.224

Table 14.3.   Relationship of factor scores with ethnicity of gynaecologists questioned

Factor	Caucasian (*n*=124)		Non-Caucasian (*n*=21)		*t*	*P*
	Mean	SD	Mean	SD		
'Efficiency'	11.8	2.6	11.9	3.3	0.18	0.856
'Complexity'	19.2	4.1	18.5	3.7	−0.67	0.502
'Liberalism'	25.5	3.5	22.6	3.4	−3.49	0.001
'Pathology'	2.2	2.8	21.5	3.1	−1.14	0.258
'Communication'	14.9	2.3	14.3	2.6	−1.08	0.281

Table 14.4.   Parameter estimates for a multiple linear regression model to show relationships between scores for 'sociocultural liberalism' as the dependent variable and sex, age and ethnicity

Variable	No. in category	Estimate	Standard error	*t* ratio	*P*
Intercept	–	24.87	0.40	62.45	<0.0001
Sex – female	44	1.05	0.32	3.34	0.0011
Ethnicity – non-Caucasian	21	−1.22	0.37	−3.25	0.0014
Age – under 38 years	52	0.9	0.90	0.30	0.0036

who would feel it worthwhile to devote extra time to follow-up consultations even in the absence of obvious disease through to those who would see their role as a mainly technical one and discharge the patient at the first opportunity. There is of course no clear evidence as to which approach is more likely to benefit the patient but the attitude of the doctor will influence the way in which care is provided.

'Complexity'

The questions involved in 'complexity' relate to the idea of CPP as a difficult condition to treat both in general and with regard to specific patients. This difficulty engenders a negative emotional response in the doctor as expressed in some of the items, or by contrast a heightened sense of satisfaction at having dealt effectively with a difficult patient. Ambivalence, frustration and inadequacy reflect the negative emotions evoked by consultations with 'heartsink' patients. When dealing with such patients more intellectual and emotional resources are required on the part of the doctor both to consider other treatment options and to overcome emotional reactions that could block more lateral or creative thinking.

'Sociocultural liberalism'

'Sociocultural liberalism' describes a scale of values ranging from opposition to change and innovation, with a wish to retain the established order, through to an openness to change and readiness to consider alternative social models. In a medical context, attitudes at the 'conservative' end of this scale could at best be described as benignly paternalistic, but at worst might signify the assumption of an authority to manage or control the lifestyles of others. Respondents in the main study sample were distributed predominantly towards the 'liberal' end of this scale with a mean score of 25/35. In contrast, a 1983 sample of British medical students[13] given some of the items included in this factor gave a much wider and more 'conservative' range of responses, perhaps reflecting some of the social changes of the intervening years. It would be of great interest to know how responses to these items might change during the course of medical education, and at what stage they become fixed. As in the above study of medical students, significant differences in response to these items were noted between men and women and, in addition in the present study, in relation to ethnicity and age. Those scoring higher on this factor tended to be female, under 38 years of age and describe themselves as Caucasian.

'Pathology'

The construct involved in 'pathology' is concerned with the observation of visible pathology and disturbance of physiological processes. Kleinman *et al.*[14] drew a distinction between disease as treated by doctors (that is, abnormalities in structures and functions of organs and systems) and illness as suffered by patients (that is, the changes in social function that make up the patient's experience of sickness). Those with high scores on this factor are rejecting a view that evidence of visible pathology is the most important aspect of treatment. In more positive terms, the patients' lived experience is fully taken into account and not relegated to a subordinate position. While it may be difficult and unwise to attempt to separate disease and illness, which are inherently intertwined, an emphasis on the latter neglected aspect is needed, especially in the hospital environment where the main focus is on diagnosis, treatment and elimination of disease, particularly of the acute variety. Younger respondents had scores on this factor indicative of greater openness to the illness model. This may signify a move in medical education during the last decades away from teaching what Kleinman and colleagues refer to as 'the veterinary practice of medicine'.

'Communication'

The final construct, 'communication', is clearly relevant to all medical consultations but may be especially important where the patient has a non-life-threatening but distressing condition which is difficult to treat, such as CPP. This factor appears to represent the confidence of the doctor, or lack of confidence, that good rapport and communication can be established even in the absence of a clearly definable pathological process that can be treated, and that this is worthwhile.

But does it matter?

It will be noted that it is not possible to draw conclusions from the above study as to which position on an attitudinal sub-scale is most likely to benefit the patient. It is possible that patients will respond to different doctors and that some will form therapeutic relationships more effectively with those manifesting certain attitudes. For example, some patients may appreciate an open and non-directive style emanating from sociocultural liberalism; others may interpret this as indicating lack of confidence, certainty or even technical competence on the part of the doctor, and prefer a doctor with a more directive consulting style that is rooted in conservative social norms and find this reassuring.

Does the medical consultation influence outcome?

Ninety-eight women referred from primary care for hospital investigation by general gynaecologists for CPP of at least six months' duration were followed up six months after the initial consultation.[15] In this cohort, 12 (11.4%) had endometriosis, 10 (9.5%) had adhesions and 15 (14.2%) had other significant gross pathology. No positive diagnosis could be deduced in 29 (27.6%). A symptom complex suggestive of IBS (three or more symptoms) was present in 15 (14.2%) but 13 of these overlapped with other diagnoses. A symptom complex suggestive of pelvic congestion syndrome, taking the presence of four or more symptoms as positive, was present in 57 (59.9%) but overlapped with seven of 12 diagnoses of endometriosis, six of adhesions and eight of other gross gynaecological pathology; nine cases shared IBS and pelvic congestion syndrome symptom complexes.

Thirty-four doctors undertook the consultations; 54 (52%) of the patients were seen by a consultant, 19 (18%) by a senior registrar, 18 (17%) by a registrar and 14 (13%) by a senior house officer. Nineteen (18%) were seen by a woman doctor. Eight doctors saw five or more patients, accounting for 64% of the patients taking part in the study. Medical consultations were rated by patient and doctor using a four-item scale.[16]

In multivariate models, as well as disease factors, the individual doctor undertaking the consultation was shown to influence the severity of pain six months later. The rating of the initial consultation by the patient predicted pain resolution ('probability'), but only in those in whom exercise was not impaired by pelvic pain (Figure 14.1).

An interpretation of the above might be that where the illness is not overwhelming there is more scope for the establishment of a useful therapeutic relationship during the consultation; where impairment is more marked, the impact of a positive consultation

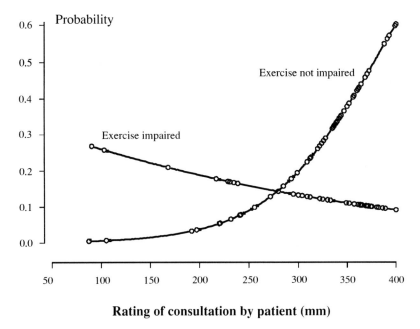

Figure 14.1.   The rating of the initial consultation by the patient predicted pain resolution ('probability'), but only in those in whom exercise was not impaired by pelvic pain. Reproduced with permission from the *Journal of Women's Health* (ref. 15)

is not likely to be sustained. The way in which patients recall the initial consultation six months later and the interaction between that recall and current pain experience is the subject of further work recently presented.[17]

Conclusions

Implications for clinical practice

Clinicians need to be aware of the importance of the initial medical consultation as a factor influencing patients' outcome from investigation and treatment. While consulting styles reflect the individual personality of the doctor, we need to be aware of our own underlying attitudes and how these might enter into the dynamics of the consultation.

Women presenting with pelvic pain in whom no clear diagnosis is present, or where diagnoses overlap, need to be given clear explanations which do not undermine the legitimacy of their experience of pain or convey a message of dismissal.

The setting in which consultations for pelvic pain take place needs adequately to reflect the referral pattern: patients with long-standing or disabling symptoms require extended consultation times and access to other advice and treatment resources, as in a multidisciplinary model.

Implications for medical education

Study guides need to emphasise the importance of due attention to the patient's needs in terms of treatment objectives and needs for explanation, rather than an exclusive pursuit of a pathological diagnosis. Consulting styles that address these needs can be taught in role play and evaluated in objective structured clinical examination (OSCE) formats, as can the communication skills required to convey diagnostic uncertainty or negative findings without undermining the patient's confidence.

Implications for research

Further studies are required of the relationship between consulting style and patient outcomes, perhaps using observational techniques such as video-recording of consultations. Research is needed to clarify the importance of elements in the patient's experience, such as continuity of care and the contribution of different members of a multidisciplinary team.

Acknowledgements

We would like to thank Dr Mark Van Vugt (a lecturer in psychology at the University of Southampton) and Dr Zoë Matthews (a lecturer in demography at the University of Southampton) for their help with this manuscript.

References

1.   Fishbein M. *Readings in Attitude Theory and Measurement*. New York: John Wiley; 1967.
2.   Zimbardo PG, Ebbessen EB, Maslach C. *Influencing Attitudes and Changing Behaviour*, 2nd edn. New York: Random House; 1977.
3.   General Medical Council. Tomorrow's Doctors: Recommendations on Undergraduate Education. London: General Medical Council; 1993.
4.   Ajzen I, Fishbein M. Attitudes and normative beliefs as factors influencing behavioural intention. *J Personal Soc Psychol* 1972;**21**: 1–9.
5.   Eagley A, Chaiken S. *The Psychology of Attitudes*. Orlando FL: Harcourt Brace; 1993.
6.   Festinger LA. *Theory of Cognitive Dissonance*. London: Tavistock Publications; 1959.
7.   Howell MC. What medical schools teach about women. *N Engl J Med* 1974;**291**: 304–7.
8.   Kelman HC. Compliance, identification and internalisation: three processes of attitude change. In: Fishbein M, editor. *Readings in Attitude Theory and Management*. New York: John Wiley and Sons; 1967. p. 469–76.
9.   Elliott TE, Murray DM, Elliott BA, *et al.* Physician knowledge and attitudes about cancer pain management – a survey from the Minnesota cancer pain project. *J Pain Symptom Manage* 1995;**10**: 494–504.
10. Turk DC, Brody MC, Okifuji EA. Physicians' attitudes and practices regarding the long-term prescribing of opioids for noncancer pain. *Pain* 1994;**59**:201–8.
11. Hart FD. The control of pain in the rheumatic disorders. In: Hart FD, editor. *The Treatment of Chronic Pain*. Lancaster: Medical and Technical Publishing Co. Ltd; 1974. p. 63–96.
12. Selfe SA, van Vugt M, Stones RW. Chronic gynaecological pain: an exploration of medical attitudes. *Pain* 1998;**77**: 215–25.
13. Savage WD, Tate P. Medical students' attitudes towards women: a sex-linked variable? *Med Educ* 1983;**17**: 159–64.

14. Kleinman A, Eisenberg L, Good B. Clinical lessons from anthropologic and cross-cultural research. *Ann Intern Med* 1978;**88**: 251–8.
15. Selfe SA, Matthews Z, Stones RW. Factors influencing outcome in consultations for chronic pelvic pain. *J Women's Health* 1998;**7**:1041–8.
16. Fry RPW, Stones RW. Hostility and doctor–patient interaction in chronic pelvic pain. *Psychother Psychosom* 1996;**65**:253–7.
17. Stones RW, Selfe SA. Dimensions of patient recollection six months after hospital consultation for chronic pelvic pain. *Abstracts of the American Pain Society Meeting Phoenix* 2001, no. 740. 2001.

Chapter 15

Surgical management of pelvic pain in endometriosis

Christopher J.G. Sutton

Introduction

Before the advent of laparoscopic surgical treatment it was necessary to perform open surgery by laparotomy in order to treat endometriosis and it was therefore reserved for advanced disease, particularly ovarian endometriomas (chocolate cysts). In the last 25 years of the 20th century a revolution occurred in surgical practice with the advent of minimal access surgery, whereby similar surgical procedures were undertaken through multiple small incisions using the optics of the laparoscope transmitted by closed circuit television cameras to one or more television monitors (Figure 15.1). This allowed a more comfortable operating position for the surgeon, since he did not have

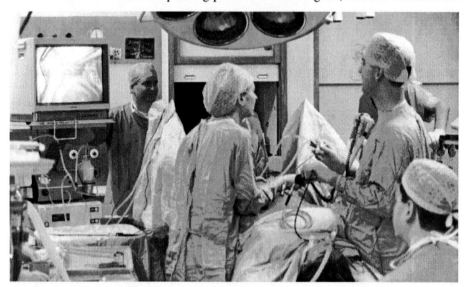

Figure 15.1. Typical operating theatre set up for laparoscopic laser surgery

to bend over to look down the laparoscope, but could stand erect looking at a television monitor on the opposite side of the patient. Equally the assistants were able to help the surgeon by looking at another television monitor on the opposite side of the patient. It also allowed the nurses and technicians to take part in the operation, allowing them to anticipate the surgeon's needs and to make equipment instantly available when needed.

This change in surgical technique occurred at a time when physicians were increasingly disillusioned with medical treatment of endometriosis, not only because it was associated with unpleasant adverse effects, but also because it was extremely expensive and in many instances the disease was suppressed by the medication but recurred after cessation of treatment, even as early as after the first two ovulatory cycles.[1] Additionally, the drugs were ineffective against ovarian endometriomas and deep infiltrating disease in the rectovaginal septum, which appears to be an increasingly common finding. A paper by Waller and Shaw[2] showed that there was a 53.4% recurrence of disease at five years' follow-up, whereas long-term follow-up following surgical excision at laparoscopy showed only 19% recurrence at five years.[3]

Aims of conservative surgery

Most patients presenting with symptoms of endometriosis do so at a relatively early age and therefore conservative surgery is essential in order to retain their potential for fertility. The aims of conservative surgery are shown in (Table 15.1).

All ectopic endometrial tissue is either vaporised with the laser or excised by electrosurgery or the ultrasonic scalpel. This means the removal of black deposits of haemosiderin; the red flame-like lesions, with their associated neoangiogenesis that implies active implants; as well as all the vesicular lesions (sagograins) and the yellow brown peritoneal areas;[4] any white infiltrating disease, which usually signifies fibromuscular hyperplasia often, but not always, around ectopic endometrial glands; and stroma, which has an appearance more in keeping with an adenomyotic nodule.[5] Most ovarian endometriomas (chocolate cysts) are densely adherent to the peritoneum of the ovarian fossa, close to the ureter and initial scissor dissection and aqua-dissection are necessary to free the endometrioma from the pelvic sidewall, which usually results in the release of old haemosiderin (chocolate fluid). This is aspirated and irrigated until the effluent runs clear and then the lining of the endometrioma is either excised or vaporised with a laser or by bipolar coagulation.

Many of these laparoscopic surgical procedures involve the interruption of afferent sensory pathways, either by uterine nerve ablation or by presacral neurectomy, to decrease dysmenorrhoea, which is the leading presenting symptom of many patients with endometriosis. The role of these denervation procedures is still controversial and will be dealt with later.

Table 15.1.   Aims of conservative surgery in endometriosis for pain

- Cytoreduction of all ectopic endometriotic implants
- Interruption of afferent sensory pathways (uterine nerve ablation or presacral neurectomy)
- Removal of ovarian endometriomas
- *En bloc* excision or laser vaporisation of deep infiltrating disease in the rectovaginal septum and uterosacral ligaments

Initial development of laparoscopic laser surgery for endometriosis

During the 1980s, centres in Europe and the USA, reporting on the effectiveness of various lasers in relieving the pain of endometriosis, gave rates for pain relief of 60–70% of women using the CO_2 laser.[6-8] Similar results were achieved with the neodymium:yttrium–aluminium–garnet (Nd:YAG) laser,[9] the argon laser[10] and the KTP/532 laser.[11]

When we started using the CO_2 laser down the laparoscope in 1982 in Guildford, we were mainly concerned with the safety of using such a high-powered energy source within the abdominal cavity. In fact it turned out to be safe and during the last 18 years, having treated well over 7000 women, we have had no accidents with the CO_2 laser. This is partly due to the fact that one has to exercise extreme caution and only activate the laser when the helium–neon aiming beam can be clearly seen and also to make absolutely sure that no vital structures are in close proximity.

Our next important goal was to look at the effectiveness of using the laser to ablate peritoneal endometriosis. We therefore followed our first 228 patients over five years (Figure 15.2) and at the end of that time 126 of the 187 patients who had previously suffered pain (70%) were pain-free. Thirty-eight of the patients were not improved, but most of these were subjected to a second-look procedure and there was no sign of any recurrent endometriosis and many of these patients subsequently had different reasons for their pelvic pain, such as irritable bowel syndrome; several also had various psychological problems, two were eventually diagnosed as having Munchausen syndrome. Seventeen of the patients suffered a relapse during the five-year follow-up and second-look laparoscopy showed that endometriosis had recurred, but almost always at different sites and six patients were lost to follow-up. Of the 56 patients with infertility due to endometriosis alone, 45 became pregnant (an 80% pregnancy rate).

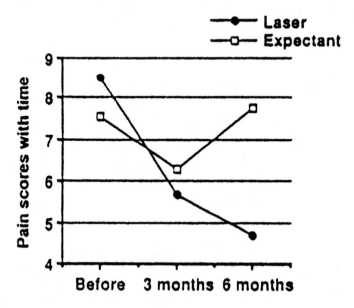

Figure 15.2.   Median visual analogue pain scores

Unfortunately this study was retrospective and although it is difficult to argue with the conception rates, the relief of pain is a highly subjective phenomenon. It would be entirely possible for a surgeon to influence the result of the pain relief, particularly when using highly technological equipment such as a laser, which tends to increase the patient's perception of the result, and in some instances the patient will indicate that pain relief has been achieved in order to please the surgeon.

The only way that this issue could be resolved was to perform a randomised controlled trial, which had to be prospective, and also had to be double-blind so that neither the patient nor the person following up the patient was aware that intervention had occurred in the form of laser surgery or whether the intervention was merely a diagnostic laparoscopy alone. In 1995, we published the results of such a trial, which remains the first and only such trial in the world literature on endometriosis.[12]

Evidence-based medicine – the Guildford laser laparoscopy trial

The aim of this study was to assess the efficacy of laser laparoscopy by the established scientific method of a prospective, randomised, double-blind controlled trial comparing the results of those women with minimal to moderate endometriosis AFS Stages I to III,[13] who were treated with the laser and those in the control arm who had diagnostic laparoscopy alone.

This study was approved by the Hospital Ethics Committee, but they reasonably felt that it was unethical to withhold treatment from patients in severe pain due to Stage IV disease, particularly because our previous experience had shown 80% pain relief in this group, most of whom had failed to respond to medical therapy.[14]

The study population was recruited from women seen in the gynaecological outpatient clinic with pain suggestive of endometriosis who had been advised to undergo a diagnostic laparoscopy. In order to be included in the study, women were between 18 and 45 years of age, were neither pregnant nor lactating and had not received any treatment (medical or surgical) for endometriosis in the previous six months.

The study was explained in detail and informed consent was obtained. This was particularly difficult because many of these women had been specifically referred for laser surgery by consultants in other hospitals and the research registrars had the unenviable task of having to explain to them that at this stage of development of laser laparoscopy we were not entirely sure whether this procedure worked and to offset any inconvenience it was agreed that if, when the code was broken at six months, the patient was still experiencing pain and was in the 'no treatment' group, then we would expedite her admission for laparoscopic laser surgery. Before the laparoscopy the patients were asked to record the intensity of their pain on a 10-cm linear analogue scale marked from 0 to 10; 0 representing no pain at all and 10 representing the worst pain they had experienced in their life.[15]

Between March 1990 and February 1993, 74 women were recruited and at the time of laparoscopy treatment were allocated randomly (computer-generated randomisation sequence) to laser treatment or expectant management. The laser treatment included vaporisation of all visible endometriotic implants, adhesiolysis and uterine nerve transection using a triple-puncture technique. The patients in the control arm had exactly the same incisions but merely had a diagnostic laparoscopy, although during this it was necessary to remove the serosanguinous fluid from the pouch of Douglas in order to perform a thorough inspection of the entire pelvic peritoneum. Patients were not informed which treatment group they had been allocated to and were followed up at three months and six months after surgery by an independent observer (research nurse), who also was unaware of the treatment that had been carried out.

Results of the study

Of 74 women who entered the study, 63 (32 laser, 31 expectant) completed the study to the six-month follow-up visit. The 11 patients who were excluded had either become pregnant or been put on the oral contraceptive by their family doctor, although both the patients and the doctors were requested not to do this during the course of the study, and three were lost to follow-up. The results can be seen in Figure 15.3 and it can clearly be seen that at three months post operation there was little difference between the two groups, but at six months the difference reached statistical significance when 62.5% of the patients who had had the laser treatment were better and only 22.6% of the patients who had received no treatment said they were better. The results were worst for Stage I disease and this is probably because some of the minimal changes seen in mild endometriosis could possibly be due to inflammatory changes or Walthard cell rests or other non-specific changes in the appearance of the peritoneum. Unfortunately the disease could not be confirmed by biopsy because that would have acted as a cyto-reductive procedure and could not truly be called expectant management. If the Stage I patients were excluded, then 73.7% of patients achieved pain relief, which is similar to the figure obtained in our retrospective study.

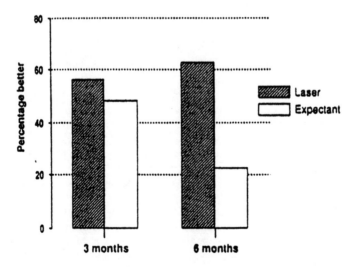

Figure 15.3.   Proportion of patients with pain symptom alleviation at all stages

Discussion

There are several interesting features of this study that merit discussion. We were surprised that the results at three months were similar for the laser group (56%) compared with the expectant group (48%). There was no significant difference between these two figures and we were surprised to find that almost half of the patients with no treatment claimed that they were better. This placebo effect has been noticed in other studies where dysmenorrhoea was reported to have improved in up to 30% of patients in the placebo arm of an Italian study comparing expectant management with gonadotrophin-releasing hormone (GnRH) analogues.[16] They found that this improvement did not last longer than three months, which was exactly the same as our finding. In particular, the visual analogue scale clearly shows that at six months in the expectant arm the patients had returned to the original score, whereas the laser-treated group had continued to improve. This has also shown us that it can take at least three months for the benefit of laparoscopic laser surgery to be noticed, so we now advise patients of this and only see them for follow-up at six months.

Another benefit of this study was to allow us to look at the natural history of endometriosis, because it had been assumed that it was invariably a progressive disease. We had the opportunity to look at a group of patients who had not received any treatment but had an established diagnosis and to report the findings of the second-look laparoscopy and compare the changes in their symptoms.[17] At second-look laparoscopy ten cases (42%) had no change in the American Fertility Society (AFS) score, seven cases (29%) had an increased score, with three patients moving to a higher stage, but we were surprised to find that one-third of the patients (seven cases) had a reduced AFS score, with three patients moving to a lower stage. These patients had improved or resolved symptoms whereas in the others, the symptomatology was the same or had become more severe while they were waiting for laparoscopic laser surgery. This study enabled us to show that the disease does progress in the majority of patients, but in up to one-third it can regress and in a few of them it disappeared altogether. This finding has also been confirmed in studies on higher primates with experimentally induced endometriosis.[18]

Long-term follow-up of the trial patients

We have now conducted a long-term follow-up on this cohort of patients by telephone interview with a mean time since the operation of 88.6 months (range 77–104).[19] Of the 32 patients who had undergone a laser laparoscopy we were able to contact 22 (68.8%). We had to remove four from the study (12.5%) because they had been taking the oral contraceptive pill, which diminishes the symptoms of endometriosis, and six (18.8%) were lost to follow-up. Nevertheless, we found that 60% of the patients had continued to have satisfactory symptom relief, one was menopausal and four needed mild analgesia only. Three of the patients had undergone repeat laser laparoscopy for new disease in different sites and five were leading pain-free lives, three of whom had conceived successful pregnancies. Of those that continued to have painful symptoms six had undergone repeat laser laparoscopy on one or more occasions, two had required psychiatric help and required strong analgesia. Interestingly, all of the six who eventually had a hysterectomy and bilateral salpingo-oophorectomy showed a normal pelvis macroscopically at the time of operation and no histological evidence of endometriosis was seen, apart from one small focus of adenomyosis in the uterus of one woman.

The conclusion from this is that regardless of treatment (all of these women had been on strong medical treatment) a certain group of patients will not get better and will continue to complain of pelvic pain, sadly even after a hysterectomy.

Nevertheless, laparoscopic laser surgery results in satisfactory symptom relief at six months and the majority of these patients continue to have symptom relief over many years. It also has the advantage that treatment can be performed at the same time as the diagnosis is made, with no extra morbidity or mortality in our experience over 18 years and it avoids the use of expensive medical treatments which often have severe and unpleasant adverse effects.

Ovarian endometriomas (chocolate cysts)

There is considerable controversy over the pathogenesis of ovarian endometriomas and some authorities consider that they are a completely different disease to peritoneal endometriosis.[20] As long ago as 1957 Hughesdon, a pathologist at University College Hospital in London, suggested that bleeding from endometriotic implants on the posterior surface of the ovary caused the ovary to adhere to the peritoneum of the ovarian fossa and because subsequent bleeding into the space enclosed by the adhesions was prevented from escaping there was invagination of the ovarian cortex as the endometrioma enlarged.[21] The majority of ovarian endometriomas would appear to fit into this category, since they are densely stuck to the peritoneum of the broad ligament close to the ureter and have to be freed by laparoscopic blunt dissection with a strong stainless steel probe and sometimes need to be divided by laparoscopic scissors. The ovary is gradually levered upwards away from the ovarian fossa and during this process it invariably ruptures. The haemosiderin-laden fluid is then aspirated and irrigated until the effluent runs clear and in our department the whole of the inside of the endometrioma is photocoagulated with the emerald green KTP/532 laser, which penetrates only a few millimetres and thus causes minimal damage to developing follicles under the surface[22,23] (Figure 15.4). If a KTP/532 laser is not available then superficial coagulation can be achieved by using a bi-cap endocoagulator (Cory Brothers, Horsham, UK), which attaches to the suction and irrigation equipment and is relatively simple and safe to use.

An alternative technique is to aspirate the endometrioma initially at the first diagnostic laparoscopy procedure or under ultrasound control and then give the patient GnRH analogues for three months, after which time the shrunken endometrioma will have a relatively avascular capsule, which can be vaporised effectively with the CO_2 laser. This particular laser will cause little damage to the developing follicles under the fibrous surface of the capsule, but would not work in the presence of the haemosiderin-laden fluid of the chocolate cyst.[24]

Some laparoscopic surgeons advocate stripping out the ovarian cyst capsule by traction and countertraction. In the case of a true endometrioma this merely results in stripping out the ovarian cortex and results in profuse bleeding, which requires bipolar coagulation to control, and the inevitable build-up of heat results in damage to the developing oocytes beneath the surface. It is important to realise that not all 'chocolate cysts' are endometriomas and the chocolate material may merely represent

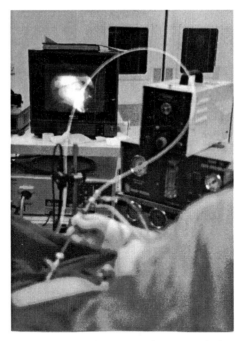

Figure 15.4.   Emerald green KTP 532 laser used to treat ovarian endometriosis

haemosiderin and be a reflection of internal bleeding into the cyst. In most of these situations the ovary is not adherent to the posterior leaf of the broad ligament, but is suspended free from the mesovarium and often represents a benign cyst adenoma with internal haemorrhage or a haemorrhagic corpus luteal cyst, or occasionally an endometrioma that has arisen from coelomic metaplasia of invaginated epithelial inclusions.[20]

However the endometrioma is dealt with by laparoscopic surgery, it is important to be certain at the end of the procedure that there is reasonable haemostasis and if this is not possible the ovary can be packed with Surgicel™ gauze (Ethicon Endosurgery, Edinburgh, UK), but on no account should there be any arterial bleeding at the end of the procedure. Sometimes it is tempting to try and restore ovarian anatomy with laparoscopic sutures, but this should be resisted because sutures are a potent cause of tissue ischaemia, which is the main initiating factor in adhesion formation.[25]

Results of laparoscopic surgery of endometriomas

Photocoagulation of the endometrioma capsule with the KTP/532 laser is associated with a low recurrence rate.[26] Daniell and colleagues, from Nashville, have reported significant relief of pain and a pregnancy rate of 37.5% in 32 patients trying for conception.[22]

At the International Society for Gynecologic Endoscopy meeting in Washington, we reported our results on our first 102 patients with large endometriomas in 1992 (between 3 cm and 18 cm) and were surprised to find that 80% of the patients had significant subjective improvement in pain and 57% of those trying to conceive became pregnant.[23] Most of the pregnancies occurred within the first few cycles and if they were to achieve a pregnancy it was most likely within the first nine months. More recently, in 1997, we reported a further 165 women who presented with large endometriomas more than 3 cm in diameter.[27] In this study we used either the CO_2 or the KTP laser and found pain resolution in 74% of the women and a pregnancy rate of 45% and noted that there was a higher recurrence rate (30%) in those treated with the CO_2 laser compared with only 12.5% in those who had been treated with the KTP laser. The slightly lower pregnancy rate than in the first series probably reflects the fact that this later group included many patients referred from other centres who had already had previous laparotomies.

It is well known that adhesions are more likely to form following laparotomy than laparoscopic surgery.[28] This experimental animal study has been supported in a clinical setting using a randomised trial in which adhesions were assessed at second-look laparoscopy following either laparotomy or laparoscopic surgery in the treatment of tubal pregnancy and there was much less adhesion formation in the laparoscopy group.[29]

Deeply infiltrating endometriosis

Deep endometriosis is almost invariably located in the rectovaginal septum, the uterosacral ligaments or sometimes in the uterovesical fold. Three distinct types of this condition have been described by Koninckx and Martin.[30] Type 1 is characterised by a large pelvic area of classical endometriosis or the subtle lesions described by Jansen and Russell[4] surrounded by white scar tissue. When these lesions are excised or vaporised with the CO_2 laser, they are usually found to infiltrate deeper than 5 mm and are in the shape of a cone, becoming progressively smaller as they deepen.

Type 2 lesions are mainly formed by retraction of the bowel and are recognised clinically as obvious bowel retraction around a small typical lesion. In some women, however, no endometriosis can be seen laparoscopically but the induration can be clearly felt by a combination of rectal and vaginal examination. Type 3 lesions are spherical endometriotic nodules in the rectovaginal septum and can be clearly felt as painful nodules at that site and colposcopic examination of the vagina tends to reveal dark blue, domed cysts, about 3 to 4 mm in diameter in the posterior vaginal fornix. These are the most severe lesions and have a tendency to spread laterally up and around the uterine artery and sometimes cause sclerosis around the ureter although, interestingly, never appear to invade the layers of the ureteric wall. The behaviour of this type of deep infiltrating disease, which is virtually unresponsive to drug therapy, is such that it can be considered an indirect argument for the hypothesis that deep endometriosis has escaped from the inhibitory influence of peritoneal fluid and is mainly under the control of the peripheral circulation.[31]

Possible environmental aetiological factors

Koninckx et al.[32] suggested that dioxin and polychlorinated biphenyl pollution is a possible co-factor in the cause and development of deep infiltrating endometriosis, which is resulting in a steadily increasing proportion of hysterectomies performed for this disease from 10% in 1965 to over 18% in 1984.[33] Using epidemiological data reported by the World Health Organization, they link the highest concentrations of dioxin in breast milk in Belgium,[34] which appears to have the highest incidence of endometriosis in the world and much of this is of the deeply infiltrating type.[35] The highest concentration of cases is in the industrial corridor running along the south of the country (J. Donnez, personal communication).

Dioxin has immunosuppressive activities and is a potent inhibitor of T-lymphocyte function.[36,37] A group of rhesus monkeys[38] that were chronically exposed to dioxin for a period of four years, followed by serial laparoscopies, were found to develop endometriosis seven years after the termination of dioxin exposure and in the majority of these cases it was of the deeply infiltrating variety. Dioxin is a potentially harmful by-product of the chlorine-bleaching process used in the wood pulp industry, which includes the manufacture of feminine hygiene products such as tampons. It is worrying that young girls are increasingly being encouraged to use tampons and therefore may be exposing the tissues of the rectovaginal septum and posterior fornix to chronic exposure with a known immunosuppressant. It has been suggested that a woman may use as many as 11 000 tampons in her lifetime and this represents a worrying level of dioxin exposure, which could result in deeply infiltrating endometriosis and it could explain the increasing incidence of this condition in young women.

Surgical treatment

Laparoscopic inspection, ultrasonography or magnetic resonance imaging are not completely adequate to delineate these lesions. This can only be properly done during surgical excision and subsequent pathological inspection of the lesion to determine its shapes and depths of penetration. Before performing any operative laparoscopy the patient should have a proctoscopy and sigmoidoscopy, preferably during menstruation, and appropriate radiological investigations. If the lesion extends laterally an intravenous urogram is required, but if it is confined to the rectovaginal septum it is necessary to perform an air-contrast barium enema, sometimes combined with a vaginogram, which should be carefully examined in the lateral views. A thorough bowel preparation is mandatory in all women suspected of having deep endometriosis and patients should be warned that there is a real risk of perforating the bowel and, if this does happen, a colonic surgeon should be available to repair such a defect, although if the bowel preparation has been satisfactory it should not be necessary to require a colostomy and indeed some of the perforations can be adequately repaired transanally, or even laparoscopically.[39]

In the past it has been necessary to resort to laparotomy for these patients but with increased experience in laparoscopic surgery, many of them can be treated by laparoscopy using CO_2 laser or electrosurgical excision or sharp dissection with scissors. In addition, it is sometimes necessary to perform vaginal excision, either from below or by laparoscopy, once the plane of cleavage has been developed between the rectum and the vagina.[39–42] Inevitably with this kind of surgery, which is probably the most difficult type of laparoscopic surgery and requires considerable skill and experience, each surgeon will use the method that is best in his hands. In our department we use a high-power, super-pulse CO_2 laser to develop the plane of cleavage between the rectum and the vagina, with special instrumentation to separate these two structures from below and careful palpation in order to avoid damaging the rectum. Even in highly skilled hands such damage is inevitable from time to time; Nezhat and Nezhat[42] reported a series of 174 women in whom there were nine bowel perforations and a further two patients required ureteric stents. Nevertheless, moderate to complete pain relief was achieved in 162 of the women. If dissection has to be very close to the rectum it is a wise precaution to fill the pelvis with warm Ringer's lactate solution and insufflate the rectum with air or methylene blue to look for any unrecognised rectal lacerations or perforations.[39] A vaginal incision is often, but not routinely, required and, when the vagina is opened, the procedure may be completed vaginally or laparoscopically. In addition, it is sometimes possible to vaporise the vaginal blue, domed cysts via a colposcope with a finger inserted in the rectum to make sure that the vaporisation does not damage the rectum.

To excise uterosacral nodules, the peritoneum is incised lateral to the uterosacral ligament. It is necessary first to identify the ureter and occasionally to dissect it out along its course. Once it is displaced laterally the uterosacral ligament is resected, beginning posteriorly and working towards the uterus. Once the nodule has been freed from the underlying tissue the anterior part of the ligament is cut and most of these deep uterosacral implants can be treated without any need for a vaginal incision.

Patients with full-thickness bowel or bladder lesions require more extensive surgery which is probably better dealt with by laparotomy, although some advanced laparoscopic surgeons have reported successful results employing transanal circular stapling devices[39] and laparoscopic and transanal or transvaginal repair with or without the help of colorectal surgeons.[43,44]

Although this type of surgery is difficult and time consuming, the results justify the effort, particularly since many of these patients are unresponsive to medical therapy. Koninckx and Martin analysed their results in 250 women in whom deep endometriosis had been excised using the CO_2 laser and showed a cure rate of pelvic pain in 70%, with the recurrence rate of less than 5% during a follow-up period of up to five years.[31] These results should be interpreted with some caution because inevitably there is a learning curve in this kind of surgery and inspection of the data revealed that the completeness of excision has steadily increased with experience and the results of the more recent years strongly suggested an almost complete cure rate with a very low recurrence rate.

Pelvic denervation procedures

Since pelvic pain and dysmenorrhoea are common symptoms among young women, it is not surprising that many attempts have been made to interrupt some of the afferent sensory nerve fibres supplying the uterus. The operation of presacral neurectomy by laparotomy has a long history and was described even before the outbreak of the Second World War. In those days it was a formidable operation with a relatively high complication rate and had a failure rate of around 11–15% in primary dysmenorrhoea and 25–40% in secondary dysmenorrhoea, which was mainly due to endometriosis.[45,46]

In 1954, Joseph Doyle of Massachusetts described the procedure of paracervical uterine denervation which bears his name.[47] Doyle's procedure involved the excision of the uterosacral ligaments, which carry most of the sensory pain fibres to the lower part of the uterus, at their attachment to the posterior aspect of the cervix. He suggested that the procedure could be performed vaginally by gynaecologists, but general surgeons would prefer a large laparotomy incision. His results were extremely impressive, with complete pain relief in 63 out of 73 women (86%), partial relief in six cases and only four failures. With such a satisfactory outcome it is difficult to see why the operation sank into obscurity but this was possibly due to the advent of the oral contraceptive and prostaglandin synthetase inhibitors, which reduced the demand for such relatively drastic forms of surgical intervention.

Since 1980, however, interest in Doyle's procedure has been revived with the advent of minimal access surgery. The laparoscopic uterine nerve ablation (LUNA) takes only a few minutes to perform with a surgical laser or electrosurgical needle and produces the same tissue effect without the need for major surgery and has an extremely low complication rate.

Anatomy of the uterine nerve supply

The perfect neuro-ablative surgical procedure for pelvic pain would interrupt all the afferent sensory nerves from all the pelvic organs and leave all other nerves unaffected. Unfortunately, this is clearly impossible because the uterus and ovaries receive their nerve supply not only through a series of nervous plexuses but also by nerves that accompany the ovarian and uterine arteries and it would be impossible to interrupt all these nervous pathways without damage to the vascular supply of the reproductive organs.[48]

The body of the uterus appears to be innervated only by sympathetic fibres.[49] The cervix is mainly supplied by parasympathetic fibres, (but also some sympathetic) which traverse the cervical division of the Lee–Frankenhauser plexus, which lies in, under and around the attachments of the uterosacral ligament to the posterolateral aspect of the cervix.[50-52] Sympathetic fibres can also be found in this area, which have reached the cervix by accompanying the uterine arteries. Excellent illustrations of Lee's dissection showing the nerves in this plexus can be seen in the Wellcome Historical Museum in London.

From the uterosacral ligaments the parasympathetic afferent fibres reach the dorsal root ganglia of the first to fourth sacral spinal nerves (S1–S4) via the pelvic splanchnic nerves (nervi erigentes) and the inferior hypogastric plexus. Theoretically therefore, division of the uterosacral ligaments at the point of their attachment to the cervix should lead to interruption of most of the cervical sensory fibres and some of the corporal sensory fibres and lead to a diminution in uterine pain at the time of menstruation. However, clearly the sympathetic afferent fibres that accompany the uterine, iliac and inferior mesenteric arteries to the sacral sympathetic trunk via the sacral splanchnic nerves will not be interrupted and therefore complete denervation is not possible.

Surgical division of the uterosacral ligaments by LUNA or resection of the presacral nerves could be reasonably expected to diminish central pain from dysmenorrhoea, but could not be expected to relieve lateral pain, especially that coming from the ovaries, because these fibres bypass the uterosacral ligament and course through the corresponding plexuses to their cells of origin in the dorsal route ganglia of the 10th and 11th thoracic spinal nerves. Indeed, some of the upper ovarian plexus afferent nerves go directly via the renal and aortic plexuses and even bypass the superior hypogastric plexus, so that even a complete presacral neurectomy would not interrupt them.

LUNA

LUNA can be performed on patients with either primary or secondary dysmenorrhoea at the same time as a diagnostic laparoscopy is performed. The pelvis is carefully inspected for associated pathology, particularly endometriosis, and if this is found the endometriotic implants should be vaporised with the CO_2 laser or electrosurgery. The broad ligaments are carefully inspected to try to identify the course of the ureters, which can rarely lie close to the uterosacral ligaments but are usually 1–2 cm laterally. The characteristic peristaltic movements can usually be recognised beneath the peritoneal surface but if there is extensive endometriosis with associated fibrosis it is sometimes necessary to dissect out the ureters, which requires considerable laparoscopic surgical expertise.

The surgeon should also be aware of some thin-walled veins lying just lateral to the uterosacral ligaments, and also the presence of an artery deep in the uterosacral ligament, which, if accidentally punctured, can cause considerable and dramatic bleeding, which can be difficult to stop with the CO_2 laser. It is essential therefore that haemostatic equipment, such as bipolar diathermy, is immediately available and should have been tested at the start of the operation. Irrigation and suction equipment should also be working in order to keep the laparoscopic field clear of blood and to allow immediate identification of the bleeding point.

The ligaments are vaporised, forming a crater about 2 cm in diameter and 1 cm deep, and the procedure should continue until all the nerve fibres have been divided and at the base of the crater there is normal retroperitoneal fat. Sometimes, in advanced endometriosis, the uterosacral ligaments are infiltrated with endometrial glands and stroma and the surrounding fibromuscular hyperplasia and it is possible that the removal of all this disease tissue is an important contributing factor to the good results of this procedure.

Over the past 18 years that we have been performing this operation in Guildford we have had no mortality and no serious morbidity, but in the world literature there has been a report of two deaths in the USA from secondary haemorrhage and also two cases of subsequent prolapse, but this is almost certainly coincidental, because the uterosacral ligaments do not play a major part in pelvic floor support.[53,54]

Presacral neurectomy

The operation of presacral neurectomy at laparotomy has been in use for at least 70 years and the first published series was in 1937.[55] Because of the relatively high incidence of complications this type of major abdominal surgery is rarely used nowadays, although in the hands of extremely experienced and skilled laparoscopic surgeons it can be performed laparoscopically, even on a day-care basis. This is an extremely difficult laparoscopic procedure because the retroperitoneal space in front of the sacral promontory is extremely vascular. It is necessary to reflect the sigmoid colon laterally aided by a left-sided tilt of the operating table and to be absolutely certain of obtaining haemostasis before dividing or excising the nerves of the superior hypergastric plexus. These have widely varying anatomical configurations[56] and the presacral space is extremely vascular. Bleeding here, particularly from the middle sacral artery, can be extremely troublesome as also can be bleeding from the periostial blood vessels. Additionally, there have been problems with certain devices, particularly the argon beam coagulator, which employs an electron channel of argon gas through which radio-frequency energy is conducted. In two operations this has reflected off the surface of the periosteum and the energy has torn the common iliac vessels with catastrophic bleeding.[57] However, in skilled hands the operation can give good long-term results.[58,59]

Unfortunately, this procedure has a high incidence of complications and in the study of Chen et al., 31 of the 33 patients who underwent laparoscopic presacral neurectomy experienced constipation, which was severe in some cases.[60] In another study reporting presacral neurectomy at laparotomy, Candiani et al.[60] reported that 13 women had long-standing constipation, three had urinary urgency and two had a completely painless first-stage of labour. There was also one patient who required a subsequent laparotomy 48 hours postoperatively because of a presacral haematoma.

Laparoscopic presacral neurectomy is regarded as an extremely advanced level IV procedure in the Royal College of Obstetricians and Gynaecologists classification, (which is the most advanced level of laparoscopic surgery) and could only be performed in highly specialised centres practising advanced laparoscopic surgery. LUNA, however, should be within the skill of any reasonably competent laparoscopic surgeon practising in most district general hospitals.

Is there any evidence base for denervation procedures?

A Cochrane review published in 2000[61] suggested that there is insufficient evidence to recommend the use of pelvic neuroablation in the management of dysmenorrhoea, regardless of cause. Considering how often LUNA has been performed in recent years, it is surprising that there has been so little in the way of well-designed randomised controlled trials. A small randomised double-blind prospective study was published in 1987 by a team from Detroit.[62] Although there were only 21 patients in this study it compared LUNA with diagnostic laparoscopy only in patients with primary dysmenorrhoea and appeared to be effective in the short term, but its effectiveness appeared to decline over time. Chen et al.[59] confirmed this suggestion and demonstrated that laparoscopic presacral neurectomy may retain its effectiveness for a longer period of time but, as mentioned above, there was a considerable number of unpleasant adverse effects.

The Guildford Birthright Trial described above had a major flaw in that all patients in the treatment arm had LUNA as well as laser vaporisation of all visible endometriotic implants. This inevitably attracted criticism on the basis that there was uncertainty as to which of these procedures contributed to the overall good results. We have since completed a further randomised double-blind prospective trial of 51 randomised patients, in which one group had LUNA plus laser vaporisation of endometriosis while the control arm merely had laparoscopic laser vaporisation of endometriosis without any denervation procedure. At the six-month follow-up it was found that the LUNA procedure did not confer any additional benefit on the overall good result, which was almost the same as in our original randomised, controlled trial.[63] A further study by Vercellini and his colleagues came to the same conclusion in a randomised, prospective study with 81 patients.[64] It is interesting to speculate on the overall good results obtained with LUNA in our original retrospective study.[65] A possible explanation is that many patients with severe dysmenorrhoea do have deep infiltration of the uterosacral ligaments and the large laser crater, measuring about 2 cm in diameter and 5–10 mm deep, must have clearly removed a lot of this abnormal tissue, which is known to give rise to severe pain. We are increasingly seeing young women with deep infiltrating endometriosis running laterally from the rectovaginal septum or a nodule posterior to the cervix, which then infiltrates laterally into the uterosacral ligaments and sometimes even into the pelvic sidewall.

Radical excision of the uterosacral ligaments, either with a CO_2 laser or with electrosurgery, is increasingly performed and because the tissue removed is similar to a bull's horn is called the Arcus Taurinus procedure. Using this technique Dubuisson and his team in Paris have produced dysmenorrhoea relief in 46 of 50 (92%) women, with dyspareunia relief in 47 of 51 (92%). They noted that the revised AFS score[13] bore no correlation with symptoms and this scale of disease severity is only really of any value in patients with infertility. They also noted that the treatment was equally efficacious whether or not the histology showed endometrial glands and stroma. In almost 50% of cases this was not present and the pathological finding was fibromuscular hyperplasia. This observation makes nonsense of the criticism of laser vaporisation of uterosacral ligament disease as being inferior to *en bloc* dissection since it does not provide a histological specimen. We disagree with this because the white fibromuscular hyperplasia is obvious and one continues vaporising until one is down to normal tissue. Using this technique we obtain similar results to those of other teams using electrosurgery, but our technique takes between 40 minutes and an hour, whereas radical excision can take two or three times this amount of operating time.

Radical surgery – total hysterectomy and bilateral salpingo-oophorectomy

Although most studies of laparoscopic laser surgery show pain relief in about 70% of treated women, there remains the difficult problem of how to manage the failures. In the long-term follow-up of the Guildford Birthright study, referred to above, we found that six patients eventually came to hysterectomy. However, there was no sign of endometriosis either macroscopically or microscopically at surgery and, sadly, their hysterectomies did not relieve their pain.

It is imperative to rule out other causes of pelvic pain, particularly when second-look laparoscopy does not show any sign of residual disease.

Most of our work has been in the development of conservative surgery, which is due to the fact that this is often a young population and many of these women have not yet completed their families. Nevertheless, in a number of patients the only realistic solution to the pain and misery inflicted by endometriosis is to perform a pelvic clearance, which includes a total abdominal hysterectomy and bilateral salpingo-oophorectomy with removal of all active deposits of endometriosis. It is illogical to conserve one ovary on the basis of a patient's young age because oestrogens are the stimulus to growth of ectopic endometrial tissue and if any ovarian tissue remains the disease is likely to recur in as many as 40% of women at five years.[66] More important is the fact that, if ovarian tissue is conserved at the time of hysterectomy for endometriosis, 25% of the women will require subsequent laparotomies, often more than one.[67] At the initial surgery the ovary is often free and mobile but as the disease process continues it becomes increasingly bound down to the ovarian fossa by dense adhesions. This is a particularly perilous location because the ureter is close, and attempts to remove the ovary are fraught with difficulty and often lead to incomplete removal – the ovarian remnant syndrome whereby a small nub of ovarian tissue remains and secretes sufficient oestrogen to encourage proliferation of further deposits of endometriosis.

It is important to explain to the patient that conservation of the ovary will often result in recurrent disease and a more logical approach is to remove the ovaries and give immediate hormone replacement, initially as an oestradiol 50 mg and testosterone 100 mg implant inserted in the abdominal fat at the time of wound closure and, subsequently, to continue with oestradiol alone in the form of implants, transdermal patches or oral medication. The addition of cyclical progesterone is unnecessary and, indeed, is positively harmful because it could lead to further growth and bleeding from any residual implants.

Conclusion

Surgical therapy for endometriosis has undergone a dramatic revival in the past 25 years, not only because it can accurately remove endometrial implants and ameliorate pain symptoms, but also because it is the only possible way to restore pelvic anatomy distorted by large ovarian endometriomas, tubo-ovarian or bowel adhesions and fibrotic infiltrative endometriosis invading the rectovaginal septum and obliterating the cul-de-sac.

The 1990s witnessed a revolution in technological progress and surgical skill in minimal access operative laparoscopy in gynaecology. Most of this effort has been directed towards conservative surgery to improve fertility but there has been a discernible trend towards performing curative radical surgery by laparoscopic hysterectomy and bilateral salpingo-oophorectomy.[68] Advanced laparoscopic surgery can also be employed in the more severe stages of the disease to remove dense fibrotic infiltrative disease of the rectovaginal septum or pelvic sidewall with retroperitoneal dissection of the ureters and even segmental resection of the colon involved with endometriosis.[69]

Such procedures take a large amount of operating theatre time, are expensive in advanced technology equipment and require a skilled and dedicated team effort to ensure a successful outcome but the benefits for the patients are enormous. The advantage lies not only in the reduced postoperative discomfort and rapid return to normal life but there is evidence that the endoscopic approach is associated with less morbidity, infection and adhesion formation, which often thwarts the best intentions of the traditional old-fashioned laparotomists.

During the first decade of the 21st century it is likely that minimal access endoscopic surgery will continue to expand and develop and is likely to become the mainstay of treatment for endometriosis until science elucidates the cause of the condition. This may then allow a more logical approach aimed at prevention of this strange and difficult disease.

References

1.   Evers J. The second look laparoscopy for the evaluation of the results of medical treatment of endometriosis should not be performed during ovarian suppression. *Fertil Steril* 1987;**47**:502–4.
2.   Waller KG, Shaw RW. Gonadatrophin-releasing hormone analogues for the treatment of endometriosis: long-term follow-up. *Fertil Steril* 1993;**59**:511–15.
3.   Redwine DB. Conservative laparoscopic excision of endometriosis by sharp dissection: life table analysis of re-operation and persistent or recurrent disease. *Fertil Steril* 1991;**56**:528–634.
4.   Jansen R, Russell P. Non-pigmented endometriosis: clinical, laparoscopic and pathological definition. *Am J Obstet Gynecol* 1986;**155**:1154–9.
5.   Donnez J, Nisolle M, Smets M, Bassil S, Casanas-Roux F. Recto-vaginal septum adenomyotic nodule: a distinct entity. A series of 460 cases. In: Sutton CJG, Diamond M, editors. *Endoscopic Surgery for Gynaecologists*. London: WB Saunders; 1998. p. 357–62.
6.   Davis GD. Management of endometriosis and its associated adhesions with the CO_2 laser laparoscope. *Obstet Gynaecol* 1986;**68**:422–5.
7.   Feste JR. Laser laparoscopy: a new modality. *J Reprod Med* 1985;**30**:413–18.
8.   Sutton CJG, Hill D. Laser laparoscopy in the treatment of endometriosis. A five-year study. *Br J Obstet Gynaecol* 1990;**97**:56–60.
9.   Lomano JM. Nd:YAG laser ablation of early pelvic endometriosis: a report of 61 cases. *Lasers Surg Med* 1987;**7**:56–60.
10.   Keye WR, Dixon J. Photocoagulation of endometriosis by the Argon laser through the laparoscope. *Obstet Gynecol* 1983;**62**:383–6.
11.   Daniell JF, Miller W, Tosh R. Initial evaluation of the use of the potassium-titanyl-phosphate (KTP/532) laser in gynaecologic laparoscopy. *Fertil Steril* 1986;**46**:373–7.
12.   Sutton CJG, Ewen SP, Whitelaw N, Haines P. Prospective, randomised, double-blind, controlled trial of laser laparoscopy in the treatment of pelvic pain associated with minimal, mild and moderate endometriosis. *Fertil Steril* 1994;**62**:696–700.
13.   The American Fertility Society. Revised American Fertility Society classification of endometriosis: 1985. *Fertil Steril* 1985;**43**:351–2.
14.   Sutton CJG, Nair S, Ewen SP, Haines P. A comparison between the CO_2 and KTP lasers in the treatment of large ovarian endometriomas. *Gynecol Endosc* 1993;**2**:113.
15.   Revill SI, Robinson JO, Rosen M, Hogg MIJ. The reliability of a linear analogue scale for evaluating pain. *Anaesthesia* 1976;**31**:1191–6.
16.   Fedele L, Bianchi S, Bocciolone L, Di Nola G, Franchi D. Buserelin acetate in the management of pelvic pain associated with minimal and mild endometriosis: a controlled study. *Fertil Steril* 1993;**59**:516–21.
17.   Sutton CJG, Pooley AS, Ewen SP, Haines P. Follow-up report on randomised controlled trial of laser laparoscopy in the treatment of pelvic pain associated with minimal to moderate endometriosis. *Fertil Steril* 1997;**68**:1070–74.
18.   D'Hoogh TM. Natural history of endometriosis in baboons: is endometriosis an intermittent and/or progressive disease? In Venturini PL, Evers JLH, editors. *Endometriosis: Basic Research and Clinical Practice*. London: Parthenon Publishing Group; 1997.
19.   Jones KD, Haines P, Sutton C. Long-term follow-up on a controlled trial of laser laparoscopy for pelvic pain. *J Soc Laparoendosc Surg* 2001;**5**:111–15.
20.   Donnez J, Nisolle M, Casanas-Roux F, Clerks F. Endometriosis: rationale for surgery. In: Brosen I, Donnez J, editors. *Current State of Endometriosis. Research and Management*. Carnforth: Parthenon Publishing; 1993. p. 385–95.
21.   Hughesdon PE. The structure of endometrial cysts of the ovary. *J Obstet Gynaecol Br Emp* 1957;**44**:69–84.
22.   Daniell JF, Kurtz BR, Gurley LD. Laser laparoscopic management of large endometriomas. *Fertil Steril* 1991;**55**:692–5.
23.   Sutton CJG. Lasers in infertility. *Hum Reprod* 1993;**8**:133–46.

24.   Sutton CJG, Hodgson R. Endoscopic cutting with lasers. *Min Invas Ther* 1992;**1**:197–205.
25.   Raftery A. The effect of peritoneal trauma on peritoneal fibrinolytic activity and intraperitoneal adhesion formation. *Eur Surg Res* 1981;**13**:397–401.
26.   Marrs RP. The use of the KTP laser for laparoscopic removal of ovarian endometrioma. *J Obstet Gynecol* 1991;**164**:1622–6.
27.   Sutton CJG, Ewen SP, Jacobs SA, Whitelaw N. Laser laparoscopic surgery in the treatment of ovarian endometriomas. *J Am Assoc Gynecol Laparosc* 1997;**4**:319–23.
28.   Luciano AA, Maier D, Coch E, Nillsen J, Whitman F. A comparative study of post-operative adhesions following laser surgery by laparoscopy versus laparotomy in the rabbit model. *Obstet Gynecol* 1989;**74**:220–24.
29.   Lundorff P, Hahlin M, Kiallfelt B, Thorburn J, Lindblom B. Adhesion formation after laparoscopic surgery in tubal pregnancy: a randomised trial versus laparotomy. *Fertil Steril* 1991;**55**:911–15.
30.   Koninckx PR, Martin DC. Deep endometriosis: a consequence of infiltration or retraction or possibly adenomyosis externa? *Fertil Steril* 1992;**58**:924–8.
31.   Koninckx PR, Martin DC. Treatment of deeply infiltrating endometriosis. *Curr Opin Obstet Gynaecol* 1994;**6**:231–41.
32.   Koninckx PR, Braet P, Kennedy S, Barlow DH. Dioxin and endometriosis. *Hum Reprod* 1994;**9**:1001–2.
33.   National Centre for Health Statistics. *Hysterectomies in the United States 1965–84, vital and health statistics.* Data from the National Health Survery; 1987. Series 13, no. 92, DHSS Publ. (PHS) 88–175. Hyattsville MD: National Centre for Health Statistics; 1987.
34.   World Health Organization (WHO). *Level of PCBs, PCDDs and PCDFs in Breast Milk: Result of WHO Co-ordinated Interlaboratory Quality Control Studies and Analytical Field Studies. WHO Environmental Health Series.* Geneva: WHO; 1989.
35.   Martin DC, Hubert GD, Van der Zwaag R, El Zeky FA. Laparoscopic appearances of peritoneal endometriosis. *Fertil Steril* 1989;**51**:63–7.
36.   Holsapple MP, Snyder NK, Wood SC, Morris DL. A review of 2, 3, 7, 8-tetrachlorodibenzo-p-dioxin-induced changes in immunocompetence *Toxicology* 1991;**69**:219–55.
37.   Neubert R, Jacob-Muller U, Stahlmann R, Helge H, Neubert D. Polyhalogenated dibenzo-p-dioxins and dibenzofurans and the immune system. *Arch Toxicol* 1992;**65**:213–19.
38.   Rier SE, Martin DC, Bowman RE, Dmowsky WP, Becker JL. Endometriosis in Rhesus monkeys (Macaca Mulatta) following chronic exposure to 2, 3,7 ,8-tetrachlorodibenzo-p-dioxin. *Fundam Appl Toxicol* 1993;**21**:433–41.
39.   Reich H, McGlynn F, Salvat J. Laparoscopic treatment of cul-de-sac obliteration secondary to retrocervical deep fibrotic endometriosis. *J Reprod Med* 1991;**3**:516–22.
40.   Martin DC. Laparoscopic treatment of advanced endometriosis. In: Sutton CJG, Diamond MWB, editors. *Endoscopic Surgery for Gynaecologists.* London: WB Saunders; 1993. p. 229–37.
41.   Martin DC. Laparoscopic and vaginal colpotomy for the excision of infiltrating cul-de-sac endometriosis. *J Reprod Med Obstet Gynaecol* 1988;**33**:806–8.
42.   Nezhat C, Nezhat F, Pennington E. Laparoscopic treatment of infiltrative rectosigmoid colon and rectovaginal septum endometriosis by the technique of video laparoscopy and the CO_2 laser. *Br J Obstet Gynaecol* 1992;**99**:664–7.
43.   Redwine DB. Non-laser resection of endometriosis. In: Sutton CJG, Diamond MWB, editors. *Endoscopic Surgery for Gynaecologists.* London: W. B. Saunders;1993, p. 220–28.
44.   Redwine DB, Sharpe DR. Laparoscopic segmental resection of the sigmoid colon for endometriosis. *J Laparoendoscop Surg* 1991;**1**:217–20.
45.   Tucker AW. Evaluation of pre-sacral neurectomy in the treatment of Dysmenorrhoea. *Am J Obstet Gynecol* 1947;**53**:336–40.
46.   Ingersoll F, Meigs JV. Pre-sacral neurectomy for dysmenorrhoea. *N Engl J Med* 1948;**238**:357–9.
47.   Doyle JB. Paracervical uterine denervation for dysmenorrhoea. *Trans N Engl Obstet Gynaecol Soc* 1954;**8**:143–6.
48.   Johnson N, Wilson M, Farquhar C. Surgical pelvic neuro-ablation for chronic pelvic pain: a systematic review. *Gynaecol Endosc* 2000;**9**:351–61.
49.   Owman C, Rosenbren E, Sjoberg NO. Adrenergic innovation of the human female reproductive organs: a histochemical and chemical investigation. *Obstet Gynecol* 1967;**30**:763–73.
50.   Frankenhauser G. Die Bewegungenerven der Gebärmutter. *Z Med Nat Wiss* 1864;**1**:35–9.
51.   Campbell RM. Anatomy and physiology of sacro-uterine ligaments. *Am J Obstet Gynecol* 1950;**59**:1–5.
52.   Latarjet A, Roget P. Le plexus hypogastrique chez la femme. *Gynecol Obstet* 1922;**6**:225–8.
53.   Davies GD. Uterine prolapse after laparoscopic uterosacral transection in nulliparous airborne

trainees: a report of three cases. *J Reprod Med* 1996;**41**:279–82.

54.   Good MC, Copas PR, Jr, Doodey MC. Uterine prolapse after laparoscopic uterosacral transection: a case report. *J Reprod Med* 1992;**37**:995–6.

55.   Cotte G. Resection of the pre-sacral nerve in the treatment of obstinate dysmenorrhoea. *Am J Obstet Gynecol* 1937;**33**:1034–40.

56.   Biggerstaff ED. Laparoscopic surgery for pelvic pain. In: Sutton CJG, Diamond MWB, editors. *Endoscopic Surgery for Gynaecologists,* 2nd edn. London: W. B. Saunders; 1998. p. 261–71.

57.   Daniell JF, Lalonde CJ. Advanced laparoscopic procedures for pelvic pain and dysmenorrhoea. *Bailliere's Clin Obstet Gynaecol Adv Laparosc Surg* 1995;**9**:795–807.

58.   Nezhat C, Nezhat F. A simplified method of laparoscopic pre-sacral neurectomy for the treatment of central pelvic pain due to endometriosis. *Br J Obstet Gynaecol* 1992;**99**:659–63.

59.   Chen FP, Chang SD, Chu KK, Soong YK. Comparison of laparoscopic Pre-sacral neurectomy and laparoscopic uterine nerve ablation for primary Dysmenorrhoea. *J Reprod Med* 1996;**41**:463–6.

60.   Candiani GB, Fedele L, Vercellini P, Bianchi S, Di Nola G. Presacral neurectomy for the treatment of pelvic pain associated with endometriosis: a controlled study. *Am J Obstet Gynecol* 1992;**167**:100–103.

61.   Johnson N, Wilson M, Farquhar C. Surgical pelvic neuroablation for chronic pelvic pain: a systematic review. *Gynaecol Endosc* 2000;**9**:351–61.

62.   Lichten EM, Bombard J. Surgical treatment of primary dysmenorrhoea with laparoscopic uterine nerve ablation. *J Reprod Med* 1987;**32**:37–41.

63.   Sutton CJG, Dover RW, Pooley A, Jones K, Haines P. Prospective, randomised, double-blind controlled trial of laparoscopic laser uterine nerve ablation in the treatment of pelvic pain associated with endometriosis. *Gynaecol Endosc* (in press).

64.   Vercellini P, Aimi G, Busacca M, Uglietti A, Viganali M, Crossignani PG. Laparoscopic uterosacral ligament resection for dysmenorrhoea associated with endometriosis: results of a randomised controlled trial (abstract). *Fertil Steril* 1997;**68** (suppl. 1):3.

65.   Sutton CJG. Laser uterine nerve ablation. In: Donnez J, Nisolle M, editors. *An Atlas of Laser Operative Laparoscopy and Hysteroscopy.* Louvain: Nauerwelaerts Publishing; 1994. p. 47–52.

66.   Wheeler JH, Malinak LR. Recurrent endometriosis: incidents, management and prognosis. *Am J Obstet Gynecol* 1983;**146**:247–53.

67.   Henderson AF, Studd JWW, Watson N. The retrospective study of oestrogen replacement therapy following hysterectomy for the treatment of endometriosis. In: Shaw RW, editor. *Advances in Reproductive Endocrinology*, Vol. 1. *Endometriosis.* Carnforth: Parthenon Publishing; 1989. p. 131–40.

68.   Sutton CJG. Laparoscopic hysterectomy. *Curr Obstet Gynaecol* 1992;**2**:225–8.

69.   Redwine DB, Sharpe DR. Laparoscopic segmental resection of the sigmoid colon for endometriosis. *J Laparoendosurg* 1991;**1**:436–8.

Chapter 16

Pelvic pain II

Discussion

Discussion following the papers of Mrs Barnard, Mr Stones and Professor Sutton

Beard: Professor Sutton, two things concern me slightly. One is that there is again an assumption that because someone has pain and is found to have endometriosis, that must be the cause of the pain. Second is this issue of how do you assess pain. All your colleagues and yourself say 'pain better' or 'pain not better', but we all know that it is a much more complex issue because not only does it involve some sort of qualitative assessment, but quality of life indicators are very important nowadays.

Sutton: Those patients were assessed on a visual analogue scale which many people find a pretty accurate way of assessing pain – not just present pain but even pain that has happened some time ago. They all have visual analogue scores, and in that recent paper[1] they had them for all of the main symptoms – dyspareunia, dysmenorrhoea and pelvic pain unrelated to periods. We also did a subjective score, which they rated themselves on a five-point scale.

We did not do quality of life, but Professor Garry has done that on some of his studies.[2] That has become the latest fashion. He found that there was an improvement in quality of life but not as great as the pain relief.

Thornton: One of the benefits of attending a meeting like this for me is that some of the talks really make you think. I hope that they will improve my practice. One of the talks that really made me think was Mrs Barnard's. I would like to ask her about a couple of points. I believe you suggested that as clinicians we should not push on patients' abdomens while making a diagnosis. I would agree with most of what you said about that, but it is important that we exclude a number of causes of pain by history and clinical examination. I would suggest that rather than not use clinical examination to make a diagnosis, we should use it perhaps more than we do at the moment but with the difference that we concentrate on correctly interpreting our findings, particularly in the patients that you describe.

Second, you made an interesting comment that mixtures of pain relief may be better than single drugs alone. If that is true, you are absolutely right that we need to let people know. This is not my major area and I do not know the background literature, but I wondered whether there was evidence that various combinations of drugs were more effective for pain relief.

Barnard: I will answer your second question first by simply referring you to Mr Stones, from whom I learned about the different strategies for approaching pain by combining different treatments. I would not pretend to know more than that.

On the abdominal pressure, I agree entirely with its use as a diagnostic tool as one of many. My question is about the context in which it was used and interpreted, bearing in mind that, like lots of women, I went with pelvic pain that was very much associated with periods and period cycles and ovulatory cycles. The point I was trying to make was that you can easily just reroute somebody into a gastroenterology pigeonhole where they should not be in the first place.

Stones: To comment on the combination therapy, there is a lack of randomised control trials in that area, given that most pharmaceutical research – surprise, surprise – is about single agents. The material with which I am particularly familiar is TENS and drug combinations.

Crowhurst: The World Health Organization as long ago as about 1988 issued a publication about broad guidelines for treating pain for use in underdeveloped countries. They had three basic steps. The first step is simple analgesics – aspirin and suchlike – together with other simple therapies. The second step is compound therapies plus stronger things such as co-dydramol and other non-steroidals. The third group is what we call serious painkillers such as opioids and things of that sort. That is a simple thing, and it is being revised at the moment, as I understand it.

Tookman: You are right, analgesic prescribing is a matter of prescribing analgesics plus co-analgesics. Combination analgesia is certainly a way forward, and there are other techniques as well to manage pain.

Berkley: It is called the pain ladder. I wanted to address another issue that Mrs Barnard raised about patient symptomatology, especially for dysmenorrhoea. There was a paper on pain about two years ago that asked women who had severe dysmenorrhoea and women who did not both to use the McGill pain questionnaire words to describe their symptoms. This was dealing with the issue of commonality of knowledge and expectations for dysmenorrhoea. The results were almost identical between the two groups. The women without dysmenorrhoea who were asked to describe what would be their dysmenorrhoeic pains used almost the same language, virtually indistinguishable from those who actually had dysmenorrhoea. It speaks to your point about the usefulness of the words in some cases, or the uselessness of the words in some cases.

Coldron: A question for Mr Stones. You talked about medical education and trying to alter the attitudes of medical students towards patients. You were talking about objective structural clinical examinations – that is a clinical examination which the students undertake in their third, fourth and fifth years. My observation has been that clinical skills *per se* are not taught these days in medical schools and biomedical molecular science has the emphasis. Clinical skills are not really emphasised, and within that the interviewing of a patient. I have found it an uphill battle to introduce clinical skills at any level within medical schools, and I wondered whether this group could look at medical education on the clinical side within the medical schools.

Stones: In Southampton we teach clinical skills from year one.

References

1. Sutton CJG, Dover RW, Pooley A, Jones K, Haines P. Prospective randomised double-blind controlled trial of laparoscopic laser uterine nerve ablation in the treatment of pelvic pain associated with endometriosis. *Gynaecol Endosc* 2001; (in press).
2. Garry R, Clayton R, Hawe J. The effect of endometriosis and its radical excision on quality of life indicators. *Br J Obstet Gynaecol* 2000;**107**:44–54.

SECTION 5

VULVAL AND ABDOMINAL PAIN

Chapter 17

Chronic vulval pain

David C. Foster

Introduction

Two general reviews of chronic vulval pain have been published since 1998 that summarise the condition, classify subtypes and propose therapy.[1,2] In contrast, this paper will briefly overview the causes of chronic vulval pain, in terms of 'primary' and 'secondary' types. Following the overview, we will propose in further detail a neuromuscular basis for three defined types of 'primary' chronic vulval pain. We hope to interweave clinical observations, relevant human research, models in animal research, therapeutic options and research areas in need of further development.

Classification

A useful classification should provide at least one of several goals: (i) to reflect understanding of the pathophysiology of the condition, (ii) to predict prognosis of defined disease subsets, or (iii) to provide insight into the choice of therapy. A useful classification of chronic vulval pain remains elusive for several reasons. First, its pathophysiology remains obscure, second, therapeutic options are not well studied, and finally, a diverse group, including gynaecologists, dermatologists, neurologists, psychiatrists and physiotherapists, manage chronic vulval pain. This diverse group hold different understandings of pathogenesis, terminology and treatment. The classification, proposed by McKay in 1989, continues to be commonly referenced in contemporary reviews.[3] McKay divided vulvodynia into five major groups: (1) vulval dermatoses, (2) cyclic candidiasis/vulvitis, (3) vulval papillomatosis, (4) essential/dysaesthetic vulvodynia, and (5) vulvar vestibulitis. Although useful for the time, the McKay classification does not reflect the current understanding of chronic vulval pain in the year 2001. For instance, the classification emphasises dermatoses but overlooks other diagnoses such as pudendal neuralgia, obstructed Bartholin's glands and desquamative vaginitis. Furthermore, the classification includes the concept of vulval papillomatosis now recognised as a normal variant found commonly in asymptomatic women.[4]

Table 17.1.   'Primary' chronic vulval pain, also known as vulval dysaesthesia

	Localised vulval dysaesthesia	Generalised vulval dysaesthesia	Circumvaginal motor spasm
Related diagnoses	Vulval vestibulitis syndrome vestibulodynia clitorodynia	Pudendal, ilio-inguinal, genitofemoral, and post-herpetic neuralgia, impingement of sacral nerve roots and 'essential' vulvodynia	Levator syndrome, vaginismus, unstable urethra, proctalgia fugax
Proposed pathophysiology	Neuro-inflammation	Neuralgia	Dystonia
Clinical finding	Localised allodynia and variable surface inflammation	Peripheral hyper-hypo-aesthesia following nerve distribution	High/unstable motor tonus affecting pelvic muscles
Other clinical findings	Commonly bilateral	More commonly unilateral, often aggravated by sitting	Midvaginal pain, urgency/frequency, rectal pain
Prevalence	Common	Less common than 'localised'	Often superimposed, less commonly isolated
Treatment	Tricyclic antidepressants, gabapentin, topical lidocaine, surgery	Tricyclic antidepressants, gabapentin, correction of nerve impingement or traction	Physical therapy, biofeedback, baclofen sympatholytics
Animal model	Cutaneous injection of formalin, Freund's or pro-inflammatory cytokines	Sciatic nerve ligation models (Bennett, Chung, Seltzer)	Urethral instability model

Table 17.2.   'Secondary' chronic vulval pain

Anatomic/ structural	Dermatoses/ mucositis	Inflammatory (systemic)	Infectious
Bartholin's gland obstruction	Contact dermatitis (esp. urinary, faecal incontinence and ectropion)	Anorectal Crohn's	Recurrent bacterial infection (mobiluncus leptothrix)
Chronic introital fissure	Lichen sclerosus	Sjogren's	Recurrent fungal infection (moniliasis)
Unruptured hymen	Lichen simplex chronicus	Atrophic	
Post-episiotomy	Erosive lichen planus	Hypo-oestrogenism	Recurrent herpes simplex
Post-surgical scar	Desquamative vaginitis, vesiculobullous conditions	Radiation-induced	

Recognising the need for an updated classification, the 1999 World Congress of the International Society for the Study of Vulvovaginal Disease (ISSVD) convened a discussion group to update the classification of chronic vulval pain.[5] The discussion group focused on the ill-defined category of chronic vulval pain *without visible dermatosis* and proposed the term 'vulval dysaesthesia, (vulvodynia)' for this category. Vulval dysaesthesia was further divided into 'generalised' and 'localised' types.

'Localised vulval dysaesthesia' was synonymous with vulval vestibulitis syndrome and included vestibulodynia and clitorodynia. Unfortunately, the ISSVD proposal is unpublished.

Due to the absence of an updated, widely accepted classification, this paper will present a working classification of chronic vulval pain. The classification excludes acute vulval pain (of less than three months' duration). Chronic vulval pain will be first divided into 'primary' (Table 17.1) and 'secondary' (Table 17.2). Primary pain conditions commonly arise from a pre-existing pathological condition, such as infection, trauma, or other inflammation, but the presence of a pre-existing condition is no longer necessary for maintenance of the chronic pain state. Secondary pain conditions, in contrast, require a chronic condition, such as lichen sclerosus, chronic/recurrent candidiasis, or vaginal fissure, to coexist in order to maintain the chronic vulval pain state. A review of the various types of secondary pain conditions will direct the clinician toward those disease states to consider before diagnosing primary chronic pain. We anticipate that the list of 'secondary' pain conditions may expand as further understanding of chronic vulval pain develops.

Prevalence of chronic vulval pain and vulval dysaesthesia (vulvodynia)

The population prevalence of chronic vulval pain is unknown. In a private gynaecological practice in the USA, Goetsch reported a 15% prevalence rate of vulvodynia.[6] Because of the intimate nature of painful intercourse, the most common symptom of chronic vulval pain, the number of cases is likely to be under-reported. According to the National Health and Social Life Survey (NHSLS), a national probability sample study of sexual behaviour, 15.6% (230/1479) of women reported sexual dysfunction secondary to 'pain during sex'.[7] Of the women with dyspareunia in the NHSLS, the proportion with vulval dysaesthesia (vulvodynia) is unknown. Studies from Binik and colleagues[8-11] using structured interviews, standardised pain measures, psychometric tests and gynaecological examinations of 105 women with dyspareunia, in Montreal, have helped to characterise dyspareunia into four diagnostic subtypes: no dyspareunia-related physical findings (24%), vulval vestibulitis (46%), vulval vaginal atrophy (13%), and mixed/other conditions (17%). The vulvar vestibulitis subset reported the highest frequency of pain to touch, pain on gynaecological examination and a unique psychosocial profile (discussed later, under Future research issues). The population prevalence rate can be estimated by combining the NHSLS and the data reported by Binik'sgroup. Approximately 7% of women between 18 and 59 years of age are estimated to have vulval vestibulitis. Based on 500 randomly chosen patients from Columbia Presbyterian Medical Center Cutaneous-Vulvar Service the most common diagnoses included vulval vestibulitis (36.2%), lichen sclerosus (19.2%) and vaginitis/vaginosis (14.8%).[12]

'Localised' vulval dysaesthesia, also known as vulval vestibulitis

Vulval vestibulitis is characterised by dyspareunia or pain to light touch associated with one or more painful foci of the vulval vestibule and no identifiable source of pain such as herpes, *Candida* or pemphigoid. Friedrich's criteria[13] remain the accepted standard for diagnosis and include: (i) severe pain on vestibular touch or attempted vaginal entry, (ii) tenderness localised within the vestibule, and (iii) physical findings of erythema of various degrees. Peckham *et al.*[14] studied 67 women with vulval vestibulitis, which they termed 'focal vulvitis'. The authors noted that vestibular inflammation was 'rarely seen with the naked eye', whereas the physical demonstration of vestibular hypersensitivity and allodynia were considered 'essential' diagnostically. Exquisite sensitivity to touch was found to be characteristically focal, reproduced with remarkable precision by independent observers, and separated from nontender areas of the vulva and vagina by a matter of millimetres. In 81% of patients all painful foci were located on the mucosa of the lower half of the vestibule, between 3 o'clock and 9 o'clock, and limited by the line of keratinisation (Hart's line) and the hymenal ring. The remaining 19% included focal areas of tenderness within defined limits of the vestibule but extending towards the urethral orifice.

Although published case–control studies of vulval vestibulitis[15–17] lack a commonly identified risk factor (Table 17.3), inflammation or trauma may act as the common denominator. The two studies that found an association between vulval vestibulitis and recurrent candidiasis also reported a frequent absence of confirmatory wet-mounts or cultures for fungus. Reports of candidiasis were assumed from symptoms of itching and burning which partially responded to antifungal therapy. Ketoconazole, a common antifungal, has been shown to have intrinsic anti-inflammatory properties, suggesting that a partial response to ketoconazole may not support a fungal causation.[18] The highest strength of association in our case–control study was found between vulval vestibulitis and the Caucasian race (Table 17.3).[17] The basis of this racial difference remains obscure. No consistent molecular evidence of an increased frequency of human papillomavirus (HPV)-associated DNA has been found in vulval vestibulitis. However, the treatments for HPV-associated infection, including application of trichloroacetic acid, podopophyllin, and laser ablation, remain clinically suspect as sources of genital injury. A two-year review (1997–99) of 201 patients from the University of Rochester Vulvar Service found that 90% of patients with vulval vestibulitis were able to identify a traumatic or inflammatory occurrence temporally associated with onset of chronic vulval pain.[19] Traumatic or inflammatory events reported included: recurrent 'yeast' (21%), an episode of unusually painful intercourse (18%), delivery of a child (18%) and laser therapy (8%).

Table 17.3.   Case–control studies of vulval vestibulitis

	Case (*n*)	Control (*n*)	Risk factor	OR (CI)
Mann *et al.* (1992)[15]	71	71	Recurrent candidiasis	15.2 (n/a)
			History of condyloma	8.0 (n/a)
Bazin *et al.* (1994)[16]	57	173	OCs started at <17 years	11.0 (1.3–97.1)
			First intercourse at <16 years	3.3 (1.4–8.0)
Foster *et al.* (1995)[17]	95	188	Caucasian	15.7 (2.47–65.2)
			Nulliparity	2.9 (1.42–3.02)
			Recurrent candidiasis	1.8 (1.06–3.16)

OR, odds ratio; CI, confidence intervals; OCs, oral contraceptives

Localised vulval dysaesthesia as a pain model

The unique anatomic position and embryological origin of the vestibule may lead to a unique inflammatory response similar to that of the lower urinary tract or rectum. The initiation of chronic pain may be based upon local injury of delicate mucosal tissue, activation of mast cells, macrophages and fibroblasts and subsequent release of pro-inflammatory cytokines such as interleukin-1β (IL-1β) and tumour necrosis factor-α (TNF-α). Because the allodynia of vulval vestibulitis appears highly demarcated and is similar in location across cases, careful study of the perineal body from external vulva to lower vagina provides a unique resource for the study of chronic pain. Perineal tissue from vestibulitis cases and pain-free controls are readily available following perineoplasty or posterior vaginal repair, respectively. Figure 17.1 illustrates the perineal tissue region collected for study by selected biopsy. Our studies have included cytokine/neurokine assay, measures of nerve fibre density and structure, *in situ* analysis of inflammatory mediators, and selective fibroblast cultures from site of pain and sites without symptoms.

Cytokine and neurokine studies

Two inflammatory cytokines IL-1α and TNF-β, were compared in selected regions of the vulva, vestibule and hymen in vulval vestibulitis cases and in pain-free controls.[20] Surgical specimens were selectively sampled according to anatomic site from 12 cases undergoing perineoplasty for vulvar vestibulitis and from ten pain-free controls undergoing posterior vaginal repair. The samples were prepared into tissue homogenates and analysed for concentrations of IL-1β and TNF-α via sandwich enzyme-linked immunosorbent assay.

Median tissue levels of IL-1β (Figure 17.2) and TNF-α (Figure 17.3) were elevated 2.3-fold and 1.8-fold, respectively, in women with vulval vestibulitis compared with pain-free women. When analysed by selected anatomic site in patients with vulval vestibulitis, highest median levels of IL-1β (5 ng/mg total protein) were found at the hymenal region. Regional elevation in inflammatory cytokines with vulval vestibulitis varied with clinical history. For example, elevated IL-1β and TNF-α tissue concentrations at the hymen were associated with painful sexual intercourse continuing from first sexual experience. In contrast, elevated tissue concentrations of cytokines at

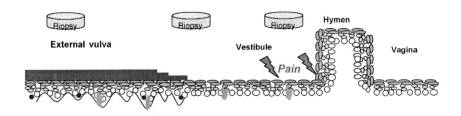

Figure 17.1. A schematic representing the perineum; areas of sampling include external vulva which is classically unaffected by allodynia in contrast to the vestibular region in vicinity to the hymen

the external vulva were associated with a history of external skin irritation. Cytokine elevations correlated poorly with inflammatory cell infiltrate and suggested cytokine production from another cell source. Furthermore, concentrations of IL-1β and TNF-α found in vulval vestibulitis cases were similar to tissue concentrations which induced peripheral nerve irritability in animal studies (see Animal research – correlates to chronic vulval pain below).

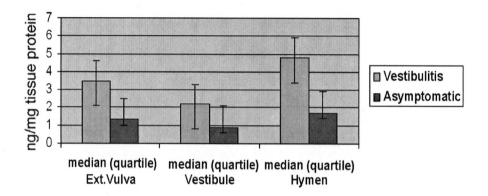

Figure 17.2.   Interleukin-1β levels in the lower genital tract of patients with vulval vestibulitis and asymptomatic controls

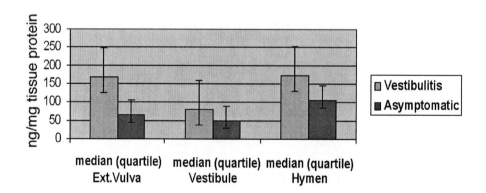

Figure 17.3.   Tumour necrosis factor-α levels in the lower genital tract of patients with vulval vestibulitis and asymptomatic controls

Nerve fibre density and morphology

Several studies have found an increase in nerve fibre density in vulval vestibulitis. Westrom *et al.*[21] reported that stromal nerve fibre density per square unit was significantly correlated with the level of inflammation. However, nerve fibre density was not significantly correlated with the presence or absence of pain. The authors used S-100 immunostain and rated inflammation and nerve fibre density on a subjective scale of none, mild, moderate, severe and extensive. Of the immunocytochemical antisera available for identification of peripheral nerves, PGP 9.5 has been demonstrated to give reliable results with particularly good staining of epidermal fibres.[22] Bohm-Starke *et al.* used PGP 9.5 to study biopsies in the vicinity of Bartholin's gland.[23] The authors reported a significantly higher number of intra-epithelial nerve fibres in vulvar vestibulitis cases than in asymptomatic controls. The technique of classification was 'less nerve fibres (0 to 3 nerve profiles)' and 'more nerve fibres (4–30 nerve profiles)'. Unfortunately, the determination of fibre density was not performed in a blinded fashion and the method of counting fibres ('nerve profiles') was not adequately defined. Improved analysis of nerve density may result with the use of validated counting techniques for epidermal nerve fibre density and nerve morphometry as described in 1999.[24] Figure 17.4 demonstrates an intra-epithelial free nerve ending in the vulval vestibule which is positively stained for substance P (sP) by avidin–biotin complex immunocytochemistry. The figure shows the characteristic 1–2-μm varicose packets of sP within presumed c-fibres that penetrate the vestibular epithelium and terminate within one to two cell layers of the surface. Substance-P-positive [sP(+)] immunoreactive fibres were significantly fewer in number in the hymenal tissues of vulval vestibulitis cases than in asymptomatic controls. The immunocytochemical findings were independently confirmed by an enzyme-linked immunosorbent assay of the tissue homogenate from the same site (Table 17.4, data submitted for publication). The paradox of elevated inflammatory mediators in the presence of decreased numbers of sP(+) immunoreactive fibres has been demonstrated in chronic constriction injury models of neuropathic pain..[25] Reduced sP levels have been suggested to be based upon continued release of sP in the absence of substantial upregulation of sP mRNA.

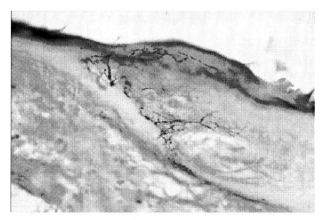

Figure 17.4.   Neural fibres of the vulval vestibule in a patient with vulval vestibulitis, stained with avidiin–biotin complex immunocytochemistry for substance P

Table 17.4. Quantification of substance P using two techniques of immunocytochemistry and enzyme-linked immunosorbent assay in the lower genital tract in vulval vestibulitis and asymptomatic controls; data shown as median (quartiles)

	External vulva	Vulval vestibule	Hymen
SP(+) nerve by ABC/CC (fibres/10 hpf)			
Vestibulitis	33.5 (26–40)**	7.5 (4–12)	9 (4–20)
Asymptomatic	76.5 (72–93)	18 (7–24)	14.5 (7–27)
SP within tissue homogenate ELISA (pmol/mg protein)			
Vestibulitis	1.77 (1.76–23.5)	1.02 (0.54–7.7)	1.07 (1.01–5.85)
Asymptomatic	7.90 (1.2–17.38)	1.08 (0.66–1.47)	3.10 (1.28–26.5)

**Wilcoxon $P < 0.002$.

Fibroblast heterogeneity in vulvar vestibulitis using fibroblast cultures

Reddy et al.,[26] from our facility, have completed preliminary studies of fibroblast heterogeneity in the vulval vestibule compared with the external vulva in cases and controls. Research, using a myriad of tissues including lung, periodontium and periostium, finds that the fibroblast acts as a central mediator of inflammation. In addition, fibroblasts demonstrate a heterogeneity in terms of surface markers Thy-1(+) and Thy-1(−) and functional phenotypes: 'fibrotic' versus 'immunogenic' types. The following observations are based upon vimentin-positive, cytokeratin-negative fibroblast cultures sampled from the anatomic regions of greatest pain (prehymenal region), from pain-free areas of the external vulva, and from corresponding anatomic regions in pain-free controls. The findings include the following:

- Fibroblasts in tissue culture sampled from the vestibule in cases and controls demonstrate increased levels of both CD-40 and CD-40 ligand on the cellular surface

- Fibroblasts in tissue culture sampled from areas of vulval vestibulitis produce 20-fold higher levels of IL-6 following IL-1β and TNF-α stimulation compared with unaffected vulval or vestibular fibroblasts

- Fibroblasts sampled from the vulvar vestibule of cases and controls, differentially produce cyclo-oxygenase-1 (COX-1) and COX-2 following stimulation with interferon-γ (IFN-γ) and CD-40 ligand. Fibroblasts in tissue culture in vulval vestibulitis cases produce significantly higher levels of COX-1 and COX-2 than fibroblasts from pain-free controls.

Assuming that consistent results are found in further studies, the presence of fibroblast heterogeneity may provide a mechanism for highly localised peripheral nerve induction of hyperalgesia through COX-induced production of prostaglandin E_2 localised to the region of the vestibule.

Genetics of vulval vestibulitis syndrome ('localised' vulval dysaesthesia)

IL-1 receptor antagonist (IL-1RA) is polymorphic in humans. Genes coding for IL-1α, IL-1β and IL-1RA are located in close proximity on chromosome 2q13-21. The presence of allele 2 of the IL-1RA gene (IL-1RA*2) has been associated with several disorders including periodontitis, Graves' disease, multiple sclerosis, Sjögren's syndrome and ulcerative colitis.[27,28] In one study, 52.9% of a sample of vulval vestibulitis cases were found to be homozygous for IL-1RA*2 compared with 8.5% of a sample of asymptomatic women.[29] Comparing the proportion of cases homozygous for the IL-1RA*2 polymorphism in terms of diseases mentioned above, vulval vestibulitis carried the highest proportion of cases homozygous for the IL-1RA*2 polymorphism. Paradoxically, the IL-1RA*2 allele is associated with increased production of IL-1β.[300] An association between IL-1RA*2 and increased production of IL-1β within affected tissue of vulval vestibulitis subjects has yet to be demonstrated.

Generalised vulval dysaesthesia (neuralgia of pudendal, ilio-inguinal, genitofemoral nerves and sacral nerve root impingement and 'essential' vulvodynia)

Injury, infection, surgical entrapment or compression of the pudendal, ilio-inguinal, genitofemoral nerves and sacral nerve roots may be the basis of a subset of vulval pain cases categorised as neuralgia. Pelvic pain secondary to neuralgia may actually result from damage or injury to the neuraxis at a variety of locations including the cerebral cortex, spinal cord, sacral plexus and peripheral nerve. Pudendal nerve injury may follow obstetric or mechanical trauma, excessive straining, post-shingles outbreak, or surgical corrections of prolapse by the vaginal approach.[31-34] Ilio-inguinal nerve injury has been associated with needle suspensions for urinary incontinence and other surgical procedures in proximity to the external inguinal ring.[35,36] Ilio-inguinal neuropathy presents as a lateralised burning or lancinating-type pain which radiates to the ipsilateral labia majora and inner thigh. Ilio-inguinal neuropathy is commonly associated with a decreased sensation to touch of the region of innervation and pain is relieved by local injection of anaesthetics in the vicinity of the ilio-inguinal nerve. In a small number of patients with perineal pain of 'obscure origin', sacral-meningeal (Tarlov's) cysts have been identified by magnetic resonance imaging.[37,38] Because this particular type of chronic vulval pain is less common than 'localised' vulval dysaesthesia (vulval vestibulitis), the reports are limited to case series and clinical trials are non-existent.

The diagnostic criteria for neuralgia-associated chronic vulval pain varies in published reviews. Neuralgia pain is characterised by episodic, lancinating, needle-like pain found in the distribution of the specific nerve or dermatome.[39] Constant burning dysaesthesia may be an accompanying symptom. Pudendal nerve terminal motor latency via St Mark's electrode has been used as a diagnostic marker of pudendal neuropathy and neuralgia. As is evident in other forms of neuralgia, however, the evidence of damage through nerve conduction defects may be minimal or impossible to document.[40] Although case reports attribute vulval pain to pudendal nerve injury, larger studies suggest that only a small proportion of patients with measurable pudendal nerve injury may suffer from vulval pain.[41] Conversely, pudendal nerve motor latency abnormalities do not appear to predict response to surgical unentrapment of the pudendal nerve.[42] Therefore, at the clinical level, the diagnosis of neuralgia is predominantly based upon a temporal relationship to a traumatic event and classical symptoms and signs.

Circumvaginal motor spasm (vaginismus, proctalgia fugax, unstable urethra)

Neuromuscular dysfunction may also contribute to the pathophysiology of chronic vulval pain. Glazer *et al.* has compared the EMG behaviour of the pelvic floor in cases of 'dysaesthetic vulvodynia' to asymptomatic women. Cases were found to have reduced ability to contract the pelvic floor, reduced ability to relax the pelvic floor and increased muscular instability at rest, compared with asymptomatic controls.[43] A study previously reported from our clinic supports Glazer's observation of increased pelvic floor motor instability. Vulval vestibulitis cases demonstrate abnormally high urethral pressure variability compared with normal controls and to controls with extragenital chronic pelvic pain (Figure 17.5).[44] Although variation in muscular tone of the urethral sphincter was felt to be the probable source of this variability, the external urethral sphincter comprises a portion of the pelvic diaphragm and commonly functions in concert with the levator muscles.

Two conditions of the anal canal, proctalgia fugax and the chronic anal fissure, appear similar to motor problems of the vaginal and urethral tracts. Rectal pressure variability has been demonstrated in proctalgia fugax, a chronic pain condition of the rectum. Proctalgia fugax cases differ from sex- and age-matched controls by the development of an increase in baseline and amplitude of rectal pressure variability during an acute episode of pain.[45] The frequency and amplitude of rectal pressure variability appears similar to the frequency and amplitude of urethral instability found in our study (Figure 17.5).[45,46] Three clinical trials for treatment of chronic anal fissures have provided additional insight into the phenomenon of chronic pain of pelvic muscle origin.[46–48] Clinical responses to botulinum toxin therapy suggest the pathogenic basis for development of a chronic anal fissure is sphincter spasm.[46] With respect to internal (smooth muscle) versus external (striated muscle) sphincter, fissure healing was most closely associated with reduced tone of the external sphincter.[48] Whether excessive urethral and rectal pressure variablility is present in all chronic vulval pain patients or only a subset remains unknown.

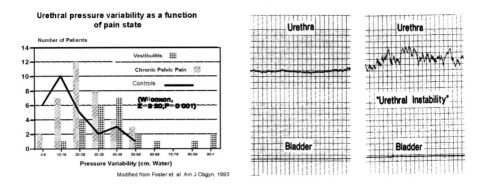

Figure 17.5. Comparison of pressure variability recorded within the urethra in vulvar vestibulitis cases, chronic pelvic pain controls and asymptomatic controls; variability was significantly higher in vulval vestibulitis cases

Animal research – correlates to 'primary' vulval dysaesthesia

Neuroinflammatory correlate: development of a cutaneous irritable nociceptor

In the rat model, a dose–response relationship has been reported between the IL-1β subcutaneous concentration and both number and latency of neural impulses following a standard mechanical stimulus.[49] Following local injection of IL-1β, the mean neural discharge from the saphenous nerve to heat, cold and touch stimuli within the defined receptive field increased up to 484%. Neural discharge to mechanical stimulation also demonstrated a reduction in the threshold by 50–60%. Prolonged cutaneous pain can be induced in animal models by peripheral injection of IL-1β or TNF-α in concentrations similar to the elevated tissue levels found in vulval vestibulitis.[20]

TNF-α and IL-1β act synergistically in most inflammatory conditions, rising and falling with identical timing of gene products and receptors.[50] Increasing concentrations of intradermally injected TNF-α result in potentiation of irritable nociceptors similar to IL-1β. Local administration of TNF-α promotes demyelination through attack upon the oligodendrocyte,[51-53] produces hyperalgesia when injected intradermally,[54] promotes reflex sympathetic dystrophy of the hand,[55] produces thermal hyperalgesia and mechanical allodynia when injected in the vicinity of a previously normal nerve,[56] and increases spontaneous activity of a delta and C fibres both at the nerve terminal and even at mid-axonal levels.[57] TNF-α polypeptides have also been shown to develop a trimer conformation with a central pore which has the ability to insert into bilaminar lipid membranes and act as a sodium channel.[58]

Neuropathy and neuralgia correlate: the sciatic nerve ligation model

Over the last decade, variations of sciatic nerve ligation in the rat (Bennet, Seltzer and Chung models)[59-61] have been shown to produce a long-term neuropathic pain state. The neuropathy is characterised by reduced hind paw withdrawal to mechanical stimuli, decreased latency to withdrawal to heat, and a characteristic behaviour complex which has been interpreted as pain behaviour. Through numerous reports ranging from behavioural to molecular, the models have been felt to mirror the phenomenon of human neuropathy. The sciatic nerve ligation models have been extremely useful in identifying potential therapeutic options. For example, the injection of neutralising antibodies to TNF-α (specifically to TNF receptor-1) produces a reduction of mechanical hyperalgesia after chronic constriction nerve injury.[62]

Muscle spasm correlate: urethral instability in the rat

A single inflammatory challenge to the lower urinary tract in the rat results in changes in pelvic floor muscle activity. In response to intravesical instillation of saline followed by a single instillation of capsaicin, the external urethral sphincter in the rat demonstrates markedly increased short-term oscillations of urethral pressure from the normal (15 mmHg ± 3 mmHg) to (70 mmHg ± 9 mmHg).[63] Selective neural blockade indicated this phenomenon to be an interaction between capsaicin-sensitive primary afferent fibres, innervating the urethra, and the somatic efferent innervation to the urethral rhabdosphincter. Repeat instillation of capsaicin, known to result in temporary loss of c-fibre density, failed to re-elicit the enhanced oscillations and this loss of responsiveness lasted more than four days. From this research, an association between pain-mediating c-fibres and motor instability of the pelvic floor is supported.

Medical and surgical treatments for chronic vulval pain

Suggested empiric therapies for chronic vulval pain have included tricyclic antidepressants such as amitriptyline and desipramine, gabapentin, intralesional interferon, systemic acyclovir, sympathectomy, acupuncture, low oxalate diet, capsaicin, psychotherapy, biofeedback and surgery.[64-71] Unfortunately, treatment efficacy has often been limited by the adverse effects of the medication and the patients' hesitancy to undergo surgery. Although the mechanism of analgesic action remains unknown, tricyclic antidepressants may interfere with injury-induced central sensitisation of the dorsal horn cells via the descending inhibitory adrenergic neural tracts.[72] In prospective randomised trials, tricyclic antidepressants reduce chronic pain in diabetic neuropathy, post-herpetic neuralgia, and post-stroke central pain.[73-79] McKay reported on a retrospective study of women with 'essential' vulvodynia who responded to low-dose amitriptyline, (20–100 mg).[69] Amitriptyline was less effective in vulvodynia patients under the age of 40 years, unless they also had symptoms of fibromyalgia or urethral syndrome. Pagano reported on a retrospective study of amitriptyline in 230 women with vulvar vestibulitis.[80] The dose of amitriptyline ranged from 10 to 75 mg and 89 women of 230 (58%) 'responded well' to treatment, with 45 of the 230 women (20%) 'cured' at six months. An alternative oral agent, gabapentin, is a structural analogue of γ-aminobutyric acid whose mechanism of action is not fully understood. Gabapentin has been demonstrated in clinical trials to be effective for post-herpetic neuralgia and diabetic neuropathy.[81,82] Although gabapentin has been used clinically as an alternative to tricyclic antidepressants for neuropathic pain, its effectiveness for vulvodynia is unconfirmed by clinical trial.

A pharmacologically distinct local effector, lidocaine (class 1_B anti-arrhythmic), has been reported to relieve neuropathic pain and suppress inflammation in conditions such as interstitial cystitis, post-herpetic neuralgia, ulcerative colitis and experimental colitis, following repeated topical applications.[83-88] The lidocaine patch has been specifically approved by the Food and Drug Administration for treatment of post-herpetic neuralgia, a 'model' neuropathic pain syndrome where a majority of patients have allodynia.[89] The neuro-inflammatory state found in vulval vestibulitis may be analogous to the 'irritable nociceptor (pain fibre)' found in post-herpetic neuralgia.[90] In terms of mechanism, lidocaine may act 'locally' to block the neuro-inflammatory process through a number of mechanisms including a reduced release of IL-1β.[88] Topical lidocaine has been found to be well tolerated at the squamomucosal junction of the lower genital tract. The predominant adverse effect is transient burning upon application, resulting in a 1–2% cessation of use.[91] The immediate analgesic effect of topical lidocaine, although different from the long-term anti-inflammatory effect described above, may additionally improve adherence to treatment.

Treatment of chronic pain conditions, such as vulval vestibulitis, through a combined 'central' and 'peripheral' approach is intuitively attractive. In an open-label study in 53 vestibulitis patients, we found 71% became fully asymptomatic or sexually functional with minimal pain with combined desipramine and topical lidocaine therapy compared with a 50% response using desipramine alone.[91] The median effective dose of desipramine was 150 mg daily. Reported adverse effects included constipation, dry mouth, nervousness, dizziness and somnolence in decreasing order of frequency with a treatment drop-out rate of 25%. The most common adverse effect, which resulted in discontinuation, was the complaint of 'nervousness'. After cessation of desipramine, two-thirds of cases continued to report pain relief for at least six months.

Surgical treatment of 'localised' vulval dysaesthesia (vulval vestibulitis)

A compiled analysis of surgical case series of vulval vestibulitis cases who underwent perineoplasty found 89% of 646 women with a 'significant decrease in pain' (complete response plus partial response).[92] We found similar favourable long-term outcomes (greater than 48 months) for perineoplasty with 51 of 93 women (54.8%) 'asymptomatic', 31 (33.3%) 'minimally symptomatic', seven (7.5%) 'unchanged', and four of the 93 women (4.3%) 'worse'.[93] Differences in surgical success across subgroups for age, parity, duration of symptoms, type of pathology, degree of partner support, psychiatric history, sexual abuse history and the patient's opinion of the postoperative appearance did not achieve statistical significance. Other than the percentage of patients who failed to have improvement of pain 11 of the 93 women (11.8%), the major postoperative complication rate was low, with only one patient (1.1%) reporting anal sphincter weakness. No patient variable studied predicted surgical success in correcting vulval vestibulitis.

Decompressive, infiltrative ablative options for neuralgia

Published data on technique and therapeutic outcome of various decompressive operations for pudendal, ilio-inguinal and sacral nerve root compression are limited to collections of case reports.[42,94] Small series on surgical management of sacromeningeal (Tarlov's) cysts have also been published.[37,38] For pudendal neuralgia, computerised tomography-guided infiltration with anaesthetic–cortisone combinations have been reported to be effective in selected cases.[94] Although local phenol injection and radio-ablation of the pudendal nerve have been clinically performed, published outcomes are not available. Particularly with injection of caustic agents such as phenol, concern must be raised with uncontrolled spread of the caustic effect into the region of the sacral plexus.

Future directions for therapy

Before industry-funded research is likely to proceed, researchers will need to clearly answer the questions of prevalence, proportions of subsets and long-term morbidity of chronic vulval pain. At the present time, research on prevalence funded by the National Institutes of Health is under way.

Local cytokine antagonism

Systemic administration of the anti-inflammatory cytokine IL-10 has been found to be well tolerated in humans, to suppress the pro-inflammatory cytokines, IL1-β and TNF-α, and, after intralesional injection, to provide prolonged symptomatic improvement of psoriasis. Huhn et al.[95] studied healthy volunteers who underwent a single intravenous bolus. Flu-like symptoms, headache, myalgias, fever and chills occurred only with the highest dose (100 μg/kg). IL-1β production was markedly suppressed (from 17% to 49%) at two hours and suppression extended to 48 hours at higher doses (from 25 μg/kg to 100 μg/kg). Inhibition of TNF-α was observed for at least 12 hours and TNF-α synthesis was suppressed at the highest dose (100 μg/kg) for more than 24 hours. In a second study, Huhn et al.[96] found pronounced suppression of lipopolysaccharide-induced TNF-α for more than 12 hours and of IL-1β for more than 24 hours. Asadullah et al.[97] found significantly lower levels of IL-10 mRNA in psoriatic skin in contrast to atopic dermatitis and mycosis fungoides. Treatment of psoriatic patients with IL-10 produced no adverse effects and all patients reported loss of skin itching. Loss of itching and a significant reduction in TNF-α extended beyond four days after cessation of IL-10 therapy. Treatment options for cytokine antagonism include antibodies to TNF-α. The injection of neutralising antibodies to TNF-α (specifically to TNF receptor-1) produces a reduction of mechanical hyperalgesia after chronic constriction nerve injury.[62] Several anti-TNF-α products are under study in humans.

Modulation of central sensitisation at the dorsal horn

The best known NMDA receptor antagonist in clinical use is ketamine, a 'dissociative' anaesthetic/analgesic. Ketamine has been used clinically for neuro-inflammation in the treatment of post-herpetic and post-traumatic neuralgia.[98,99] The use of ketamine in cases of trigeminal neuralgia found an NMDA-dependent and an NMDA-independent pattern of response.[100] Ketamine, and the shorter-acting NMDA receptor antagonist phencyclidine ('angel dust') are known for their hallucinatory adverse effects and abuse potential. Selective NMDA NR2B antagonists, such as ifenprodil, have been developed to exploit the benefits of anti-nociception combined with a reduced adverse effect profile. Earlier clinical reports focused on the utility of ifenprodil in elderly individuals with arterial occlusive disease, demonstrating enhanced walking distance and improved quality of life.[101,102]

Implantable nerve stimulation for pudendal neuralgia

Sub-chronic, implantable sacral nerve root stimulation (Interstim®, Medtronic, Inc.) has been approved by the Food and Drug Adminstration for the management of severe urgency/frequency disorders of the bladder. Following release, interest has developed in the use of the Interstim device for difficult neuropathies such as pudendal neuralgia.[103] The technique of S1 to S4 trans-foramenal stimulation requires patience and a significant time for precise positioning. Early experience using the technique has been favourable in terms of pain relief. Problematically, the trans-foramenal leads tend to migrate away from the point of effective stimulation with body movement.

Botulinum toxin therapy for levator syndrome (circumvaginal muscle spasm)

Botulinum toxin A (Botox®, Allergan, Inc.) has been reported to relieve myofascial neck, and upper back pain in two double-blind studies.[104,105] Botulinum toxin has also been shown to permit spontaneous healing of chronic anal fissures in a dose–response fashion, particularly when injection is directed towards the external anal sphincter. Long-term follow-up, however finds a significant recurrence rate of chronic anal fissures associated with recovery of sphincter tonus. Clinical use for disorders of pelvic floor musculature, such as levator syndrome, vaginismus or proctalgia fugax has not yet been published. Because the levator muscles are situated deep from the perineal surface, botulinum toxin injection may be facilitated by electromyographic guidance of injection.[106]

Future research issues: development of outcome measures for clinical trials research in genital pain

Outcome measures remain problematic for clinical trials of chronic vulval pain because of a relative deficiency of easily administered, clinically relevant, quantifiable, reliable and valid measures of pain and sexual dysfunction. Three categories of outcome measures for generic pain research include the visual analogue scale (VAS), psychometric testing and quantitative sensory threshold (QST) testing. The VAS is considered one of the best methods with which to assess pain response to therapy. Reliability and validity testing has been demonstrated in many studies.[107,108] However, controversy remains as to what degree of numerical change should be considered a 'clinical response', in terms of VAS.[109,110] The standard threshold of 50% relief of pain (50% reduction of VAS) has generally become accepted as minimal evidence of clinical response, in spite of lack of trials to evaluate validity. In terms of primary outcome variables, the VAS-based 'global pain scale' has become an accepted standard through widely published randomised clinical trials in post-herpetic neuralgia, diabetic neuropathy and human immunodeficiency virus-related peripheral neuropathy.[81,82]

Multidimensional psychometric tests may provide a more comprehensive assessment of the pain and sexual dysfunction than the simple VAS. Psychometric measures including the Brief Symptom Inventory, the Sexual Opinion Survey and the Locke Wallace Adjustment Scale have compared vulvar vestibulitis to other forms of dyspareunia and to normal controls in cross-sectional studies.[8,10] Vulval vestibulitis did not differ significantly from controls on psychological symptomatology. On indices of sexual functioning, vulval vestibulitis cases showed a lower overall level of sexual functioning, lower sexual desire, lower frequencies of intercourse, lower ability to achieve orgasm with penetration or oral genital contact, and were significantly more 'erotophobic' than controls. However, use of these instruments as outcome measures has been criticised as unsuitable for repeated measures analysis.

The vulval algesiometer, developed by Curnow et al.,[111] provides QST tracking of pain intensity, particularly in terms of response to therapy. A pilot study of 25 vulval vestibulitis cases tested four sites of the vulval vestibule, before and after therapy.[112] Algesiometer scores were calculated by adding the maximally tolerated pulse without pain at the four anatomic sites of the vestibule. 'Clinically improved' cases reported a pretreatment median score of 21/32 and a post-treatment median score of 32/32, a difference that was statistically significant. In contrast, 'clinically unimproved' cases reported median of 18/32 post-treatment. The major criticism concerning QST techniques, in general, concerns the clinical relevance of 'improvement' in QST. Thus, similar to the VAS score, QST may be best interpreted within the context of patient 'satisfaction with outcome'.

Conclusion

It is hoped that this review of chronic vulval pain will provide both a background for clinicians and stimulate the interest of researchers. A further 'basic science' understanding of pain and novel forms of therapy is needed for women suffering with chronic vulval pain. Perhaps some of the suggested therapeutic directions may spur interest in future clinical trials.

References

1.   Ridley CM. Vulvodynia, Theory and management. *Dermatol Clin* 1998;**16**:775–8.
2.   Masheb RM, Nash JM, Brondolo E, Kerns RD. Vulvodynia: an introduction and critical review of a chronic pain condition. *Pain* 2000;**86**:3–10.
3.   McKay M. Vulvodynia: a multifactorial problem. *Arch Dermatol* 1989;**125**:256–62.
4.   Moyal-Barracco M, Leibowitch M, Orth G. Vestibular papillae of the vulva. Lack of evidence for human papillomavirus etiology. *Arch Dermatol* 1990;**126**:1594–8.
5.   Foster DC. Personal communication.
6.   Goetsch MF. Vulvar vestibulitis: prevalence and historic features in a general gynecologic practice population. *Am J Obstet Gynecol* 1991;**164**:1609–14.
7.   Laumann EO, Paik A, Rosen RC. Sexual dysfunction in the United States: prevalence and predictors. *JAMA* 1999;**281**:537–44.
8.   Meana M, Binik YM, Khalife S, Cohen DR. Biopsychosocial profile of women with dyspareunia. *Obstet Gynecol* 1997;**90**:583–9.
9.   Meana M, Binik YM, Khalife S, Cohen DR. Dyspareunia: sexual dysfunction or pain syndrome? *J Nervous Mental Dis* 1977;**185**:561–9.
10. Meana M, Binik YM, Khalife S, Cohen DR. Affect and marital adjustment rating of dyspareunic pain. *Can J Psychol* 1998;**43**:381–5.
11. Reissing ED, Binik YM, Khalife S. Does vaginismus exist? A critical review of the literature. *J Nervous Mental Dis* 1999;**187**:261–74.
12. Heller DS, Randolph P, Young A, Tancer ML, Fromer D. The cutaneous-vulvar clinic revisited: a 5 year experience of the Columbia Presbyterian Medical Center Cutaneous-Vulvar Service. *Dermatology* 1997;**195**:26–9.
13. Friedrich EG. Vulvar vestibulitis syndrome. *J Reprod Med* 1987;**32**:110–14.
14. Peckham BM, Maki DG, Patterson JJ, Hafez GR. Focal vulvitis: A characteristic syndrome and cause of dyspareunia. *Am J Obstet Gynecol* 1986;**154**:855–64.
15. Mann MS, Kaufman RH, Brown D, Adam E. Vulvar vestibulitis: significant clinical variables and treatment outcomes. *Obstet Gynecol* 1992;**79**:122–5.
16. Bazin S, Bouchard C, Brisson J, Morin C, Meisels A, Fortier M. Vulvar vestibulitis syndrome: an exploratory case-control study. *Obstet Gynecol* 1994;**83**:47–50.
17. Foster DC. Case–control study of vulvar vestibulitis. *J Women's Health* 1995;**6**:677–80.
18. Morrison GD, Adams S, Curnow JS, Parsons RJ, Sargeant P, Frost TAA. A preliminary study of topical ketoconazole in vulvar vestibulitis syndrome. *J Dermatol Treat* 1996;**7**:219–21.
19. Foster DC. Unpublished data.
20. Foster DC, Hasday JD Elevated tissue levels of inflammatory cytokines: Interleukin 1 beta and tumor necrosis factor alpha in vulvar vestibulitis. *Obstet Gynecol* 1997;**89**:291–5.

21. Westrom LV, Willen R. Vestibular nerve fiber proliferation in vulvar vestibulitis syndrome. *Obstet Gynecol* 1998;**91**:572–6.

22. Karanth SS, Springall DR, Kuhn DM, Levene MM, Polak JM. An immunocytochemical study of cutaneous innervation and the distribution of neuropeptides and protein gene product 9.5 in man and commonly employed laboratory animals. *Am J Anat* 1991;**191**:369–83.

23. Bohm-Starke N, Hilliges M, Falconer C, Rylander E. Neurochemical characterization of the vestibular nerves in women with vulvar vestibulitis syndrome. *Gynecol Obstet Invest* 1999;**48**:270–75.

24. Herrmann DN, Griffin JW, Hauer P, Cornblath DR, McArthur JC. Epidermal nerve fiber density and sural nerve morphometry in peripheral neuropathies. *Neurology* 1999;**53**:1634–40.

25. Xu J, Pollock CH, Kajander KC. Chromic gut suture reduces calcitonin-gene-related peptide and substance P levels in the spinal cord following chronic constriction injury in the rat. *Pain* 1996;**64**:503–9.

26. Reddy S. Foster DC, Phipps R. Difference in cytokine and PGE$_2$ production between vulvar and vestibular fibroblasts. Abstract#377, 48th Annual Meeting of Society for Gynecologic Investigation, Toronto, CA. 2001. (Submitted for publication).

27. Hurme M, Lahdenpohja N, Santtila S. Gene polymorphisms of interleukins 1 and 10 in infectious and autoimmune diseases. *Ann Med* 1998;**30**:469–73.

28. Perrier S, Coussediere C, Dubost JJ, Albuisson E, Sauvezie B. IL-1 receptor antagonist (IL-1RA) gene polymorphism in Sjogren's syndrome and rheumatoid arthritis. *Clin Immun Innumopathol* 1998;**87**:309–13.

29. Jeremias J, Ledger WJ, Witkin SS. Interleukin 1 receptor antagonist gene polymorphism in women with vulvar vestibulitis. *Am J Obstet Gynecol* 2000;**182**:283–5.

30. Santtila S, Savinainen K, Hurme M. Presence of the IL-RA allele 2 (IL1RN*2) is associated with enhanced IL-1 beta production *in vitro. Scand J Immunol* 1998;**47**:195–8.

31. Sangwan YP, Coller JA, Barrett MS, Murray JJ, Roberts PL, Schoetz DJ. Unilateral pudendal neuropathy. Significance and implications. *Dis Colon Rectum* 1996;**39**:249–51.

32. Alevizon SJ, Finan MA. Sacrospinous colpopexy: management of postoperative pudendal nerve entrapment. *Obstet Gynecol* 1996;**88**:713–15.

33. Benson T, McClellan E. The effect of vaginal dissection on the pudendal nerve. *Obstet Gynecol* 1993;**82**:387–9.

34. Jorge JM, Wexner SD, Ehrenpreis ED, Nogueras JJ, Jagelman DG. Does perineal descent correlate with pudendal neuropathy? *Dis Colon Rectum* 1993;**36**:475–83.

35. Monga M, Ghoniem G. Ilioinguinal nerve entrapment following needle bladder suspension procedures. *Urology* 1994;**44**:447–50.

36. Miyazaki F, Shook G. Ilioinguinal nerve entrapment during needle suspension for stress incontinence. *Obstet Gynecol* 1992;**80**:246–8.

37. Van de Kleft E, Van Vyve M. Chronic perineal pain related to sacral meningeal cysts. *Neurosurgery* 1991;**29**:223–6.

38. Davis SW, Levy LM, LeBihan DJ, Rajan S, Schellinger D. Sacral meningeal cysts: evaluation with MR imaging. *Radiology* 1993;**187**:445–8.

39. Hagen NA. Sharp, shooting neuropathic pain in the rectum or genitals: pudendal neuralgia. *J Pain Symptom Management* 1993;**8**:496–501.

40. Selby G. Diseases of the fifth cranial nerve. In: Dyck PJ, Thomas PK, Lambert FH, Bunge R, editors. *Peripheral Neuropathy*, 2nd edn. Philadelphia: WB Saunders, 1984, p. 1256–9.

41. Amarenco G, Le Cocquen-Amarenco A, Kerdraon J, Lacroix P, Abda MA, Lanoe Y. Les nervalgies perinales. *Press Med* 1991;**20**:71–4.

42. Mauillon J, Thoumas D, Leroi AM, Freger P, Michot F, Denis P. Results of pudendal nerve neurolysis transposition in twelve patients suffering from pudendal neuralgia. *Dis Colon Rectum* 1999;**42**:186–92.

43. Glazer HI, Jantos M, Hartmann EH, Swencionis C. Electromyographic comparisons of the pelvic floor in women with dysesthetic vulvodynia and asymptomatic women. *J Reprod Med* 1998;**43**:959–62.

44. Foster DC, Robinson JC, Davis KM. Urethral pressure variation in women with vulvar vestibulitis. *Am J Obstet Gynecol* 1993;**169**:107–12.

45. Eckardt VF, Dodt O, Kanzler G, Bernhard G. Anorectal function and morphology in patients with sporadic proctalgia fugax. *Dis Colon Rectum* 1996;**39**:755–62.

46. Kennedy ML, Sowter S, Nguyen H, Lubowski DZ. Glyceryl trinitrate ointment for the treatment of chronic anal fissure: results of a placebo controlled trial and long-term follow-up. *Dis Colon Rectum* 1999;**42**:1000–1006.

47. Dorfman G. Levitt M, Platell C. Treatment of chronic anal fissure with topical glyceryl trinitrate. *Dis Colon Rectum* 1999;**42**:1007–10.

48. Minguez M, Melo F, Espi A, Garcia-Granero E, Mora F, Lledo S, *et al.* Therapeutic effects of different doses of botulinum toxin in chronic anal fissure. *Dis Colon Rectum* 1999;**42**:1016–21.

49. Fukuoka H, Kawatani M, Hisamitsu T, Takeshige C. Cutaneous hyperalgesia induced by peripheral injection of interleukin-1beta in the rat. *Brain Res* 1994;**657**:133–40.

50. Sundy JS, Patel DD, Haynes BF. Cytokines in normal and pathogenic inflammatory responses. In: Gallin JI, Snyderman R, editors. *Inflammation: Basic Principles and Clinical Correlates.* Philadelphia: Lippincott, Williams and Wilkins; 1999. p. 433–41.

51. Probert L, Akassoaglou K, Pasparakis M, Kontogeorgos G, Kollias G. Spontaneous inflammatory demyelinating disease in transgenic mice showing central nervous system-specific expression of tumor necrosis factor alpha. *Proc Natl Acad Sci USA* 1995;**92**:11294–8.

52. Selmaj KW, Raine CS. Tumor necrosis factor mediates myelin and oligodendrocyte damage *in vitro. Ann Neurol* 1988;**23**:339–46.

53. Soliven B, Szuchet S. Signal transduction pathways in oligodendrocytes: role of tumor necrosis factor-alpha. *Int J Dev Neurosci* 1995;**13**:351–67.

54. Poole S, Cunha FQ, Selkirk S, Lorenzetti BB, Ferreira SH. Cytokine-mediated inflammatory hyperalgesia limited by interleukin-10. *Br J Pharmacol* 1995;**115**:684–8.

55. Oyen WJ, Arntz IE, Claessens RM, Van der Meer JW, Corstens FH, Goris RJ. Reflex sympathetic dystrophy of the hand:an excessive inflammatory response? *Pain* 1993;**55**:151–7.

56. Wagner R, Myers RR. Endoneural injection of TNF-alpha produces neuropathic pain behaviors. *Neuro Report* 1996;**7**:2897–901.

57. Sorkin LS, Xiao WH, Wagner R, Myers RR. Tumor necrosis factor alpha induces ectopic activity in nociceptive primary afferent fibers. *Neuroscience* 1997;**81**:255–62.

58. Kagan BL, Baldwin RL, Munoz D, Wisnieski BJ. Formation of ion permeable channels by tumor necrosis factor alpha. *Science* 1992;**255**:1427–30.

59. Bennett GJ, Xie YK. A peripheral neuropathy in rat that produces disorders of pain sensation like those seen in man. *Pain* 1988;**33**:87–107.

60. Seltzer Z, Dubner R, Shir Y. A novel behavioral model of neuropathic pain disorders produced in rats by partial sciatic nerve injury. *Pain* 1990;**43**:205–18.

61. Kim SH, Chung JM. An experimental model for peripheral neuropathy produced by segmental spinal nerve ligation in the rat. *Pain* 1992;**50**:355–63.

62. Sommer C, Schmidt C, George A. Hyperalgesia in experimental neuropathy is dependent on the TNF receptor 1. *Exp Neurol* 1998;**151**:138–42.

63. Conte B, Maggi CA, Giachetti A, Parlani M, Lopez G, Manzini S. Intraurethral capsaicin produces reflex activation of the striated urethral sphincter in urethane-anesthetized male rats. *J Urol* 1993;**150**:271–77.

64. Woodruff JD, Parmley TH. Infection of the minor vestibular gland. *Obstet Gynecol* 1983;**62**:609–12.

65. Sarrel PM, Steege JF, Maltzer M, Bolinsky D. Pain during sex response due to occlusion of the Bartholin's gland duct. *Obstet Gynecol* 1983;**62**:261–4.

66. Friedrich E. Therapeutic studies on vulvar vestibulitis. *J Reprod Med* 1988;**33**:514–18.

67. Stewart DE, Whelan CI, Fong IW, Tessler KM. Psychosocial aspects of chronic, clinically unconfirmed vulvovaginitis. *Obstet Gynecol* 1990;**76**:852–6.

68. Solomons CC, Melmed MH, Heitler SM. Calcium citrate for vulvar vestibulitis: a case report. *J Reprod Med* 1991;**36**:879–82.

69. McKay M. Dysesthetic ('essential') vulvodynia: Treatment with amitriptyline. *J Reprod Med* 1993;**38**:9–13.

70. Marinoff SC, Turner ML, Hirsch RP, Richard G. Intralesional alpha interferon: cost-effective therapy for vulvar vestibulitis syndrome. *J Reprod Med* 1993;**38**:19–24.

71. Bornstein J, Pascal B, Abramovici H. Intramuscular beta-interferon for severe vulvar vestibulitis. *J Reprod Med* 1993;**38**:117–20.

72. Baldessarini RJ. Drugs and the treatment of psychiatric disorders. In: Gilman A, Rall TW, Nies AS, Taylor P, editors. *The Pharmacologic Basis of Therapeutics.* Elmsford, NY: Pergamon Press Inc.; 1990. p. 408.

73. Max MB, Culnane M, Schafer SC, Gracely RH, Walther DJ, Smoller B, *et al.* Amitriptyline relieves diabetic neuropathy pain in patients with normal or depressed mood. *Neurology* 1987;**37**:589–96.

74. Max MB, Schafer SC, Culnane M, Smoller B, Dubner R, Gracely RH. Amitriptyline but not lorazepam relieves postherpetic neuralgia. *Neurology* 1988;**38**:1427–32.

75. Sindrup SH, Gram LF, Skjold T, Grodum E, Brosen K, Beck-Nielsen H. Clomipramine vs. desipramine vs. placebo in the treatment of diabetic neuropathy symptoms: a double blind cross-over study. *Br J Clin Pharmacol* 1990;**30**:683–91.

76. Max MB, Kishore-Kumar R, Schafer SC, Meister B, Gracely RH, Smoller B, *et al.* Efficacy of desipramine in painful diabetic neuropathy: a placebo controlled trial. *Pain* 1991;**45**:3–9.

77. Max MB, Lynch SA, Muir J, Shoaf SE, Smoller B, Dubner R. Effects of desipramine, amitriptyline, and fluoxetine on pain in diabetic neuropathy. *N Engl J Med* 1992;**326**:1250–56.

78. Watson CP, Chipman M, Reed K, Evans RJ, Birkett N. Amitryptyline versus maprotiline in postherpetic neuralgia: a randomized double blind crossover trial. *Pain* 1992;**48**:29–36.

79. Leijon G, Boivie J. Central post-stroke pain – a controlled trial of amitriptyline and carbamazine. *Pain* 1989;**36**:27–36.

80. Pagano R. Vulvar vestibulitis syndrome: an often unrecognized cause of dyspareunia. *Aust N Z J Obstet Gynaecol* 1999;**39**:79–83.

81. Rowbotham M, Harden N, Stacey B, Bernstein P, Mangus-Miller L, for the Gabapentin Postherpetic Neuralgia Study Group. Gabapentin for the treatment of post-herpetic neuralgia, a randomized controlled trial. *JAMA* 1998;**280**:1837–42.

82. Backonja M, Beydoun A, Edwards KR, Schwartz SL, Fonseca V, Hes M, LaMoreaux L, Garofalo E, for the Gabapentin Diabetic Neuropathy Study Group. Gabapentin for the symptomatic treatment of painful neuropathy in patients with diabetes mellitus, a randomized controlled trial. *JAMA* 1998;**280**:1831–6.

83. Asklin B, Cassuto J. Intravesical lidocaine in severe interstitial cystitis. Case report. *Scand J Urol Nephrol* 1989;**23**:311–12.

84. Bjorck S, Dahlstrom A, Johansson L, Ahlman H. Treatment of the mucosa with local anaesthetics in ulcerative colitis. *Agents Actions Special Conference Issue* 1992;C60–C72.

85. McCafferty DM, Sharkey KA, Wallace JL. Beneficial effects of local or systemic lidocaine in experimental colitis. *Am J Physiol* 1994;**266**:G560–G567.

86. Li Y, Wingrove DE, Too HP, Marnerakis M, Stimson ER, Strichartz GR, *et al.* Local anesthetics inhibit substance P binding and evoked increases in intracellular Ca^{2+}. *Anesthesiology* 1995;**82**:166–73.

87. Rowbotham MC, Davies PS, Verkempinck CV, Galer BS. Lidocaine patch: double-blind controlled study of a new treatment method for post-herpetic neuralgia. *Pain* 1996;**65**:39–44.

88. Sinclair R, Eriksson AS, Gretzer C, Cassuto J, Thomsen P. Inhibitory effects of amide local anaesthetics on stimulus-induced human leukocyte metabolic activation, LTB4 release and IL-1 secretion *in vitro*. *Acta Anaesthesiol Scand* 1993;**37**:159–65.

89. Galer BS, Rowbotham MC, Perander J, Friedman E. Topical lidocaine patch relieves postherpetic neuralgia more effectively than a vehicle topical patch: results of an enriched enrollment study. *Pain* 1999;**80**:533–8.

90. Rowbotham MC, Fields HL. Post-herpetic neuralgia the relation of pain complaint, sensory disturbance, and skin temperature. *Pain* 1989;**39**:129–44.

91. Foster DC, Duguid KM. Open label study of oral amitriptyline and topical lidocaine for the treatment of vulvar vestibulitis. *Abstract, International Conference on Mechanism and Treatment of Neuropathic Pain*. Rochester, NY, 1998.

92. Bornstein J, Zarfati D, Goldik Z, Abramovici H. Vulvar vestibulitis: physical or psychosocial problem? *Obstet Gynecol* 1999;**93**:876–80.

93. Foster DC, Butts C, Woodruff JD. Long-term outcome of perineoplasty for vulvar vestibulitis. *J Women's Health* 1995;**6**:669–75.

94. Pisani R, Stubinski R, Datti R. Entrapment neuropathy of the internal pudendal nerve, report of two cases. *Scand J Urol Nephrol* 1997;**31**:407–10.

95. Huhn RD, Radwanski E, O'Connell SM, Sturgill MG, Clarke L, Cody RP, Affrime MB, Cutler DL. Pharmacokinetics and immunomodulatory properties of intravenously administered recombinant human interleukin 10 in healthy volunteers. *Blood* 1996;**87**:699–705.

96. Huhn RD, Radwanski E, Gallo J, Affrime MB, Sabo R, Gonyo G, *et al.* Pharmacodynamics of subcutaneous recombinant human interleukin-10 in healthy volunteers. *Clin Pharmacol Ther* 1997;**62**:171–80.

97. Asadullah K, Sterry W, Stephanek K, Jasulaitis D, Leupold M, Audring H, *et al.* IL-10 is a key cytokine in psoriasis. Proof of principle by IL-10 therapy: a new therapeutic approach. *J Clin Invest* 1998;**101**:783–94.

98. Eide PK, Stubhaug A, Oye I, Breivik H. Continuous subcutaneous administration of the N-methyl-D-aspartic acid (NMDA) receptor antagonist ketamine in the treatment of post-herpetic neuralgia. *Pain* 1995;**61**:221–8.

99. Max MB, Byas-Smith MG, Gracely RH, Bennett GJ. Intravenous infusion of the NMDA antagonist, ketamine, in chronic post-traumatic pain with allodynia: a double-blind comparison to alfentanil and placebo. *Clin Neuropharmacol* 1995;**18**:360–68.

100. Rabben T, Skjelbred P, Oye I. Prolonged analgesic effect of ketamine, an N-methyl-D-aspartate receptor inhibitor, in patients with chronic pain. *J Pharm Exp Therap* 1999;**289**:1060–66.

101. Branchereau A, Rouffy J. [Double blind randomized controlled trial of ifenprodil tartrate versus placebo in chronic arterial occlusive disease in the legs at stage II of the Leriche and Fontaine classification.] (in French). *Journal des Maladies Vasculaires* 1995;**20**:21–7.

102. Marquis P, Lecasble M, Passa P. [Quality of life of patient with peripheral arterial obliterative disease treated with ifenprodil tartrate. Results of an ARTEMIS study] (in French). *Drug* 1998;**56** suppl. 13:37–48.

103. Lou L. Uncommon areas of electrical stimulation for pain relief. *Curr Rev Pain* 2000;**4**:407–12.

104. Cheshire WP, Abashian SW, Mann JD. Botulinum toxin in the treatment of myofascial pain syndrome. *Pain* 1994;**59**:65–9.

105. Wheeler AH, Goolkasian P, Gretz SS. A randomized double-blind prospective pilot study of botulinum toxin injection for refractory, unilateral, cervicothroacic, paraspinal, myofascial pain syndrome. *Spine* 1998;**23**:1662–7.

106. Finsterer J, Fuchs I, Mamoli B. Automatic EMG-guided botulinum toxin treatment of spasticity. *Clin Neuropharmacol* 1997;**20**:195–203.

107. Joyce CR, Zutshi DW, Hrubes V, Mason RM. Comparison of fixed interval and visual analog scale for rating chronic pain. *Eur J Clin Pharmacol* 1975;**8**:415–20.

108. Scott J, Huskisson EC. Graphic representation of pain. *Pain* 1976;**2**:175–84.

109. Seres JL. The fallacy of using 50% pain relief as a standard for satisfactory pain treatment outcome. *Pain Forum* 1999;**8**:183–8.

110. North RB. The glass is half full. *Pain Forum* 1999;**8**:195–7.

111. Curnow JS, Barron L, Morrison G, Sergeant P. Vulval algesiometer. *Med Biol Eng Comput* 1996;**34**:266–9.

112. Eva LJ, Reid WM, MacLean AB, Morrison GD. Assessment of response to treatment in vulvar vestibulitis syndrome by means of the vulvar algesiometer. *Am J Obstet Gynecol* 1999;**181**:99–102.

Chapter 18

Abdominal pain

Peter J. Whorwell

The vast majority of patients presenting to both general practitioners and gastroenterologists with chronic abdominal pain are suffering from irritable bowel syndrome (IBS). Furthermore, because the condition is so common, it accounts for an extremely large number of consultations, both in the primary- and secondary-care settings. Organic causes need to be considered and ruled out, but unfortunately this approach has led to the tradition of diagnosing the condition by a process of exclusion. Thus, patients can often be subjected to a wide range of negative investigations, only to be told there is nothing wrong with them and it must just be IBS. Not only does this trivialise the diagnosis; it also leaves the patient with the concept that they must be imagining the condition in some way, especially as IBS is often thought of as a purely 'psychosomatic' illness.

It is far better to attempt to diagnose the condition positively and only undertake investigation when necessary. Thus, a young person presenting with the classic symptoms of abdominal pain (any location), abdominal distension and a disturbed bowel habit (constipation, diarrhoea or alternating) with no family history of inflammatory bowel disease or cancer needs little investigation initially, and it is entirely reasonable to treat on the basis of symptoms. 'Alarm' symptoms, such as rectal bleeding or persistent watery diarrhoea (the diarrhoea of IBS is usually loose rather than watery), should obviously be investigated further. Somewhat surprisingly, the intensity of pain should not necessarily raise doubts about the diagnosis as in some cases this can be extremely severe.

Some years ago, a consensus working party met in Rome in order to try and improve the definition of functional gastrointestinal disorders. This led to the production of the Rome diagnostic criteria for IBS, which were updated in 1999 and are usually referred to as the Rome II Criteria.[1] Such criteria are extremely useful for research purposes, where they ensure homogeneity of patients entering various studies. However, they have so far not been widely adopted in clinical practice and there are some concerns that they may be somewhat too restrictive for routine work.

IBS is associated with a number of other symptoms that are critically important from both a management and a diagnostic point of view.[2] These consist of nausea, early satiety, backache, lethargy and urinary symptoms, and it has been shown that the presence of one or more of these features helps to substantiate the diagnosis of IBS even further.[3] In addition, women with IBS often complain of dyspareunia,[1] but the pain is more reminiscent of their IBS pain and quite often arises some time after intercourse, even the next day. It has also been shown that this problem can have a profound effect on the patient's sexual function.[4] The presence of multiple symptoms in these patients is often interpreted as meaning that they are either psychologically disturbed or hypersensitive to pain in some way. There is no doubt that patients attending secondary-care facilities with IBS tend to exhibit a high prevalence of psychopathology. However, it has also been shown that non-complaining patients in the community do not show this trend, which suggests that the presence of psychopathology makes them consult but does not necessarily cause their problem in the first place.[5,6] Furthermore, because IBS tends to be regarded as a 'psychological' disorder, this serves to cause considerable frustration in the patient when they are constantly confronted with explanations for their problems which have a strong psychological flavour. With regard to pain sensitivity, it has been shown that patients with IBS do undoubtedly tend to exhibit visceral hypersensitivity (see below), particularly when this is assessed by balloon distension techniques. However, this should not necessarily lead to the conclusion that these patients have a generally low pain threshold, as it has been shown that patients with IBS paradoxically tend to have a better tolerance of somatic pain than healthy controls.[7]

The aetiology of IBS remains unclear but it seems likely that there is a genetic predisposition to the disorder which becomes manifest when such an individual meets one or more triggering factors. These are probably numerous but well-recognised events and include infections such as gastroenteritis, antibiotics, abdominal surgery and stress.

From a pathophysiological point of view, hypersensitivity of the gut (visceral hypersensitivity) is thought to be important.[8] Although this probably occurs throughout the whole gastrointestinal tract,[9] it is most conveniently measured in the rectum by a variety of balloon distension techniques. The traditional hypothesis that IBS represents some form of motility disorder is no longer fashionable. However, this does not necessarily mean that contractions should be ignored, as in the presence of hypersensitivity even normal amplitude contractions may be sensed as excessively painful. It is also extremely likely that the central nervous system plays an important role in the perception of gastrointestinal physiological function and with the advent of functional magnetic resonance imaging, this concept is currently being actively explored.

A positive approach to diagnosing IBS with minimal investigation has been shown to be remarkably robust, with little fear of serious disease being missed.[10] However, because of the polysymptomatology of the disorder, there is a considerable risk of these patients being referred to other specialties where the diagnosis may be overlooked with the potential for multiple, often unnecessary, investigations and possibly even inappropriate interventions, especially of a surgical nature. To assess this aspect, we have assessed the prevalence of IBS in urological[11] and gynaecological[12] outpatients and found there to be a considerable excess of this disorder in such patients. This would suggest that patients with pain from their IBS who happen, for instance, to have menstrual problems, may be referred to a gynaecological rather than a gastroenterological clinic. Furthermore, if dyspareunia is also present, this might make this route of referral even more likely to happen. We also have previously shown that up to 50% of patients with IBS have urodynamic abnormalities[13] in addition to an excess of urinary symptoms.[2] Thus, it is hardly surprising that referral to urologists is also a frequent observation, with those suffering from unexplained loin pain and bladder symptoms most likely to be referred this way. Anecdotally, we have additionally seen patients who have had multiple investigations for unexplained back problems who have sometimes had questionable surgical interventions.

The importance of identifying IBS in the gynaecological setting is extremely high, not only because it may prevent unnecessary surgery but also because such surgery possibly exacerbates the underlying IBS symptoms.[14-18] We have shown, not surprisingly, that the prevalence of IBS in the gynaecological clinic varies considerably, depending on the reason for the referral.[12] For instance, it is relatively low in patients presenting with cervical abnormalities but is most frequently observed in those with abdominal pain. We have also prospectively examined the one-year outcome of patients referred to a gynaecological clinic with abdominal pain.[19] IBS was relatively rare in patients in whom a definitive gynaecological diagnosis was made, whereas in the remainder it was much more common. In addition, the prognosis in those patients with IBS was much worse than in their gynaecological counterparts, with their problems remaining unresolved after one year. These results strongly suggest that a large component of their problem emanated from their bowel rather their gynaecological system. Thus, undoubtedly, IBS patients are finding their way into gynaecological outpatient departments where they are at risk of a poor outcome. The question of whether patients with a gynaecological cause of their pain are being referred to, and possibly overlooked, in gastroenterological clinics, has not been well addressed. It seems reasonable to assume that there must be considerable overlap in the symptomatology of some gynaecological conditions and IBS and we have some preliminary data to suggest that this is the case, particularly for pelvic inflammatory disease and endometriosis. This raises the issue of whether gastroenterologists should be assessing patients with presumed IBS for potential gynaecological problems. With respect to pelvic inflammatory disease, we have looked at the prevalence of chlamydial antibodies in patients with IBS and normal controls and found no differences.[20] Thus it would appear that this condition is probably not being significantly overlooked. We have also undertaken routine abdominal and pelvic ultrasound investigations in consecutive IBS patients attending the outpatient department and have not found a significant excess of gynaecological problems.[21] However, a report published in 2000, stating that a worrying proportion of patients with ovarian cancer can present with gastrointestinal symptoms,[22] suggested that there is certainly no room for complacency.

Another facet of the overlap between gastrointestinal and gynaecological symptomatology is the role of gender and sex hormones in gastrointestinal physiology. It is a common observation that even normal women experience changes in bowel habit at the time of menses and this appears to be more exaggerated in patients with IBS.[23] The cause of this is not known but is probably more likely to be due to prostaglandin release than to fluctuation in female sex hormones. However, female hormones could well be involved in the changes in rectal sensitivity to balloon distension observed during the menstrual cycle in patients with IBS.[24] Interestingly, this is not seen in normal controls,[25] which suggests that patients with IBS are more susceptible to 'gut sensitising' events for some reason. It is also of interest that females without IBS can exhibit rectal sensitivity following polyethylene glycol-induced diarrhoea, whereas this is not induced in men.[26] This could be interpreted as indicating that the female gender predisposes to sensitisation but additional factors such as genetic predisposition are responsible for its failure to resolve and the subsequent development of IBS.

IBS is more common in females and this has always been taken as indicating some form of predisposition. However, the opposite possibility, that something about being male is protective, also needs to be considered. In 2000, we compared serum testosterone levels in male patients with and without IBS.[27] Although levels were within the normal range in IBS patients, there was a trend for them to be lower than in their healthy counterparts. In addition, luteinising hormone levels were significantly depressed in patients with IBS, suggesting that these changes had a more central origin. Thus, the question of the relationship between male hormones and the development of IBS certainly requires further attention.

The problem of overlap between gynaecological and gastroenterological symptomatology needs continuing evaluation. It would be advantageous if specialists in these two disciplines worked more closely together to ensure that such patients are offered the best possible management.

References

1. Rome II: A multinational consensus document on functional gastrointestinal disorders. *Gut* 1999; **45**: suppl. II.
2. Whorwell PJ, McCallum M, Creed FH, Roberts CT. Non-colonic features of irritable bowel syndrome. *Gut* 1986; **27**:37–40.
3. Maxton Dg, Morris J, Whorwell PJ. More accurate diagnosis of irritable bowel syndrome by the use of non-colonic symptomatology. *Gut* 1991; **32**:784–6.
4. Guthrie E, Creed FH, Whorwell PJ. Severe sexual dysfunction in females with irritable bowel syndrome: a comparison with inflammatory bowel disease and peptic ulceration. *Br Med J* 1987; **295**:577–8.
5. Drossman DA, McKee DC, Sanders RS, Mitchell CM, Cramer EM, Lowman BC, *et al.* Psychosocial factors in the irritable bowel syndrome. *Gastroenterology* 1988; **95**:701–8.
6. Whitehead WE, Bosmajian L, Zanderman AB, Costa PT, Schuster MM. Symptoms of psychologic distress associated with irritable bowel syndrome. *Gastroenterology* 1988; **95**:709–14.
7. Cook JJ, Eeden A, Collins SM. Patients with IBS have greater pain tolerance than normal subjects. *Gastroenterology* 1987; **93**:727–33.
8. Houghton LA, Whorwell PJ. Opening the door of perception in irritable bowel syndrome. *Gut* 1997; **41**:567–8.
9. Francis CY, Houghton LA, Whorwell PJ, Morris J. Enhanced sensitivity of the whole gut in patients with IBS. *Gastroenterology* 1995; **108**:A601.
10. Holmes KM, Salter RH. Irritable bowel syndrome – a safe diagnosis. *BMJ* 1982; **285**:1533–4.
11. Francis CY, Duffy J, Whorwell PJ, Morris J. High prevalence of irritable bowel syndrome in patients attending urological outpatient departments. *Digest Dis Sci* 1997; **42(ii)**:404–7.
12. Prior A, Wilson K, Whorwell PJ, Faragher EB. Irritable bowel syndrome in the gynaecological clinic: a survey of 798 new referrals. *Digest Dis Sci* 1989;**34**:1820–24.
13. Whorwell PJ, Lupton EW, Erduran D, Wilson K. Bladder smooth muscle abnormalities in patients with irritable bowel syndrome. *Gut* 1986;**27**:1014–17.
14. Prior A, Stanley KM, Smith ARB, Read NW. Relation between hysterectomy and the irritable bowel: a prospective study. *Gut* 1992;**33**:814–17.
15. Heaton KW, Parker D, Cripps H. Bowel function and irritable bowel symptoms after hysterectomy and cholecystectomy – a population-based study. *Gut* 1993;**34**:1108–11.
16. Thakar R, Manyonda I, Stanton SL, Clarkson P, Robinson G. Bladder, bowel and sexual function after hysterectomy for benign conditions. *Br J Obstet Gynaecol* 1997;**104**:983–7.
17. Radley S, Keighley MRB, Radley SC, Mann CH. Bowel dysfunction following hysterectomy. *Br J Obstet Gynaecol* 1999;**106**:1120–25.
18. Kelly JL, O'Riordain DS, Jones E, Alawi E, O'Riordain MG, Kirwan WO. The effect of hysterectomy on ano-rectal physiology. *Int J Colorect Dis* 1998;**13**:116–18.
19. Prior A, Whorwell PJ. Gynaecological consultations in patients with irritable bowel syndrome. *Gut* 1989;**30**:996–8.
20. Francis CY, Prior A, Whorwell PJ. Chlamydial infection in irritable bowel syndrome. Is it relevant?

Digestion 1998;**59**:157–9.

21. Francis CY, Martin DF, Whorwell PJ. Does routine ultrasound enhance diagnostic accuracy in irritable bowel syndrome. *Am J Gastroenterol* 1996;**91**:1348–50.
22. Goff BA, Mandel L, Muntz HG, Melancon CH. Ovarian cancer diagnosis. *Cancer* 2000;**89**:2068–75.
23. Whitehead WE, Cheskin LJ, Heller BR, Robinson JC, Crowell MD, Benjamin C, Schuster MM. Evidence for exacerbation of irritable bowel syndrome during menses. *Gastroenterology* 1990;**98**:1485–9.
24. Houghton LA, Lea R, Jackson N, Whorwell PJ. The menstrual cycle affects rectal sensitivity in patients with IBS but not healthy volunteers. Submitted to *Gut.*
25. Jackson NA, Houghton LA, Whorwell PJ. Does the menstrual cycle effect anorectal physiology? *Dig Dis Sci* 1994;**39**:2607–11.
26. Houghton LA, Wych J, Whorwell PJ. Acute diarrhoea induces rectal sensitivity in women but not men. *Gut* 1995;**37**:270–74.
27. Houghton LA, Jackson NA, Whorwell PJ, Morris J. Do male sex hormones protect from the irritable bowel syndrome? *Am J Gastroenterol* 2000;**95**:2296–300.

Chapter 19

Clinical significance of adhesions in patients with chronic pelvic pain

Alexander A.W. Peters, Erica A. Bakkum and Bart W.J. Hellebrekers

Introduction

The evaluation of chronic pelvic pain (CPP) is a common and puzzling clinical problem for every gynaecologist, surgeon and GP. Every medical doctor recognises the individual patient who complains about continuous low abdominal or pelvic pain that hinders her in her daily activities and for which, in spite of a regimen of diagnostic procedures and therapies, no definitive diagnosis or successful treatment has been proposed.

The actual prevalence of this chronic pelvic pain syndrome is estimated by Reiter to account for 10% of all office visits to a gynaecologist.[1] Howard claims in his review that over 40% of all diagnostic and therapeutic laparoscopies are performed for chronic pelvic pain.[2] In this review he also reports that there is a tendency for an increase in laparoscopies performed for CPP, due to either an increase in the prevalence of CPP or the awareness that in women with CPP the physical examination is not a good predictor of laparoscopic findings.[3,4]

To understand the significance of CPP and the underlying possible aetiologies, such as adhesions, one should first be able to define chronic pelvic pain. The character of the pain, the time frame in which the pain occurs and associated symptoms, such as deep dyspareunia or dysmenorrhoea, are all important factors that should be defined exactly before any clinical relevance can be assumed.

Too many generalisations are already made about aetiology or treatment due to varying definitions of CPP and thus varying groups of women. Furthermore, one should keep in mind that pain is a subjective experience and that a lack of physical findings does not negate the significance of a patient's pain. Endometriosis and adhesions are the pathological conditions that are mostly mentioned in relation to CPP.[2] This review will deal mainly with the relationship between aetiology and treatment of adhesions and CPP.

Model: adhesions and chronic pelvic pain

Adhesion formation

Adhesion formation occurs after a trauma to the visceral or parietal peritoneum. This trauma is either caused by surgical lesions, infections, endometriosis, inflammatory pathologies, chemical irritation during continuous ambulatory peritoneal dialysis and others. Adhesion formation after surgical intervention accounts for the highest percentage of adhesions, with 70–85% of all adhesions being attributed to operative procedures in the literature.[5] The remaining adhesions are ascribed to endometriosis and/or inflammatory causes (18%).[6] Congenital adhesions are also sometimes mentioned but are rarely described as a separate entity.[5]

Adhesions are formed when the parietal or visceral peritoneum is damaged and the basal membrane of the mesothelial layer is exposed to the surrounding tissues. This injury to the peritoneum, due to either surgery, infection or irritation, causes a local inflammatory reaction that leads to the formation of a serosanguineous exudate that is rich in fibrin. The fibrinous exudate is part of the haemostatic process and facilitates tissue repair by providing a matrix for invading fibroblasts and new blood vessels. On the one hand, this deposition of fibrin is an essential component of normal tissue repair, but on the other hand, resolution of this fibrin deposit is required to restore the pre-operative conditions or conditions before inflammation.

The dissolution of fibrin is mediated by the fibrinolytic system. In this system, the inactive pro-enzyme plasminogen is converted into active plasmin by tissue-plasminogen activator or urokinase-plasminogen activator. This plasmin degrades fibrin, the matrix structure of fibrinous adhesions. When the fibrinolytic capacity is insufficient, persistence of deposited fibrin may occur and fibrinous adhesions may develop. The fibrinous adhesions become organised, characterised by deposition of collagen and concomitant vascular ingrowth, as a consequence of which the adhesions are changed into fibrous, permanent adhesions. Formation of adhesions by foreign body granulomas, such as talc, gauzes or suture material, also occurs at this stage. Thus, an imbalance between fibrin deposition and fibrin dissolution is the key event in the development of adhesion formation.[7-10] Re-peritonealisation covers the defect and adhering structures with a new mesothelial layer within eight days of the initial injury.

Pain mechanisms in CPP – chemical pathway

In following the chronologic development of adhesions one might be able to discern how adhesion formation might be related to CPP. In the acute phase of adhesion formation different mediators like bradykinin, serotonin, histamine, prostaglandins, acetylcholine and proteolytic enzymes are released. All these mediators are known to be part of the pain sensation mechanism as well. However, CPP is a chronic condition. When taking into account the time frame in which adhesions are formed permanently the above-mentioned mediators will probably all have disappeared by the time the patient still observes chronic pain complaints. While adhesions are described to be stable within one month[11] after the initial injury, CPP certainly extends beyond this time interval. Prostaglandins are inconsistently related to CPP. Zhen-hai found significantly higher 6-keto-PGF10 levels in the peritoneal fluid of ten sterilised women that had pelvic pain without pathological findings compared with 15 healthy controls;[12] Rapkin and Dawood however concluded from independent studies that there was no correlation between the concentration of prostaglandins in the peritoneal fluid and the underlying diagnoses of pelvic pain or adhesions.[13,14]

Pain mechanisms in CPP – mechanical pathway

Mechanical components have also been proposed to be the underlying mechanism of pain sensation in relation to adhesions. By means of mechanical stretching of internal organs the patient will experience pain. Kresch et al.,[15] for example, observed that pain was caused by adhesion formation and the following restricted mobility of the pelvic organs. Stout et al. claim that a direct mechanical stimulation of the visceral nocireceptors is the underlying aetiology of the pain sensation.[16]

While trauma to the parietal peritoneum is painful, trauma to the visceral peritoneum is described as causing no such sensation. This is probably due to the different innervation pathways in the two structures. The parietal peritoneum is innervated by sensory and motor nerves, while the visceral peritoneum is innervated only by sensory receptors. Damage to the parietal peritoneum will be recognised at the exact localisation due to the direct pathway of innervation. Sharp, localised trauma to the visceral peritoneum seldom causes severe pain. However, diffuse stimulation of nerve endings may cause pain of the visceral peritoneum due to a summation effect. This might explain the sensation of pain in cases of adhesion formation when a diffuse area is covered with adhesions. It might also be the cause of pain in ischaemic conditions, which may occur after a trauma when a diffuse area is involved and which is known to be the underlying mechanism for adhesion formation.

An interesting discussion point might be whether different types of adhesions are related to different types of pain. Several studies were able to demonstrate the presence of nerve fibres in pelvic adhesions.[17-19] Do vascularised and innervated adhesions induce more severe pain as opposed to filmy adhesions? Or perhaps the other way around, will non-vascularised and non-innervated adhesions induce more severe pain due to the ischaemia that occurs? Another interesting point is the non-adapting nature of pain receptors. In case of continuous stimulation the threshold of the pain receptors is described as being reduced. Due to this phenomenon, hyperalgesia may occur, which might be the underlying mechanism of the chronic component of the pain sensation, as is observed in CPP.

Clinics: significance of adhesions and CPP

Definitions of chronic pelvic pain and adhesions

In order to analyse the relation between adhesions and CPP both conditions have to be defined precisely. As was stated in the introduction many generalisations have already been made about aetiology or treatment due to varying definitions of CPP and thus varying groups of women. Different ways of defining CPP have been used in the literature.[2] Important factors that are mostly part of these definitions are:

1.   Time frame in which the pain occurs; relation to the menstrual cycle;

2.   Character of the pain;

3.   Location of the pain; constant or varying;

4.   Interference with daily activities or life; severity;

5.   Associated symptoms; e.g. dysmenorrhoea, deep dyspareunia;

6.   Objectiveness of the pain, the use of questionnaires.

Howard concludes in his extensive review on CPP that duration, pattern, location and severity of the pain should all be specifically addressed in any evaluation of CPP. He advises caution with inconsistencies in defining pain, which will certainly have clinical relevance because our understanding of CPP is far from complete. When different definitions are used, dissimilar distributions of diseases will be compared. He proposes the following definition of CPP: non-menstrual pain of three or more months' duration that is localised to the anatomic pelvis and is severe enough to cause functional disability and requires medical or surgical treatment.

Another concern is the definition of adhesions. Most scoring systems are developed for defining extent and type of adhesions in relation to fertility surgery. These scoring systems are not only developed with a different goal in mind but also mostly exclude other intraperitoneal structures, especially the bowel. A revised American Fertility Score devised by Stout *et al.* proved to be significantly higher in 90 women with self-reported pelvic pain as opposed to 12 women without pelvic pain.[16] Peters also proposes a modified scoring system that includes other intraperitoneal structures, especially the bowel.[20]

Diagnostic procedures

As in every diagnostic procedure, information should at first be obtained from the history and physical examination of the patient. The history of the patient is, however, mostly not valuable in obtaining a diagnosis. Besides the above-mentioned difficulties in defining CPP the history of the patient with CPP mostly turns out to be non-specific. Stout *et al.* report that radiating pain in the leg and menstrual cycle variations are contraindications of the presence of adhesions in CPP.[16] When taking a patient's history, attention must be paid to non-gynaecological causes of pain, including psychological and social factors, but these do not assist in obtaining the diagnosis of adhesions. Previous pelvic surgery turns out to be a strong indicator of adhesions in patients with CPP, but half of the patients have no historical reason for the presence of adhesions.[2]

The physical examination is also not very specific.[3,4] A quarter of the patients with adhesions show no pre-operative findings by physical examination that suggest the presence of adhesions, according to Howard. Lundberg concluded from a study of 95 patients with pelvic pain that there was a poor correlation between pelvic examination and the existence of pelvic disease.[21] Sometimes a lessened uterine mobility or the palpation of an adnexal mass are described as being related to adhesions in a patient with CPP but both observations are very aspecific.

Blood examination will also mostly not reveal any additional information as to whether adhesions are present or not. Martin *et al.* suggested, from a study with 60 patients, that there is a relationship between *Chlamydia trachomatis* immunoglobulin G titres and dystrophic calcification, hydrosalpinges and adhesions. He concluded that this might identify those infertility patients, and maybe also those with CPP, who might benefit from a laparoscopy.[22]

Another new interesting technique to diagnose adhesions is described by Maroulis *et al.* They reported on an ultrasonography technique to visualise adhesions called hydrogynaecography. With this technique, vaginal ultrasonography, performed after the injection of isotonic saline into the cul-de-sac, was capable of identifying pelvic adhesions in 84% of infertility and pelvic pain patients, as confirmed by laparoscopy.[23]

Peters *et al.* stresses the importance of radiographic examination of the small bowel when severe, multiple vascularised adhesions involving the bowel are suspected. Especially patients who tend to have periods of exacerbation of the pain with symptoms and physical findings of small bowel obstruction (sub) ileus should undergo such an examination.[20]

Last, but certainly not least, laparoscopy should be evaluated as a diagnostic tool in patients with CPP and adhesions. Attention should be paid, when analysing these data, to inclusion and diagnostic criteria of the study groups and to the laparoscopic techniques, especially whether double or multiple puncture techniques are used to ensure adequate vision.

Cunanan *et al.*[3] reviewed 1194 charts of consecutive patients who had a diagnostic laparoscopy for pelvic pain. He found that 63% of the patients with a normal pelvic examination prior to the laparoscopy showed abnormal findings on the diagnostic laparoscopy, whereas 17.5% of the patients who had abnormal pelvic examination showed normal findings on the laparoscopy. An adhesion percentage of 19.2% was found in this study. Levitan *et al.* concluded that patients with pelvic pain who had a pathological underlying condition experienced more severe pain compared with patients without a pathologic condition,[24] thus suggesting a relationship between the presence of pathology and pain.

A study performed by Kresch *et al.* showed that 83% of the patients with pelvic pain showed some kind of pathology, of which 38% showed adhesion formation. They followed detailed inclusion criteria, which might explain the high percentage of pathology found. Although this study dealt with only 50 patients, it was a prospective study and even included a control group.[15] Stout *et al.* reported that the localisation of the pain was concomitant with the localisation of the adhesions in 97% of the patients, although extent of adhesion formation and severity of the pain showed no relation.[16] Stovall *et al.*[25] found 49% of patients with adhesions and CPP, as against 34% of the controls without CPP, showed adhesion formation. Twenty-five per cent of the patients who showed adhesions did not have any complaints of pain. One should compare the above mentioned percentages found in women with CPP with the percentages of pathology found in asymptomatic women. For example, 29% pathology was found in a control group of asymptomatic women at the time of tubal ligation.[15] Trimbos *et al.*[26] recorded laparoscopic findings in 200 asymptomatic women undergoing sterilisation. In 26% of these patients, abnormalities were found, including 14% with pelvic adhesions. Rapkin found a percentage of 39% adhesions with laparoscopy, of which 12% showed CPP. In this study group, 26% of the adhesions were found in the patients who had pain.[4]

Howard summarised all these cumulative data from the different studies and concluded that laparoscopy in patients with CPP revealed a detectable pathological condition in 61% of the patients. Twenty-five percent of these pathological conditions were adhesions. In women without CPP a pathological condition was detectable in 28%, of which adhesions accounted for 17%.[2] He concluded that women without CPP have a significant incidence of abnormal laparoscopic findings but that women with CPP have twice the incidence of laparoscopically detected pathology. Therefore, we conclude that there seems to be the suggestion of an aetiological relationship between adhesions and CPP, which is, however, not proven sufficiently.

Treatment of adhesions and chronic pelvic pain

Prevention of adhesion formation

By following the consecutive stages in the formation of adhesions one can discern different treatment modalities to prevent adhesion formation.[27] These modalities are:

1. Minimisation of trauma to the peritoneum by employing microsurgical techniques;

2. Reduction of the inflammatory reaction by means of corticosteroids, calcium-channel blockers and antihistamines, or non-steroidal anti-inflammatories, selective immunosuppressors (i.e. tumour necrosis factor-α and interleukin-1) etc.

3. Augmentation of the fibrinolysis by means of fibrinolytic agents;[10]

4. Mechanical separation of adjacent structures by means of liquid or solid barriers, such as Hyskon (32% Dextran 70), Ringer's lactate, carboxymethylcellulose, Interceed (oxidised regenerated cellulose), Poloxamer 407, Polyactive (composed of a polyethyleneglycol and polybuthyleneterephthalate co-polymer), PRECLUDE Peritoneal Membrane (expanded polytetrafluoroethylene), fibrin glue (Tissucol), ADCON (composed of polyglycan esters in phosphate-buffered saline), Seprafilm (bioresorbable membrane based on a chemically modified form of hyaluronic acid and carboxymethylcellulose), etc.[28]

Many inconsistencies have been described with all these methods. Limitation of trauma to the peritoneum, by using microsurgical techniques together with continuous irrigation and meticulous haemostasis is probably still the most effective technique.

Integrated approach to CPP

CPP requires a multidisciplinary approach because of its complex aetiology. Although the scope of this chapter is to try to elucidate the significance of adhesions and their treatment in CPP, a few words should be given to the integrated approach to CPP, as employed in our hospital. In the integrated approach equal attention is devoted to somatic, psychological, dietary, environmental and physiotherapeutic factors. This method was first analysed in a study group of 106 patients with CPP.[29] In the standard-approach group, organic causes of pain were excluded first and diagnostic laparoscopy was routinely performed. If no somatic cause could be found, attention was given to other causes, such as psychological disturbances. In the second group, an integrated approach was chosen and equal attention was paid to the above-mentioned factors. In this group laparoscopy was thus not routinely performed. Evaluation of the pain one year after the institution of the treatment revealed that the integrated approach improved pelvic pain significantly more often than the standard approach. Laparoscopy was found to play no important role in the treatment of pelvic pain.

Additionally, Steege and Stout found in a study of 30 patients that the patients without a so-called chronic pain syndrome are more likely to improve after lysis of adhesions.[30] They thus concluded that the presence of psychosocial compromise warrants pre-operative evaluation and supports the notion that lysis of adhesions is useful but should be accompanied by additional psychological evaluation and treatment.

Adhesiolysis

Most of the studies dealing with adhesiolysis address infertility or adhesion reformation. Howard's review summarises the studies on adhesiolysis and relief of CPP.[2] Many authors conclude that there is a substantial positive benefit of adhesiolysis on pelvic pain. Percentages of improvement vary from 67% (follow-up four months[31]) to 84% (follow-up one to five years[32]) or 89%.[33] When analysing these data one should take into account that in many of the studies the evaluation of pain was not blinded, no control groups were included and follow-up times differed significantly. Steege and Stout also found a positive effect of adhesiolysis in a prospective study of 30 women.[30] An improvement of 75% was found at 6–12 months after surgery in the women without a chronic pelvic pain syndrome. In women with a chronic pain syndrome 40% improvement was achieved. Seven patients had initial relief but a return of pain within three to five months, thereby stressing the importance of longer follow-up intervals. Chan and Wood also concluded that adhesiolysis was of value in patients with CPP and claimed that 65.1% of the patients with CPP were cured or experienced reduced pain.[34] Their study comprised 43 patients with CPP and 68 patients with dysmenorrhoea who were operated upon within a time frame of 5.5 years; the follow-up interval thus varied significantly. The dysmenorrhoea was also found to be improved in 47.1 % of the patients.

In our clinic, a prospective, randomised clinical trial was performed in 48 women with stage II to IV pelvic adhesions. Surgical treatment (adhesiolysis) was compared with a non-surgery group. Nine to 12 months after adhesiolysis no significant differences were found between the two groups with regard to pelvic pain. A subgroup of women with severe, vascularised and dense adhesions involving the bowel (stage IV) had significantly less pain after adhesiolysis.[29]

Laparoscopic adhesiolysis is sometimes thought to be superior to adhesiolysis by means of a laparotomy. This theory could not be confirmed by the Operative Laparoscopy Study Group, who found that adhesion reformation is a frequent occurrence after operative laparoscopy.[35] Pittaway *et al.* also concluded that laparoscopic adnexectomy was not superior to conventional adnexal excision with a laparotomy with regard to adhesion formation.[36] Lastly, Saravelos *et al.* compared open microsurgical adhesiolysis to laparoscopic adhesioslysis for pain relief in 123 women with CPP.[37] Sustained postoperative pain relief was seen in 71% of the 72 microsurgical cases and in 61% of the 51 laparoscopy cases (not statistically significant). Mean length of follow-up was 13.7 months.

Placebo effects

Psychological effects have frequently been discussed in relation to both CPP and laparoscopy in CPP. The reassurance derived from the results with laparoscopy might contribute to the beneficial effect so that prejudiced conclusions are drawn. Peters *et al.* suggest postponement of surgical assessment to more than 16 months after treatment due to the influence of the placebo effect, which seldom lasts longer.[29] Baker and Symonds performed a study in 60 patients with CPP who underwent a laparoscopy that excluded obvious pelvic pathology. At a six-month follow-up period 58% reported that they were pain free and 39% reported that their pain had diminished. Baker and Symonds concluded that treatment of pelvic pain should concentrate on the small minority of patients whose symptoms remain six months after laparoscopy.[38]

Future of adhesions and CPP

Although significant beneficial effects on CPP are obtained in many different studies with adhesiolysis we believe that surgical intervention, whether diagnostic or therapeutic, in a patient with CPP should only be performed in certain well-defined cases. As discussed extensively, too many generalisations are made about aetiology or treatment due to varying definitions of CPP, and thus varying groups of women. In addition, many conclusions are drawn from study groups that comprised women with a remarkable history of pelvic pain and/or treatment modalities for CPP that had up to then failed. High percentages of these women showed relief of symptoms. However, follow-up periods were mostly short in these studies. Furthermore severe cases of CPP and/or adhesions are liable to react positively to surgical intervention. Jansen explains this phenomenon by stressing the importance of controlling for the initial extent of the adhesions.[39] He reveals that the higher the initial score, the more likely it is that the improvement score will be positive.

From the literature and from the two studies performed in our hospital we believe that surgical intervention should be exercised in only a minority of the patients with CPP. Intervention might, for example, be beneficial in patients with CPP who show severe adhesions involving the intestinal tract or in patients with CPP who show elevated titres for *Chlamydia* immunoglobulin G. Surgical intervention might also be justified when, according to Steege and Stout, a differentiation is made between patients with or without the presence of a chronic pain syndrome. Additionally, we believe that diagnostic laparoscopy plays no important role in the treatment of pelvic pain. This is confirmed by Howard, who concluded from cumulative data that a significant percentage of pathology is also found in women without CPP. Instead, an integrated approach including psychological, somatic, environmental and physiotherapeutic aspects is recommended. More studies that analyse the effect of adhesiolysis on CPP in a randomised and controlled way should be carried out, similar to the studies analysing the effect of adhesiolysis and fertility. Primary prevention of adhesion formation is probably the most efficacious surgical method for the prevention and treatment of CPP that is caused by adhesion formation.

References

1. Reiter RC. A profile of women with chronic pelvic pain. *Clin Obstet Gynecol* 1990;**33**:130–36.
2. Howard FM. The role of laparoscopy in chronic pelvic pain: promise and pitfalls. *Obstet Gynecol Surv* 1993;**48**:357–87.
3. Cunanan RG, Courey NG, Lippes J. Laparoscopic findings in patients with pelvic pain. *Am J Obstet Gynecol* 1983;**146**:589–91.

4.   Rapkin AJ. Adhesions and pelvic pain: a retrospective study. *Obstet Gynecol* 1986;**68**:13–15.
5.   Weibel MA, Majno G. Peritoneal adhesions and their relation to abdominal surgery. A postmortem study. *Am J Surg* 1973;**126**:345–53.
6.   Brosens IA, Puttemans PJ, Deprest JD. The endoscopic localization of endometrial implants in the ovarian chocolate cyst. *Fertil Steril* 1994;**61**:1034–8.
7.   Raftery AT. Effect of peritoneal trauma on peritoneal fibrinolytic activity and intraperitoneal adhesion formation. *Eur Surg Res* 1981;**13**:337–41.
8.   Montz FJ, Shimanuki T, DiZerega GS. Postsurgical mesothelial re-epithelialization. In: DeCherney AH, Polan ML, editors. *Reproductive Surgery*. Chicago: Year Book Medical Publishers; 1987. p. 31–47.
9.   Hellebrekers BWJ, Trimbos-Kemper GCM, Bakkum EA, Trimbos JB, Declerck P, Kooistra T, *et al.* Short-term effect of surgical trauma on rat peritoneal fibrinolytic activity and its role in adhesion formation. *Thrombosis & Haemostasis* 2000;**84**:876–81.
10. Hellebrekers BWJ, Trimbos-Kemper GCM, Trimbos JB, Emeis JJ, Kooistra T. Use of fibrinolytic agents in the prevention of postsurgical adhesion formation. *Fertil Steril* 2000;**74**:203–12.
11. Bakkum EA, Trimbos-Kemper GCM. Natural course of postsurgical adhesions. *Microsurgery* 1995;**16**:650–54.
12. Wang ZH, Wu RF, Ge XL, *et al.* Relationships between pelvic pain and prostaglandin levels in plasma and peritoneal fluid collected from women after sterilization. *Contraception* 1992;**45**:67–71.
13. Rapkin A, Bhattacherjee P. Peritoneal fluid eicosanoids in chronic pelvic pain. *Prostaglandins* 1989;**38**:447–52.
14. Dawood MY, Khan-Dawood FS, Wilson L. Peritoneal fluid prostaglandins and prostanoids in women with endometriosis, chronic pelvic inflammatory disease, and pelvic pain. *Am J Obstet Gynecol* 1984;**148**:391–5.
15. Kresch AJ, Seifer DB, Sachs LB, Barrese I. Laparoscopy in 100 women with chronic pelvic pain. *Obstet Gynecol* 1984;**64**:672–4.
16. Stout AL, Steege JF, Dodson WC, Hughes CL. Relationship of laparoscopic findings to self-report of pelvic pain. *Am J Obstet Gynecol* 1991;**164**:73–9.
17. Kligman I, Drachenberg C, Papadimitriou J, Katz E. Immunohistochemical demonstration of nerve fibers in pelvic adhesions. *Obstet Gynecol* 1993;**82**:566–8.
18. Tulandi T, Chen MF, Al-Took S, Watkin K. A study of nerve fibers and histopathology of postsurgical, postinfectious, and endometriosis related adhesions. *Obstet Gynecol* 1998;**92**:766–8.
19. Herrick SE, Mutsaers SE, Ozua P, Sulaiman H, Omer A, Boulos P, *et al.* Human peritoneal adhesions are highly cellular, innervated, and vascularized. *J Pathol* 2000;**192**:67–72.
20. Peters AAW, Trimbos-Kemper GCM, Admiraal C, Trimbos JB. A randomized clinical trial on the benefit of adhesiolysis in patients with intraperitoneal adhesions and chronic pelvic pain. *Br J Obstet Gynaecol* 1992;**99**:59–62.
21. Lundberg WI, Wall JE, Mathers JE. Laparoscopy in evaluation of pelvic pain. *Obstet Gynecol* 1973;**42**:872–6.
22. Martin DC, Khare VK, Miller BE. Association of *Chlamydia trachomatis* immunoglobulin gamma titers with dystrophic peritoneal calcification, psammoma bodies, adhesions, and hydrosalpinges. *Fertil Steril* 1995;**63**:39–44.
23. Maroulis GB, Parsons AK, Yeko TR. Hydrogynecography: a new technique enables vaginal sonography to visualize pelvic adhesions and other pelvic structures. *Fertil Steril* 1992;**58**:1073–5.
24. Levitan Z, Eibschitz I, de Vries K, Hakim M, Sharf M. The value of laparoscopy in women with chronic pelvic pain and a 'normal pelvis'. *Int J Gynecol Obstet* 1985;**23**:71–4.
25. Stovall TG, Elder RF, Ling FW. Predictors of pelvic adhesions. *J Reprod Med* 1989;**34**:345–8.
26. Trimbos JB, Trimbos-Kemper GCM, Peters AAW, Van der Does CD, Van Hall EV. Findings in 200 consecutive asymptomatic women, having a laparoscopic sterilization. *Arch Gynecol Obstet* 1990;**247**:121–4.
27. Bakkum EA, Trimbos JB, Trimbos-Kemper GCM. Postsurgical adhesion formation and prevention, – recent developments. *Reprod Med Rev* 1996;**5**:1–13.
28. Hellebrekers BWJ, Trimbos-Kemper GCM, van Blitterswijk CA, Bakkum EA, Trimbos JB. Effects of five different barrier materials on postsurgical adhesion formation in the rat. *Hum Reprod* 2000;**15**:1358–63.
29. Peters AAW, van Dorst E, Jellis B, van Zuuren E, Hermans J, Trimbos JB. A randomized clinical trial to compare two different approaches in women with chronic pelvic pain. *Obstet Gynecol* 1991;**77**:740–44.
30. Steege JF, Stout A. Resolution of chronic pelvic pain after laparoscopic lysis of adhesions. *Am J Obstet Gynecol* 1991;**165**:278–83.

31. Daniell JF. Laparoscopic enterolysis for chronic abdominal pain. *J Gynecol Surg* 1989;**5**:61–6.
32. Sutton C. Macdonald R. Laser laparoscopic adhesiolysis. *J Gynecol Surg* 1990;**6**:155–9.
33. Goldstein DP, deCholnoky C, Emans SJ, Leventhal JM. Laparoscopy in the diagnosis and management of pelvic pain in adolescents. *J Reprod Med* 1980;**24**:251–6.
34. Chan CLK, Wood C. Pelvic adhesiolysis – the assessment of symptom relief by 100 patients. *Aust N Z J Obstet Gynaecol* 1985;**25**:295–8.
35. Operative Laparoscopy Study Group. Postoperative adhesion development after operative laparoscopy: evaluation at early second-look procedures. *Fertil Steril* 1991;**55**:700–704.
36. Pittaway DE, Takacs P, Bauguess P. Laparoscopic adnexectomy. A comparison with laparotomy. *Am J Obstet Gynecol* 1994;**171**:385–91.
37. Saravelos HG, Li TC, Cooke ID. An analysis of the outcome of microsurgical and laparoscopic adhesiolysis for chronic pelvic pain. *Hum Reprod* 1995;**10**:2895–901.
38. Baker PN, Symonds EM. The resolution of chronic pelvic pain after normal laparoscopy findings. *Am J Obstet Gynecol* 1992;**166**:835–6.
39. Jansen RPS. Controlled clinical approaches to investigating the prevention of peritoneal adhesions. In: DiZerega GS, Malinak LR, Diamond MP, Linsky CB, editors. *Treatment of Postsurgical Adhesions*. New York: Wiley-Liss; 1990. p. 177–92.

Chapter 20

Vulval and abdominal pain

Discussion

Discussion following the papers of Professor Foster, Dr Whorwell and Dr Peters

Kennedy: I have a question for Professor Foster. You talked about polymorphism in interleukin-1 (IL-1). What sort of numbers of cases and controls did you test and how were the controls chosen?

Foster: This work was done through Steve Witkin's laboratory at Cornell University. I believe he had approximately 50 vulval vestibulitis patients, a similar number of human papillomavirus (HPV)-infected patients and about twice as many controls. The significance of the HPV-infected patients was that they found that the polymorphism was lower in that population than it was in the uninfected controls, so there was an implication that not having that polymorphism made them more susceptible to infection.

Kennedy: Has the polymorphism been associated with any other conditions?

Foster: It has been associated with multiple sclerosis, with alopecia areata, with all sorts of colitis and rheumatoid arthritis, but every one of those only has about half of the percentage incidence of homozygosity as the vestibulitis has.

Stones: I would like to ask Dr Foster to give us a little clinical description of what he means by vestibulitis. In my practice, since hearing about vestibulitis, I have started routinely testing all my patients for allodynia with a cotton tip swab and I am finding it very frequently present, even in people where that is not their primary complaint. It seems to me that in many cases that is probably referred pain from some site elsewhere in the pelvis.

Foster: You are certainly describing the finding of allodynia exactly as I would find it. The precision of the allodynia is important. Most of these people will have tenderness just in front of the hymenal remnants and it rapidly drops off when you get out to the external vulva. I often use a visual analogue scale or a visual analogue thermometer, and I would anticipate a greater than 50% drop off within a centimetre of the hymenal ring. You can certainly see other types of conditions associated with vestibulitis, and that is an issue that needs to be clarified as far as the relationship between them. We have seen it in the urinary tract, as I have mentioned.

Stones: Would you require the presence of some erythema there as well as tenderness, or not necessarily?

Foster: No. That has been a discussion of the International Society for the Study of Vulvovaginal Disease (ISSVD): does erythema need to be present? What has been observed by people who see large numbers of vestibulitis is that the erythema changes from time to time. This may be related to substance P, or a number of the other mediators that have intermittent release may cause erythema to change from one time to the next.

Thornton: Following on from what you have just said about substance P, you also presented data for one of the interleukins and for tumour necrosis factor-α (TNF-α) and the implication is always that the changes you demonstrated are causing the vestibulitis. Do you know that there is cause and effect, or could it be that those changes in TNF-α and the like are an effect of vestibulitis?

Foster: That is an excellent question. The connection that we are suggesting is more in the area of prostaglandin E_2 and the fact that the fibroblasts are producing very large amounts of prostaglandin E_2, either with stimulation with IL1β or with interferon-γ CD40 ligand. There is very good evidence that the presence of prostaglandin E_2 with the tetrodotoxin-resistant sodium channel actually induces a greater leakiness of the tetrodotoxin-resistant sodium channel, leading to the nerve having a tendency to fire. At least there is a direction to look between prostaglandin E_2 and some of the sodium channels we see at the end of free nerve endings.

Beard: Dr Foster, I am plagued in my pelvic pain clinic with women in the old age group who have an apparently normal vulva but absolutely crippling pain which presents clinically in a very predictable way. Curiously, it presents in completely the opposite direction to pelvic congestion. They find that the pain is relieved by walking around. But they have one thing in common: often they have had a crisis in their life when the pain actually starts. I wonder whether you have a view on that group?

Foster: I have seen this group as well and they are quite different from the vestibulitis patients where we have a mean age of about 35 years. Many of these people tend to have a much more diffuse location of pain and it is often more of a dynamic allodynia where you actually rub across the skin and produce tenderness in contrast to the punctate type of allodynia that we see in vestibulitis. It is in that more generalised vulvodynia category and I am not sure that I can prove that it is actually a neuralgia. At this point I put that as a working diagnosis. We can now look at things such as St Mark's electrode sacral reflex latency abnormalities as a diagnostic tool, but that has not been found to be very effective. I still tend to place those patients in the generalised rather than localised vulval dysaesthesia category and treat them similarly to others with that condition. The first line would be tricyclic antidepressants and often I would try to do a specific nerve block on either pudendal, or the genitofemoral nerve in different areas.

Beard: We would agree that they are therapeutically very disappointing as a group.

Foster: Often the older women will have unilateral pain, and as soon as I hear 'My pain is mostly on one side' I shudder, because they are much more difficult to treat.

Thornton: Can I follow up on your answer to my question? I either misheard or did not understand the role of prostaglandin E_2. Did you say that it has a tetrodotoxin-like effect on the sodium channels?

Foster: Through EP, the receptor for prostaglandin E_2, and through pyruvate kinase A there appears to be a phosphorylation of the β subunit of the tetrodotoxin-resistant sodium channel. That phosphorylation results in a rapid leakage of the tetrodotoxin receptor. It has nothing to do with the prostaglandin E_2 specifically but it is active induction of a leaky receptor through the tetrodotoxin-resistant sodium channel.

Kennedy: There is a need to develop a proforma questionnaire or history sheet for common use in both gynaecology and gastroenterology clinics, and the gynaecology contribution to that questionnaire should be based upon an analysis of the negative and predictive values of symptom clusters. The potential use for this tool is in primary-care, going back to what we were discussing earlier about the need for evidence-based guidelines for referral. Ideally in neurology as well.

Sutton: Can I address a question to Dr Peters? You did not quote the study of Russell MacDonald and myself.[1] Our experience is rather different from yours. We published in 1985 and we found that in 80% of patients who had an adhesiolysis, as long as it was a tight bank of adhesions that was immobilising a loop of, usually, small bowel – occasionally large bowel – and as long as it corresponded to the site of the pain, those 80% at the end of a year were pain-free and there was not much recurrence, as far as we could see, clinically. The real question is, did you use anti-adhesion barriers or fluids? We now use icodextrin 4%, which is broken down by amylase, and since there is normally no amylase in the perineal cavity, it stays in there for seven days, so that by the time the surfaces have healed adhesions are much less likely to occur.

Peters: In this last study we did not, but we have had experience with barriers such as Interceed and Gore-Tex™ for a long time and we used all kinds of materials. I have a slide with me of what was used over time, and so many things were used with different effects. But I agree with you that it is possible, but I believe the patients have specific bowel problems if there is one strong adhesion holding part of the small intestine. That is why we have taken a lot of X-rays in the past. But they have very specific symptoms. They feel a sensation of release after the bowel contents have gone through. It is a colic-type of pain. Then it would be very effective to remove the adhesions.

Sutton: I agree with you. We tried to publish this study in the *British Medical Journal* but there was the most brilliant bit of peer review I have ever heard. They said unless we did a similar number of men they could not consider it. For a gynaecologist that is quite a difficult study!

Stones: I would like to ask Dr Whorwell about dyspareunia and irritable bowel syndrome. Clearly, dyspareunia is a very common symptom in a gynae clinic and we would probably be over-diagnosing irritable bowel syndrome (IBS) if we ascribed it to IBS. How would you sort that one out?

Whorwell: This work was done by a female psychiatrist. She went to the homes of these patients looking at the effect of IBS on sexual function.[2] I have not quoted that paper. The interesting thing about the pain is that it is never there at the time of intercourse and it is seldom there even just after intercourse. Classically it comes on the next day, and it resembles their IBS pain. It sounds as though it is provoking – I was about to say spasms, but as you know, spasm is a dirty word in IBS at the moment.

That is what it sounds as though it is provoking – the bowel problem.

Stones: The way I teach my trainees is that if it is dyspareunia with no pain afterwards, that may point more towards endometriosis, and if it is dyspareunia with immediate and intense post-coital pain, that is pointing to pelvic congestion. As you say, if there is a gap, then IBS. I would be interested in other people's comments on that.

Steege: There may be a link there. In analysing the numbers on the last almost 1000 pain patients we have seen in the last seven or eight years, if you have IBS in our patient population the odds ratio of having endometriosis is 1.8. So it is conceivable that a person with dyspareunia is getting the dyspareunia from their endometriosis at the time, and then their IBS is kicking in the next day. Both could be present in the same unfortunate individual, so there may be a linkage there.

In terms of Professor Foster's work, we have been doing something a little bit different with our vestibulitis patients. We see a large population, looking at sensitivity in other areas of the vulva in people who have vestibulitis. If you take a Q-tip and break it in half and use a sharp and dull comparison, a sizeable fraction of the vestibulitis patients, although they do not have symptoms elsewhere in the vulva, have an altered ability to discriminate sharp and dull in those areas. We are finding that if they have that altered sensation that predicts a less good response to the overnight topical xylocaine regimen that we have been using, which is interesting. It speaks to the neuropathic origin of the pain.

Foster: I interpret that as essentially what Dr Berkley was talking about – this central spreading effect that we will see at the cord when you have a local pain phenomenon. We believe that there are individuals who tend to start to get an expansion of the receptive field. It may not be limited to the vulva. We are presently doing a study looking at that capsaicin sensitivity in the dorsum of the foot. The data are not complete yet but because the foot, dermatome-wise, is fairly close to the vulva, we are at least hypothesising that we will see an altered sensitivity to the dorsum of the foot.

Steege: It connects with some of the Israeli data from the vestibulectomy procedure.[3] They are finding that if people have pain during daily activities as opposed to pain during intercourse, that predicts a less favourable outcome to the surgical procedure via the spread, if you will.

Sutton: I was just thinking of a wonderful dogmatic line in Jeffcoate's textbook. In those days they did not need evidence-based medicine, they just spoke from vast clinical experience. He says that if dyspareunia does last the following day there is definitely no gynaecological pathology, which fits in with what Dr Whorwell said.

Beard: Are you suggesting that post-coital pain is not a gynaecological symptom?

Sutton: If it is there the following day.

Beard: I am sorry, I would think that about one-third of patients who have post-coital pain will tell you it lasts into the following day.

Sutton: But most of your patients have no gynaecological pathology – that is what I am saying.

Beard: We would say that they have if you call functional disturbance, which is what we are talking about…

Sutton: No recognisable pathology…

Beard: You mean no visible pathology…

Sutton: Absolutely.

Barnard: Perhaps I could invite comments on what the pathology might be for pain lasting four or five days continuously. I would agree wholeheartedly, speaking to women with endometriosis, that many of them experience pain at the time of intercourse, not diminishing perhaps for another 48 hours or more. So I am not quite sure where that model has come from.

Berkley: Perhaps I could mention some of the results that were found by Maria Giamberardino and myself five or six years ago.[4] We looked at muscle pain thresholds and skin pain thresholds at four different sites in the body: the deltoid area and muscle, gastrocnemius area and muscle and two sites on the abdomen. We looked at this across the menstrual cycle in two groups of women, with and without severe dysmenorrhoea – on a scale of 0–100 they had to be over 60–70. What we expected was referred hyperalgesia mainly in the muscle, in the abdominal muscle more on the left side than the right side, perimenstrually in the dysmenorrhoeic women and not the non-dysmenorrhoeic women. What we found was the greatest referred hyperalgesia not in the skin but in the muscle in the abdomen on both sides, but we also found muscle hyperalgesia in all four sites that we tested throughout the cycle. In other words, two things had happened in these women with severe dysmenorrhoeia. It exacerbated the cycling of their tenderness, more so in the abdomen than in the rest of their body, but it also produced a generalised muscle but not skin hyperalgesia.

We did not know whether any of the women in this group had any kind of endometriosis that was producing their severe dysmenorrhoea but the likelihood is that there was some endometriosis in some of them, given the prevalence of endometriosis.

What are the mechanisms for something like that? We thought that what was producing it had to do with extra-strong uterine contractions when women were menstruating and therefore we would see the hyperalgesia just during the time of menstruation. Instead, what we saw was an exacerbation of a timing aspect of pain at other times with respect to their cycling – exacerbation of cyclical patterns of pain elsewhere and a generalised muscle hyperalgesia.

That is what led to all the work afterwards on viscero-visceral interactions and viscero-somatic interactions. What does it mean clinically when you are presented with a patient, or you yourself as a patient are tender all over the place – how is this happening? It pushes you to thinking about some kind of remote referred central sensitisation that has to be approached and treated polytherapeutically. We were really surprised by these data. I do not know if anyone wants to comment on how that kind of information would apply to your diagnostic strategies in the clinic.

MacLean: Mrs Barnard made a comment about persistent pain following intercourse and going on for more than 24 hours, and there is no doubt among some of the vulval vestibulitis syndrome patients – they can be totally pain-free until they attempt to have intercourse the next time. These patients avoid the situation where they would have to indulge in intercourse and once they have had intercourse will have pain that persists for some days. When Howard Glazer was over here he spoke at a meeting in Plymouth,[5] and some of the physiotherapists were there. The use of biofeedback techniques has not caught on extensively in this country, but I know that one or two of the patients have gone to physiotherapists and have been taught biofeedback and been able to control what I am sure relates more to levator muscle activity rather than uterine muscle. There is no doubt that by being able to control what is happening to their pelvic floor they seem to get better resolution of their provoked pain, and although intercourse is uncomfortable, by the following morning they are getting back to normal and being able to do things, and there is perhaps not the same dread about the next time they are going to have intercourse.

Vits: One of the reasons that biofeedback has not been taken up as widely here as it is in America is pure cost. The equipment that I have cost £8500 when I bought it a few years ago; it is now £12,500. The other thing is that I have found that I do not actually need the equipment. For a lot of the patients you just need to be very good at what you do and how you do it. You can instruct people on reduction of levator spasm without having biofeedback equipment. You can instruct them in levator contraction, and the way to do that is not with equipment, it is with one's fingers. I would still only see a limited use for the equipment, which makes the patient centre-dependent – 'I have to come in here to have this treatment' – rather than doing it for themselves at home.

Foster: In spite of the fact that we hook on to the idea that biofeedback requires a computer and pressure transducer, I would say that having a practitioner who performs a palpation of muscle tone and then gives the patient information is biofeedback. In fact, it is probably better biofeedback because there is a human touch.

Newton-John: Can I ask for some clarification on where we are standing on the issue of sexual abuse in chronic pelvic pain? Dr Peters, as I understand it, your interpretation of your data was that the incidence is no greater in pelvic pain women than in chronic pain generally, with or without pathology. We heard earlier this morning that sexual abuse is very important but is not causative. I am just wondering about recommendations or perhaps just general consensus on where we stand on the issue.

Beard: May I explain my position in what I said this morning? It seems to me that what is emerging is that if you look at general population studies or women with chronic pelvic pain, a lot of this psychopathology does not emerge. In fact, there is some evidence that there is no significant difference between control groups. But the pathology that we are seeing is in groups who have come as far as the referral to the hospital clinic, and that might account for some of the differences. Certainly, in all the hospital-based studies on which the psychology literature mostly relies sexual abuse does feature as a significant factor. Dr Collett has done quite a lot of work on this.

Steege: We did a survey of 581 women attending primary-care practices in a community in central North Carolina and found that the percentage of prevalence of abuse in that population was the same as the national surveys. We found that if women had been abused only as children there was no association of that with pelvic pain as an adult. However, if they were abused both as children and as adults – that was 13% of the population – that was correlated with a variety of different pain disorders including pelvic pain. If they were abused as adults only there was also association with pelvic pain. So the emphasis should be on degree and chronicity and severity of abuse, not so much whether it was in childhood. That is probably not associated.

Berkley: How do you relate this to Andrea Rapkin's work on the issue of 'sexual abuse' versus physical abuse and her finding that it was not sexual abuse *per se* but any kind of violent attack that was correlated with pelvic pain?[6]

Steege: In our community survey the prevalence of violent attack was much lower. In the 1000 people we are looking at now, 28% of them had some physical abuse, so that may be more cogent. That would agree with what Dr Rapkin was saying. Many of the earlier studies looking at abuse had small numbers so they combined all of those forms of abuse together. That is one of the confusing factors.

Newton-John: Correlation does not show causality. With large enough numbers we can find correlations for lots of different things, but with events that have happened 30 or 40 years ago to be able to draw a direct causal link is spurious.

Steege: I agree. The next question is always, is it relevant now? That is what I was showing in the percentages of people seen by those 15 specialists – the prevalence of abuse in their populations, including mine, is no higher than general population.

Collett: In Leicester we took our group of chronic pelvic pain women,[7] some of whom had pathology and some of whom did not, and we found that we had a higher incidence of sexual and physical abuse than in our pain population and in non-pain controls, so we need to investigate the data in a bigger series more carefully.

Berkley: One of the most important things for me as a newcomer was Dr Peters' statement about how asking those questions is not uninvasive. It is one thing to try to get at those data about how many people have had a past history of any kind of violence or abuse, but how do you go about doing that, given the assumption that it is an invasive question, as invasive as surgery?

Peters: We work in the context that if it is causing any problem at that moment with the patient – because it can – there is a context in which we can provide some care at that moment. It is not appropriate in the outpatients clinic where I have ten minutes per patient. We have seen terrible rape cases or incest cases in the Netherlands recently. I was involved in the care of some of the victims, and at the age of 25 they had prolapse plastic surgery, operations on the vagina and vulva, again and again at an age when we hardly see those kinds of problems. So abuse may not be causal, but we should realise its importance; we teach our students that before you do a pelvic examination perhaps you should not ask about negative sexual experience but you should ask if they are very much against undergoing the pelvic examination. And if they say yes – we have had patients responding strongly because there are events that they remember. So it is important. I was amazed that so many patients were referred who had had so many surgical interventions, yet the question 'Were you abused in your youth?' was not asked. But I do not believe there is a causal relationship with pelvic pain.

Smith: As a psychotherapist and having worked with these women for the last six years, I believe the issue of sexual abuse is significant. I also find it a bit of a red herring. I am very open to working with the sexually abused but with this client group I have found that I have not really had to and I rarely get into discussing or working with any issues from the sexual abuse history. If it comes up, fine, but it rarely does. What I find is that women who have been sexually abused are more likely to get a whole host of different conditions, but it is more that they lack coping skills – coping skills which would be more effective for pain management. They may find it harder to relax physically and emotionally. Again I feel that the whole coping skills approach seems to be very effective with them.

Barnard: May I endorse that? From my own limited experience of this whole realm, it is an absolute minefield. By asking an innocent question at entirely the wrong time, you may open a can of worms that will take possibly many months and sometimes years to put back in the can. I would urge strongly that that line of investigation be left very much to the realm of contracted counselling people who are really used to it. I would urge you to stay away from it because I have seen some horrendous damage done by the wrong question, innocently put, at the wrong time. It is an absolutely lethal area.

Smith: There are a lot more useful and effective questions that could be asked before the doctor asks about sexual abuse, to do with beliefs and meaning and around education. When I ask women if they have ever been asked about the stresses in their life that may trigger off these events, a lot say, 'no, but the doctor kept asking, have I ever been sexually abused?' So even when they have not, that seemed to be the only line of questioning that the doctor went down. So there can be quite a bias here that needs to be addressed and changed.

Barnard: At the risk of labouring a point, something that has occurred to me that might be useful is that what people pick up sometimes is not so much a message about abuse, although that may be in there, but you can pick up very strongly messages of being a victim and having dependency. The syndrome is there of victim, oppressor, rescuer and you need to be very skilled to unpick exactly what is going on. Lots of the women we are talking about will be sending out quite strong messages about being a victim and about being oppressed, but those are not necessarily related to sexuality in the obvious sense but sexuality in the sense of their identity and their inability to overcome problems that touch on that.

Berkley: Would you see as one possible recommendation out of this fascinating discussion developing or convening a group within the Royal College to develop ways of dealing with the issue of physical or sexual abuse within the clinical setting? Would that be something that would be meaningful?

MacLean: There was a scientific meeting convened several years ago that looked at this, and there is a publication from that meeting that I am sure is available at the RCOG bookshop.[8] It is a subject that has been addressed relatively recently.

Berkley: Conclusions?

MacLean: I would not attempt to summarise it. They realised that there were many issues that were revealed as they started to investigate both sexual and physical abuse, problems associated with pregnancy, problems associated with a variety of gynaecological conditions. It was diverse and extensive.

Steege: One of the issues that we are struggling with is that the apprehension of the meaning of physical and sexual abuse is a moving target – at least, in good old North Carolina. Fifteen years ago if you asked somebody about physical or sexual abuse they looked at you as if to say 'What kind of a person do you think I am?' Now we ask it and it is so much a part of everyday conversation that the reception of the question is very different. Certainly in the vulnerable individual it could come in the wrong way at the wrong time, but I believe the probability of that happening now seems so much less than it did 10–15 years ago. I would be right on board with you in saying that if you do ask it needs to be done extremely carefully and skilfully. It also has to be done in a context which says this is just one of many things I am asking about, I am not assuming causality here.

When I teach medical students about this, I give them a session on pelvic pain. I give them a stereotypical patient profile and I say, 'OK, what historical questions do you want to ask?' By question three they are into sexual abuse. I say, 'wait, you have to finish the whole of the rest of the history first and put it into context, because if you come out with that at question three you can cancel the rest of the interview, because you are not going to learn much'.

The other thing that chastens me in pursuing this as a matter of practicality is that for all of the literature on prevalence and impact and so on, the literature on treatment of people who have had sexual abuse in the past and how that may impact their lives is tiny and not very encouraging. Granted, we may get the information, but is there practical value to doing anything about it? This speaks to the point that if it is on the back shelf, painful as it may remain, that is probably a good place for it.

Beard: I would agree with Dr Steege that if you are working in the pain field and you are used to these problems, a gynaecologist can perfectly well ask this question. What is important is that there are back-up facilities in that clinic, as Dr Peters has suggested that there should be facilities for dealing with it. I would not want to see a barrier put into this exchange of skills that is going to be necessary if we are to treat these women both psychologically and somatically for chronic pelvic pain.

Steege: I draw a commonality between what Mrs Smith is doing with your folks and what Dr Peters' folks are doing. I will take a placebo any day if it lasts five years – I am happy. But whatever window of time it may give you, that may be the golden moment of opportunity that as surgeons we have not yet capitalised on to do the kinds of things that you are doing to prepare them for remission of symptoms and the impact on their lives.

References

1. Sutton CJG, MacDonald R. Laser laparoscopic adhesiolysis. *J Gynecol Surg* 1990;**6**:155–9.
2. Di Sebastiano P, Fink T, Di Mola FF, Weihe E, Innocenti P, Friess H, *et al.* Neuroimmune appendicitis. *Lancet* 1999;**354**:461–6.
3. Bornstein J, Goldik Z, Stolar Z, Zarfati D, Abramovici H. Predicting the outcome of surgical treatment for vestibular vestibulitis. *Obstet Gynecol* 1997;**89**:695–8.
4. Giamberardino MA, Berklet KJ, Iezzi S, de Bigotina P, Vecchiet L. Pain threshold variations in somatic wall tissues as a function of menstrual cycle, segmental site and tissue depth in non-dysmenorrheic women, dysmenorrheic women and men. *Pain* 1997;**71**:187–97.
5. McKay E, Kaufman RH, Doctor U, Berkova Z, Glazer H, Redko V. Treating vulvar vestibilitis with electromyographic biofeedback of pelvic floor musculature. *J Reprod Med* 2001;**46**:337–42.
6. Rapkin AJ, Kames LD, Darke LL, Stampler FM, Naliboff BD. History of physical and sexual abuse in women with chronic pelvic pain. *Obstet Gynecol* 1990;**76**:92–6.
7. Collett BJ, Cordle CJ, Stewart CR, Jagger C. A comparative study of women with chronic pelvic pain, chronic nonpelvic pain and those with no history of pain attending general practitioners. *Br J Obstet Gynaecol* 1998;**105**:87–92.
8. Bewley S, Friend J, Mezey G, editors. *Violence Against Women.* London: RCOG Press;1997.

SECTION 6

PAIN IN CANCER AND POSTOPERATIVE PAIN

Chapter 21

Pain control and palliative care in gynaecology

Adrian Tookman

Introduction

Palliative care has an important role to play in the management of patients with gynaecological illness who have pain. The perception that palliation should be reserved for patients who are imminently dying is common and misjudged. By adopting a palliative approach the quality of pain control will be enhanced for a far wider population of patients.

The following groups of patients should be considered:

- Patients with cancer pain undergoing treatment (surgery, radiotherapy and chemotherapy);

- Patients who have pain following definitive treatment (some of these patients will be cured);

- Patients who have advanced cancer;

- Patients who have advanced cancer and are imminently dying;

- Patients with chronic progressive painful nonmalignant conditions;

- Patients with chronic pain.

Many of these patients will benefit from a palliative approach to care, and some of these patients will need referral to a specialist palliative care physician (See Box A). A close and collaborative relationship between the palliative care team and the gynaecologist will enhance the ability to address the complex issues that arise when a patient with advanced disease has acute or chronic pain.

Assessment of pain

Pain can be alleviated or modified in most patients. A proper pain assessment leads to effective management.

Box A. Palliative care

- **Specialist palliative care services:** are those services with palliative care as their core speciality. Specialist palliative care services are needed by a significant minority of people whose deaths are anticipated, and may be provided:
  - Directly through specialist palliative care services
  - Indirectly through advice to a patient's present professional advisers/carers
- **Palliative approach:** aims to promote both physical and psychosocial wellbeing. It is a vital and integral part of all clinical practice, whatever the illness or its stage, informed by a knowledge of palliative care principles.

Definition from National Hospice Council for Hospice and Specialist Palliative Care Services: *Specialist Palliative Care: A Statement of Definitions* October 1995.[16]

It is easy to fall into the trap of focusing exclusively on the physical problems causing pain. However, non-physical factors can influence the patient's perception of pain. Patients with advanced illness have multiple needs when faced with pain, debility and possible death. Thus, for many patients, their experience of pain can be a complex one. Ignoring these complex needs can lead to inadequate pain control. The management of physical pain is pivotal in achieving optimal control but all aspects of a patient's pain experience must be considered to enable that patient to have total pain control.

Pain can be caused by:

- *Physical problems* – from the pathophysiological process of the illness itself, from the effects of treatment or from disability caused by treatment and/or illness. The majority of patients have pain at more than one site and often from many causes. Each pain should be evaluated individually. In order to establish the cause of the pain it is essential to take a careful history noting:

  - the site of pain and any radiation,

  - the type and severity of pain,

  - the onset of pain,

  - response to analgesics, and

  - exacerbating and alleviating factors.

  Physical examination often confirms the diagnosis. However, it is occasionally necessary to perform investigations such as X-rays, isotope bone scans, computerised tomography scans etc.

- *Emotional problems* – When faced with advanced illness, patients frequently experience depression, despair, anger and fear. It is important to acknowledge these emotions because it will be easier for the patient to express and discuss their problems if they are given weight and value.

- *Social problems* – Socially isolated patients can feel unsafe, and those patients who are financially insecure can feel threatened.

- *Spiritual problems* – Patients with advanced illness often search for meaning. For some, this meaning may be embedded in a religious framework. Spiritual distress can occur during this search and can significantly affect a patient's perception of pain.

- *Sexual problems* – Untoward effects of illness and treatment can affect a patient's sexuality and this is commonly seen in gynaecological practice. Physical problems from disease or treatment may be obvious but patients with gynaecological illness can experience emotional and social problems related to their sexuality. For example, they may no longer see themselves as a 'woman' or a 'mother'; they may have problems related to drugs they are taking; they may feel 'dirty' if they have a stoma. Sexual problems and problems related to body image are common, underestimated and often not discussed by the patient or clinician. Often simple explanations and support are all that is needed.

Treatment of pain with analgesics

The World Health Organization describes a three-step ladder for the prescription of analgesics:

- Step 1 Non-opioid +/– adjuvant
- Step 2 Weak opioid +/– non-opioid +/– adjuvant
- Step 3 Strong opioid +/– non-opioid +/– adjuvant.

Analgesics should be prescribed regularly. Inadequate pain control at one step requires a move to the next step rather than to an alternative drug of similar potency. Adjuvant co-analgesics can be used at each step for treating that element of the pain which is opioid-insensitive.

The correct use of opioids has made a major impact on the management of pain in patients with advanced disease, yet pain continues to be badly managed by many doctors. Unfounded fears by professionals and patients about the use of strong opioids, lack of understanding about how opioids should be prescribed correctly and an inability to recognise pain that is opioid resistant all contribute to this problem[1] (see Figure 21.1).

Oral morphine is the mainstay of the treatment of pain in advanced disease. It is available in two forms; immediate acting (4-hourly) preparations (tablets and liquids) and slow-release (12-hourly and 24-hourly) preparations (tablets, dissolvable granules and suppositories). It is safe, predictable and reliable when prescribed correctly (see Figure 21.2). This can be achieved by adhering to the following guidelines:

- Morphine should be given orally unless the patient cannot tolerate oral medication,
- It must be prescribed regularly to pre-empt pain (use on an 'as required' basis will result in poor pain control and increased incidence of adverse effects).
- Extra doses for breakthrough and incident pain must be co-prescribed to be used as necessary – i.e. *rescue analgesia*.
- It must be given an adequate trial at an adequate dose.
- Adverse effects should be anticipated so that they can be prevented (see Box B).

Figure 21.3 shows a typical prescription for morphine, breakthrough doses and laxatives.

For patients who are unable to take oral morphine, injectable diamorphine is the drug of choice. It is highly soluble and therefore smaller volumes are needed. Because

Professional and lay fears about the use of opioids have always been a barrier to their effective use. Clear communication with patients is important to allay these anxieties.

Fear of addiction
Addiction, in the sense of psychological dependence and craving, does not occur. A large drug surveillance programme of the medical use of strong opioids (12 000 patients) found only four patients (0.03%) who were considered to be addicted to morphine. Chemical dependence does occur with opioids. Withdrawal should be gradual when the patient no longer needs the opioid because the pain has been controlled by some other means (for example the pain of a bony metastasis treated by radiotherapy).

Fear of tolerance
Tolerance is the progressive increase of dose to achieve the same effect in chronic treatment. There can be an anxiety that if a patient 'gets used to' an opioid then that opioid will be ineffective when the patient is in the final phase of the illness. There is little evidence of this with respect to the analgesic effect of opioids. In chronic pain management, when patients are treated over long periods with oral opioids, the rate of rise in dose is slow and there are long periods without any dose increase. Morphine doses that escalate in patients with cancer are invariably due to disease progression and not to opioid tolerance. Tolerance does develop to some of the side effects – notably nausea and sedation – to the benefit of the patient.

Fear of respiratory depression
In cancer patients where the opioid dose is titrated against the patients' pain, clinically significant respiratory depression does not occur. Indeed a double dose at bedtime can be given safely. Pain appears to be a physiological antagonist of the depressant effects of opioids on respiration. Respiratory depression can and does occur if the underlying cause of the pain is removed and the morphine dose is not adjusted.

Fear that morphine hastens death
Morphine is often not started until the patient is virtually moribund, hence the erroneous assumption that morphine hastens death, because of the close conjunction of the two events. Early prescribing of morphine may in fact prolong life. Control of pain enables the patient to sleep, to eat better and to increase physical activity. Despite some awareness that morphine can significantly improve an individual's quality of life there remains a public misconception that starting morphine signals to the patient and their carers that death is imminent. Unfortunately this misconception is fuelled by the frequent reports in the press of morphine being given to patients when they reach a terminal stage to ease their suffering and, perhaps, hasten their death. If morphine is prescribed correctly then this is a very unlikely scenario. It is vital that patients are reassured that morphine is safe, is given for pain and does not imply that death is imminent.

Fear that morphine is sedative and hallucinogenic
In the past, morphine was often prescribed in the form of a cocktail (usually with chlorpromazine as anti-emetic and/or cocaine for enhanced sense of wellbeing). Unfortunately, as the dose of morphine was titrated upwards, the toxic effects of the other drugs emerged – sedation and hallucinations. Hence the common misconception that morphine has significant sedative and hallucinogenic properties.

Figure 21.1.   Fears about use of strong opioids[17]

OPIOIDS IN ACUTE CANCER PAIN
Acute pain needs rapid action
- rapid titration of dose against pain is best achieved using 4-hourly, normal release, opioid preparations
- use the 4-hourly, normal release, preparations for rescue doses
- prescribe rescue (breakthrough) analgesia for pain that 'breaks through' the background analgesia. Daily use of breakthrough analgesia implies that the regular dose is not adequately controlling the pain and should be increased accordingly
- prescribe rescue (incident) analgesia for pain that is precipitated by painful 'incidents', e.g. when mobilising or for dressing changes. Using incident analgesia does not imply that the pain is not being controlled by the regular medication. The regular dose of opioid need not be increased. An increase in the regular opioid could lead to increased adverse effects.
- increases in regular dose can be made:
EITHER
By calculating the amount of breakthrough medication used in the previous 24 hours and incorporating it into the regular dose (this step should be repeated until maximum analgesia is achieved)
OR
By using a 'look back' technique. The regular dose of opioid can be increased by looking back at the effect of the previous dose of opioid. If the previous dose was not adequate the next dose is incrementally increased (providing there were no untoward adverse effects)

OPIOIDS IN CHRONIC CANCER PAIN
- Ideally follow steps outlined for acute pain. When analgesia is maximum convert to a slow-release preparation, e.g. controlled-release morphine sulphate.
- In some patients, especially in the outpatient setting, it may be possible and more practical to start with slow-release preparations.
- Always prescribe rescue doses of the 4-hourly preparation as well as the regular medication.

OPIOIDS IN CHRONIC NON-CANCER PAIN
This is a controversial issue and the following are guidelines. Specialist supervision is advisable.
- Careful patient selection is crucial.
- The pain must be opioid sensitive (a trial of opioids is a reasonable approach to assess this).
- Use controlled-release preparations.
- There should be clear ground rules about the maximum dose of opioid and the amount of rescue medication.
- Strictly limit the use of rescue doses of opioids and where possible do not prescribe them. In chronic non-cancer pain it is easy for a patient to escalate the doses of both regular and rescue medication simultaneously.
- Titrate slowly, assessing effectiveness and adverse effects. It can be difficult to assess effect. A functional assessment, rather than subjective reporting of pain control, is often the best guide.
- Be prepared to switch or rotate opioids – it is believed that receptor tolerance develops in very long-term use in some patients. Receptor tolerance can also cause problems when assessing relative potencies of different opioids. Great caution is therefore advised when switching opioids in these situations. The new opioid may be far more potent than anticipated.[18]
- Long-term and regular follow-up is mandatory.

Figure 21.2.   Approaches to prescribing opioids in palliative care

---

Box B.   Side effects of morphine

- **Constipation** is virtually universal. A laxative should always be co-prescribed with regular opioids unless there is a specific contraindication such as bowel obstruction.
- **Nausea and vomiting** are less common (35% of patients). If the patient has a predisposition to vomiting then regular antiemetics should be started. Opioid-induced nausea is self limiting and anti-emetics can often be stopped after 14 days.
- **Drowsiness** occurs in about 50% of patients. This wears off after a week on a stable dose. Explanation and reassurance are usually all that is necessary.
- **Other adverse effects** include confusion, sweating, dry mouth, itch, hallucinations and myoclonus. If severe they may be an indication to use an alternative strong opioid.

---

of the 'first-pass effect' in the liver, the dose of parenteral morphine is one-half to one-third the dose of oral morphine (Figure 21.4). Subcutaneous injection is the preferred route of administration because it is less painful. If the patient needs regular injections a subcutaneous infusion pump should be used (Box C).

Other medications can be mixed with the diamorphine as needed. The most commonly used additives are anti-emetics (cyclizine, haloperidol, or low-dose levomepromazine), sedatives (midazolam and/or levomepromazine) and/or anticholinergics (hyoscine).

Alternative opioids

Morphine sulphate has always been regarded as the standard step 3 opioid. However, morphine metabolites can be responsible for adverse effects and morphine is highly dependent on the kidney for excretion. Moderate renal failure can result in morphine toxicity. Renal problems are not uncommon in patients with advanced gynaecological malignancy. Pelvic disease can cause ureteric obstruction and chemotherapy can result in temporary or permanent renal dysfunction. In these situations alternative opioids have a role. There is increasing experience in the use of alternative opioids, mainly based on clinical rather than scientific evaluation. These drugs are generally used when opioid-sensitive pain exists but morphine is causing excessive adverse effects. Alternative opioids are used in long-term pain management when pain has become resistant to morphine and when morphine has been unsuccessful for presumed opioid-

---

MORPHINE SULPHATE 10 mg orally 4-hourly
(when on a stable analgesic regimen the early morning dose can be omitted and a double dose is prescribed at bedtime)

plus

MORPHINE SULPHATE 10 mg 4-hourly when required
(this is for breakthrough pain or incidents of pain and is the same as the 4-hourly dose)

plus

CODANTHRAMER 10 ml daily
(licensed for cancer patients only)
(regular laxatives should always be co-prescribed)

Figure 21.3.   Typical morphine prescription

EQUIVALENT DOSES OF OPIOIDS
(Dose of oral morphine: dose of injected diamorphine = 2:1 or 3:1)
l0 mg of morphine sulphate orally 4-hourly
(60 mg oral morphine in 24 hours)

is equivalent to

30 mg slow-release morphine twice a day
(60 mg oral morphine in 24 hours)

is equivalent to

5 mg of diamorphine hydrochloride subcutaneously 4-hourly
(30 mg subcutaneous diamorphine in 24 hrs)

is equivalent to

30 mg diamorphine in a 24 hour subcutaneous infusion (syringe driver)

Figure 21.4. Equivalent doses of opioids

sensitive pain. There appears to be individual variability in the response to different opioids and success may sometimes be seen only once an opioid has been switched.[2] Alternative step 3 opioids are usually second-line agents.

Step 3 opioids that are being used as alternatives to morphine

Fentanyl

Fentanyl is a transdermal preparation, the patch being applied every third day. It has a biological half-life of 17 hours and can take several days to reach steady state. It is not the drug of choice where patients need quick titration or in the opioid naive. It is particularly useful in patients who cannot swallow, have absorption problems or are poorly compliant with oral medication. It is metabolised in the liver to inactive metabolites. Thus it is a useful drug in patients with renal problems. It is said to cause less constipation than morphine.[3] Switching between transdermal fentanyl and other opioids can be difficult. There are conversion tables but they are only a guide.

Box C.   When to consider a continuous subcutaneous infusion

Consider a continuous subcutaneous infusion when:

THE PATIENT IS UNABLE TO TAKE ORAL MEDICATION
• Problems swallowing
• Dysphagia – due to tumour obstruction or neuromuscular incoordination
• Aspiration
• Nausea or vomiting
• Drowsiness or unconscious
• In the terminal phase of the illness

THE PATIENT IS UNABLE TO TAKE LARGE NUMBERS OF TABLETS

PARENTERAL ROUTE IS PREFERRED
• Absorption problems in the gastrointestinal tract
• Pain responds better to injections than oral opioid (UNUSUAL)

Box D.   A 'good death'

This is considered to have occurred when the symptoms have been well controlled and the patient is at peace with himself or herself.

In a study of healthcare workers a good death had occurred when the patient was at peace with themselves, had lived life to the full, was dying in a place of their choice, was with people close to them and was comfortable physically. Conversely a bad death occurred when there was severe physical or psychological distress and the patient had incomplete or unfinished business.[19]

A new preparation, oral transmucosal fentanyl citrate, is available. It is a lozenge that is absorbed buccally. It is likely to be particularly useful in the management of incident and breakthrough pain, when a rapid onset of action is required.

Methadone

This is a long-acting opioid. Opioids are said to be ineffective in neuropathic pain. However, clinical experience challenges this. Methadone, in particular, has a role in neuropathic pain by its action on delta opioid receptors (and its postulated action on *N*-methyl D-aspartate (NMDA) receptors and seratoninergic pathways).[4] Therefore it is a useful agent in its own right or combined with morphine in pelvic pain, a complex pain frequently exhibiting a neuropathic component. Its long half-life and affinity for storage in fat make it a difficult drug to use since adverse effects, such as sedation, may appear only when significant amounts of the drug have accumulated. Following dose adjustment it will take some time for the drug to be cleared. Consequently, methadone administration should be supervised by clinicians with experience in its use.

Oxycodone

This was introduced into the UK in 2000. Extensive experience in the USA suggests that this opioid may be useful because of its lipophilicity, suggesting a role in neuropathic pain. Its metabolites are inactive. It is recommended as an agent that can be used when step 2 or step 3 opioids are required. Escalating the dose increases the potency of this opioid. It has less active metabolites than morphine, and it is widely used for both malignant and non-malignant pain.[5]

Hydromorphone

Hydromorphone is similar to, but 7.5 times more potent than, morphine with metabolites that may be less active. There have been no good comparative studies with morphine, most data coming from anecdotal and retrospective reports.

Failure of opioid therapy

There are many reasons why opioids fail[6]. They may be incorrectly prescribed, i.e. with an inadequate dose, the wrong interval or the wrong route of administration (such as oral route in a patient who is vomiting). There may be poor compliance, either noncompliance or because the regimen is too complicated to follow. Finally, the pain may be opioid resistant. This last reason is probably the most common cause of failure, when an opioid is used for a pain that is in fact opioid resistant or only partially opioid sensitive. In these circumstances co-analgesics should be considered. The likelihood of opioid sensitivity should always be assessed. If the pain is not fully sensitive to opioids then co-analgesics in addition to the opioid should be considered. In some instances opioids have no role at all.

Pains that are resistant or partially resistant to morphine and the use of co-analgesics

Pain due to a large tumour mass

This is usually due to a pelvic mass infiltrating structures in the pelvis. It produces complex pain with somatic, visceral and neuropathic components, all of which must be treated. There are elements of this pain that are frequently only partially opioid responsive.

- *Primary treatment*: opioids and treatment of coexisting neuropathic pain and bone pain. nonsteroidal anti-inflammatory drugs* (NSAIDs) and steroids** have a role;
- *Consider other treatments:* treat tumour bulk with radiotherapy, chemotherapy, surgery, or embolisation.

Musculoskeletal pain

Commonly seen secondary to weakness and debility, this pain is opioid insensitive.

- *Primary treatment:* programme of rehabilitation, physiotherapy and massage are important modalities;
- *Consider other treatments:* benzodiazepines, joint injections or acupuncture.

Colic

Partial and complete bowel obstruction are common with advanced pelvic malignancies. Management strategies are dependent on the stage of illness, the performance status of the patient and whether there are further treatment options. In

---

*Nonsteroidal anti-inflammatories: Many palliative care patients may be predisposed to gastric problems, especially those on steroids. In these cases a 'gastroprotective agent' should be co-prescribed or a NSAID/Misoprostol combination should be used. Cyclo-oxygenase-2 inhibitors are said to cause less gastric irritation.[20]

**Steroids: Steroids can have serious adverse effects so it is essential to time the initiation of therapy and to assess the benefits versus risks carefully. Steroids often produce disabling proximal myopathy, and this can be confused with cancer-induced weakness. Wound healing can be particularly troublesome in bed-bound patients, who can rapidly develop pressure sores on steroids. Cushingoid appearance can cause problems with body image.

advanced disease it is common to manage patients conservatively. Pain can occur in bowel obstruction due to tumour and distension secondary to obstruction. Tumour pain is opioid sensitive but colicky pain is opioid insensitive. It must not be forgotten that constipation can present with colic.

- *Primary treatment:* treat constipation; stop/reduce drugs causing hyperperistalsis, antispasmodics – anticholinergics;

- *Consider other treatments:* treat obstruction with surgery or chemotherapy. Reverse obstruction with steroids. Reduce distension and high volume vomiting with octreotide.

Bone pain

Direct infiltration of the pelvis by local tumour can occur. Bone pain can be due to direct tumour involvement and infiltration causing mechanical disruption to bone which can lead to fracture. In addition, bone deposits can stimulate chemical mediators which activate osteoclasts and result in pain and bone destruction. Bone metastases are uncommon with gynaecological malignancies, but patients with pelvic malignancy are now surviving longer and there is an altered pattern of disease and metastatic spread. Subsequently, there needs to be an increased awareness that bony metastases can occur in gynaecological malignancy. Bone pain is partially opioid sensitive.

- *Primary treatment:* NSAIDs, opioids;

- *Consider other treatments:* radiotherapy (local to deposit); surgical fixation of fractures and prophylactic fixation to bones likely to fracture (long bones with greater than 50% erosion of one cortex); bisphosphonates if there are widespread deposits.

Capsular pain

Capsular stretching is commonly seen with metastatic liver disease. It is partially sensitive to opioids.

- *Primary treatment:* NSAIDs, opioids; steroids;

- *Consider other treatments:* chemotherapy; radiotherapy (rarely).

Nerve pain

Neuropathic pain is common in both malignant and nonmalignant conditions. It is usually caused by nerve compression, infiltration, irritation and/or destruction. It often coexists with visceral and somatic pain, e.g. a large pelvic mass may involve pelvic viscera, bone and sacral nerve plexus. Neuropathic pain is difficult to treat. Tricyclic antidepressants have a proven benefit and are probably still the drugs of first choice. They should be used initially at low doses (e.g. amitryptyline initially 10–25 mg daily) and then titrated upwards to standard antidepressant doses.

The management of neuropathic pain is particularly difficult because of the complex changes that occur in the nervous system when there is nerve damage and neuronal loss. When peripheral nerves are destroyed they degenerate their axons, 'dying back' to the spinal cord. This is a process known as deafferentation. The resultant pain is generated in the dorsal horn of the spinal cord and can be exceptionally difficult to control. Usually it is a dysaesthetic type of pain that can be difficult for the patient to describe. Allodynia can also occur (pain evoked by stimuli that would not usually produce pain, e.g. light touch). This is thought to be due to activation of the NMDA receptors in the spinal cord, causing 'wind up'.[7] This type of hyperalgesia sometimes responds to the agents used for neuropathic pain. Drugs which act on the NMDA receptor (e.g. ketamine and 'ketamine-like' drugs) may have a role in helping this type of pain.[8] It is 'classically' opioid insensitive,[9] however, this view is now challenged. High-dose morphine and alternative opioids appear to have an important role in its management. Therefore a trial of opioids, especially alternative opioids such as methadone, is reasonable.

- *Primary treatment:* amitriptylline; antiepileptics (gabapentin, valproate); membrane stabilisers (flecainide, mexilitine); opioids and alternative opioids (methadone);
- *Consider other treatments:* Steroids; nerve blocks; radiotherapy; chemotherapy.

Managing pain – nonpharmacological approaches

The pharmacological management of pain is important; however, pain is a total experience. A management strategy that takes into account all of the needs of the patient is essential if the goal is to achieve total pain control. This may include employing a wide range of nonpharmacological interventions, entailing a multiprofessional approach to the management of pain.

Physicians, surgeons, nurses, physiotherapists, occupational therapists, psychologists, social workers, counsellors and aromatherapists are examples of professionals who have a role in the diagnosis, assessment, treatment and monitoring of patients in pain. Teamwork is vital for optimal care.

Patients with pain problems often need emotional support, especially when they have life-threatening disease. Counselling can be a valuable part of the pain management programme: if emotional, social and spiritual needs of patients are disregarded then analgesics alone will fail.

Many patients seek complementary therapies for their pain. Indeed, the use of complementary and alternative medicine has become the norm for many cancer patients.[10] Large surveys suggest that over half of all cancer patients are engaged in some form of complementary and alternative practice. There has been a steady increase in the numbers of patients receiving complementary therapies among the general population and among cancer patients.[11]

This increasing request for complementary and alternative therapies could be viewed as a reflection of our inability to address adequately all the complex issues with which our patients present. On the other hand, a more positive approach could be adopted. Although many complementary treatments are unproven there is little doubt that some patients obtain significant relief from them. There is a high demand for these therapies from the public and a political pressure to integrate these therapies into health care. Our role is to ensure that patients are treated safely and not exploited at a vulnerable time in their lives. Many therapies are now considered to be part of mainstream medicine and specialist palliative care units often employ the skills of aromatherapists, diversional therapists, acupuncturists etc. to help manage patients with pain and advancing illness. By integrating a broad range of therapeutic approaches in our treatment plans we can enhance the patient's experience.

In 1993, the British Medical Association defined these therapies as 'unconventional therapies'. They can also be described as complementary therapies, which can work alongside and in conjunction with orthodox medical treatment. The term alternative therapies is usually reserved for when they are given in place of orthodox treatment. In the USA the Office of Alternative Medicine of the National Institutes of Health has coined the term 'complementary and alternative medicine' (CAM) to encompass both of these approaches. The term integrated health care describes the provision of complementary treatments alongside orthodox medicine

Pain in the terminal phase of illness

When a patient is dying, a healthcare professional has a clear responsibility to enable that person to have a 'good death'. To make this feasible the professional must be aware of the complex problems that can occur at this time and understand that physical symptoms need to be seen in the context of the patient's psychosocial circumstances. Physical symptoms, including pain, must be controlled effectively and wider issues, such as the needs of the patient's family, should be appreciated.

The three most common symptoms are: pain; noisy, moist breathing; and restlessness and agitation.[12]

Management of the dying patient

Recognise that the patient is dying

Recognising that a patient is in fact dying can be particularly difficult when a patient has been receiving 'active' treatment. To enable there to be a 'change of gear' in treatment the carers need to acknowledge that the patient is undergoing an irreversible process and that death is imminent.[13]

Communicate

Religious and cultural needs should be identified. There should be opportunities made to enable a patient to complete tasks, to say important things and to make endings. Although it may be difficult to have a meaningful conversation at this stage, many patients are conscious when close to death. Communication with the patient to discuss their symptoms, psychological needs, anxieties and fears continues to be important. It is always less frightening when patients are aware of the changes that are happening.

Communicating with the 'family', informing them of likely changes, is important and reassuring.

Stop unnecessary medication

Unnecessary medication, e.g. insulin, steroids, antibiotics, antihypertensives etc., should be stopped.

Control pain and other symptoms

The management of the patient at this stage should follow the basic principles of symptom control. An active approach to the patient's symptom control should be taken, with treatment decisions always being made in the context of the patient's overall clinical state. General measures, such as regular and meticulous mouth care, are vital for patient comfort. Pressure area care is important, the patient's position should be continually reviewed and the patient must be on the optimal mattress to ensure comfort. A flexible approach to the needs of the patient is essential. It may be inappropriate to turn an uncomfortable patient who is close to death. Drugs must be given by the correct route. In a patient who is too weak or drowsy to take oral medication drugs should be administered subcutaneously. Symptoms can invariably be controlled with analgesics, sedatives and anti-secretory drugs.

Anticipate crises

In some cases crises can be anticipated. A large bleed may occur as a result of the tumour eroding a major artery. Acute respiratory distress might develop in a person who has stridor. In such cases 'crisis medication', usually a combination of diamorphine and midazolam, should be available to be given if an acute distressing life-threatening event occurs. This can be administered by nursing staff for urgent symptom control without delay that inevitably occurs if a doctor has to be contacted at the time of the event.

Common symptoms in the terminal phase and their management

Pain

Where possible patients should be asked about their pain. However, pain can be difficult to assess in a patient whose level of consciousness has fallen. Facial grimacing, tachypnoea and groaning when moved are all indicators that a patient may be in pain. Check for retention of urine, which is an easily reversible cause of pain and agitation.

Some patients may need to start oral or parenteral opioids at this stage. Patients who are already on regular opioids will need the equivalent dose parenterally if they are unable to manage oral medication. Opioids should always be continued even if the patient becomes unconscious. A physical withdrawal reaction will be precipitated if opioids are stopped abruptly. The parenteral route of choice is subcutaneous injection. It is safe and reliable. If more than two or three injections will be needed a continuous infusion should be started. A 24-hour subcutaneous infusion can be used in any setting (home, hospital or hospice). Diamorphine is the opioid of choice for parenteral use. It has a rapid onset of action, 5–10 minutes after a subcutaneous injection. It is highly soluble and can be combined with other drugs that are commonly needed at this time.

If a patient who is imminently dying is on transdermal fentanyl this should be continued with the current patch strength. If additional analgesia is required, injections of diamorphine or a 24-hour subcutaneous infusion of diamorphine are given in addition to the fentanyl. The fentanyl could be changed to an equivalent dose of subcutaneous diamorphine, but this switch can be difficult due to the variability in potencies and half-lives between these two drugs in individual patients

Breathing

When a patient's condition deteriorates there are many predictable changes in their respiration. Often the pattern of breathing alters and it is reassuring to the relatives to be warned of these potential changes. As the patient weakens the ability to cough up secretions is lost. This gives rise to noisy moist breathing known colloquially as the 'death rattle', which can cause much distress to relatives. It should be explained that this phenomenon is more distressing to the people looking after the patient than to the patient themselves. It can usually be relieved by anticholinergic drugs (hyoscine hydrobromide, hyoscine butylbromide, glycopyronium). It is better to start the anticholinergic drug sooner rather than later as it does not dry up existing secretions. If pulmonary oedema is felt to be a contributory factor a diuretic can be tried. Rarely, in resistant cases, suction is necessary. Sometimes changing the position of a patient can be enough to reduce noisy, grunting breathing.

Restlessness and distress

Terminal distress, preterminal agitation, terminal restlessness, terminal anguish are all terms used to describe agitation and distress in patients close to death. Terminal restlessness reflects significant suffering on the part of the patient and causes considerable distress to the relatives who witness it. It is particularly important to assess the patient and rule out easily reversible causes. Urinary retention will require catheterisation. Pain, hypoxia, constipation and pruritis can usually be easily dealt with. Sometimes just changing the position of a patient can reduce the restlessness.

Infection, hypercalcaemia, renal failure, liver failure, cerebral metastases and, in some cases, hypoxia and hypercapnia can make a patient agitated. In the context of a dying patient these are often terminal events, and active treatment might therefore be considered inappropriate.

It is often not possible to control the restlessness without also compromising consciousness. Sedation should be offered to ease a patient's distress. There are three sedatives that have an important role in terminal restlessness: midazolam, levomepromazine and phenobarbitone.[14,15]

A 'good death'

A 'good death' is important for all persons involved with the care of a patient. The professional (nurse or doctor) needs to feel rewarded and have a sense that they have done the best for the patient. The patient should have had a good death with their symptoms well controlled. The family should be satisfied that their relative was well managed. They should display appropriate grief and if the death was a 'good death' this will minimise any abnormal bereavement problems.

References

1. Zenz M, Willweber-Strumpf A. Opiophobia and cancer pain in Europe. *Lancet* 1993;**311**:1075–6.
2. Galer BS, Coyle N, Pasteniak GW, Portenoy RK. Individual variability in the response to different opioids: report of five cases. *Pain* 1992;**49**:87–91.
3. Ahmedzai S, Brooks D. Transdermal fentanyl versus sustained-release morphine in cancer pain: preference, efficacy, and quality of life. TTS-Fentanyl Comparative Trial Group. *J Pain Symptom Manage* 1997;**13**:254–61.
4. Dickenson AH. Pain and analgesia: new light on mechanism and therapy. *CME Bulletin Palliative Medicine* 1999;**1(4)**:98–103.
5. Heiskanen T, Kalso E. Controlled-release Oxycodone and Morphine in cancer related pain. *Pain* 1997;**73**:37–45.
6. Tookman A, Kurowska A. Management of cancer and neuropathic pain: management of pain in palliative care. *Prescriber* 1998;**19**:90–98.
7. Dickenson AH. NMDA receptor antagonists: interactions with opioids. *Acta Anaesthesiol Scand* 1997;**41**:112–15.
8. Dickenson AH. A cure for wind-up: NMDA receptor antagonists as potential analgesics. *Trends Pharmacol Sci* 1990;**11**:307–9.
9. Besse D, Lombard MC, Zajac JM. Pre- and postsynaptic distribution of mu, delta and kappa opioid receptors in the superficial layers of the cervical dorsal horn of the rat spinal cord: a quantitative autoradiographic study. *Brain Res* 1990;**521**:15–22.
10. Kohn M. *Complementary Therapies in Cancer Care* (Abridged report of a study produced for Macmillan Cancer Relief). London: Macmillan Cancer Relief, 1999.
11. Burnstein HJ Discussing complementary therapies with cancer patients: what should we be talking about? *J Clin Oncol* 2000;**18**:2501–4.
12. Enck RE. The last few days. *Am J Hospice and Palliative Care* Aug. 1992; July/August:11–13.
13. National Council for Hospice and Specialist Palliative Care Services. *Changing Gear – Guidelines for Managing the Last Days of Life in Adults.* London: National Council for Hospice and Specialist Palliative Care Services; December 1997.
14. McNamara P, Minton M, Twycross RG. Use of midazolam in palliative care. *Palliative Med* 1991;**5**:244–9.
15. Stirling C. Kurowska A, Tookman A. The use of phenobarbitone in the management of agitation and seizures at the end of life. *J Pain Symptom Manage* 1999;**17**:363–8.
16. National Hospice Council for Hospice and Specialist Palliative Care Services. *Specialist Palliative Care: A Statement of Definitions.* London: National Hospice Council for Hospice and Specialist Palliative Care Services; 1995
17. Tookman A, Kurowska A. Management of terminal pain and distress. *Prescriber* 1999;**10**:29–41.
18. A retrospective comparison of dose ratios between methadone, hydromorphone and morphine. *Cancer* 1996;**78**:852–7.
19. Low J, Payne S. The good and bad death perceptions of health professionals working in palliative care. *Europ J Cancer Care* 1996;**5**:237–41.
20. Cox S, Tookman A. Management of cancer and neuropathic pain: mode of action, side effects and interactions. *Prescriber* 1998;**19**:85–8.

Chapter 22

Pain and cancer – other options

Beverly Jane Collett

Although more than 70% of cancer patients with moderate to severe pain will achieve adequate control of their symptoms with routine systemic pharmacotherapy, between 10% and 30% of patients may require additional treatment.[1,2] Anaesthetic or neurosurgical techniques in selected patients may reduce or eliminate the requirement for systemic opioids.

Decision making

The use of invasive and neurodestructive techniques should be based on an evaluation of the likelihood and duration of analgesic benefit, the immediate and long-term risks, the likely survival, the availability of expertise, the duration of hospital stay and the fully informed consent of the patient.

For most pain syndromes a range of techniques exist that may be applied. In choosing between a range of procedures, the following principles are important.

- Ablative procedures are deferred for as long as the pain is controlled by nonablative techniques.

- The procedure most likely to be effective is selected. If there is a choice, the one with the fewest and least serious adverse effects is preferred.

- In the progressive stages of cancer, pain is likely to be multifocal and a procedure aimed at a single locus of pain is unlikely to yield complete relief of pain. A realistic and sound goal is to decrease pain to a level that is manageable by pharmacotherapy with minimal adverse effects.

- Whenever possible, neurolysis is preceded by the demonstration of effective analgesia with a local anaesthetic block.

- Individual clinician bias can influence decision making and a case conference is prudent when assessing a challenging case. The views of the patient are paramount.

Gynaecological pain

Pain resulting from gynaecological cancer may be due to the disease, both primary and metastatic, but about 22% is associated with treatment or concurrent disease.[3] Comprehensive assessment of the patient and the pain sites is essential.

Gynaecological cancer tends to spread locally by direct invasion or metastasises to regional lymph nodes. Pelvic pain can be difficult to manage because it is poorly localised and tends to be bilateral.

Some distinct syndromes can occur in gynaecological cancer and are discussed below.

Lumbosacral plexopathy

Lumbosacral plexopathy can be due either to tumour invasion or as a result of radiation.

Tumour invasion

Lumbosacral plexopathy most commonly occurs in association with tumours of the rectum, cervix, breast, sarcoma and lymphoma (when local intra-abdominal disease spread is responsible). Jaekle et al. investigated the natural history of lumbosacral plexopathy in 85 patients with documented pelvic tumours.[4] In 70% of patients, pain occurred in the form of pelvic or radicular leg pain and was the presenting complaint, followed by sensory symptoms and weakness some weeks to months later. Weakness in a pattern that involved more than one nerve root was the most consistent clinical finding. Sensory loss and reflex asymmetry were present in the majority of patients. The lower part of the plexus, containing innervation from L5 to S3 nerve roots is most commonly involved, with signs of foot-drop, a pelvic tilt, pelvic lordosis and numbness of the thigh, sole and perineum. Upper plexus compression causes hip flexor weakness with difficulty in climbing stairs and numbness in the anterior thigh. The most sensitive test to delineate the lesion and evaluate possible compression into the epidural space is a computerised tomography (CT) scan of the pelvis. Electromyography (EMG) may also be useful to differentiate a plexopathy from neuropathy or radiculopathy. The presence of metastatic lumbosacral plexopathy suggests advanced disease with a median survival of 5.5 months.

Specific cancer treatment, such as radiation therapy or chemotherapy, may bring about improvement of the neurological dysfunction, including pain. Oral opioid analgesics and adjuvant drugs may provide pain relief, but often spinal opioids and local anaesthetics may be needed to control this neuropathic pain syndrome.

Tumour-induced reflex sympathetic dystrophy

Reflex sympathetic dystrophy, or complex regional pain syndrome, is a term used to describe a spectrum of incompletely understood syndromes characterised by neuropathic pain and vasomotor disturbance. Classically, this is a post-traumatic process, but variations induced by tumour invasion and/or anti-tumour therapy have been recognised.

Reflex sympathetic dystrophy can occur with tumour infiltration of the lumbosacral plexus.

The quality of the pain tends to be neuralgic and/or dysaesthetic and, when constant, is characterised as burning, numbing, tingling, pressing or squeezing. Patients may complain of a sharp, stabbing, shooting pain. Evoked pain and alterations in resting sensory thresholds (allodynia, hyperaesthesia and hyperpathia) are common.

Associated findings may include a combination of vasomotor and sudomotor (sweating) abnormalities, including intermittent cyanosis, rubor or pallor, oedema, atrophy of muscle, skin, subcutaneous tissue and nails, hypohydrosis and hyperhydrosis and increased or decreased temperature (Table 22.1).

Several cases of painful hot foot due to tumour involvement of the lumbar sympathetic chain have been described in patients with cervical and rectal cancer.[5,6]

A trial of local anaesthetic blockade of the sympathetic nervous system should be considered early, even in ambiguous cases. In experienced hands, the effects of treatment are relatively innocuous and they may affect resolution of otherwise intractable symptoms.

Radiation-induced lumbosacral plexopathy

Radiation-induced lumbosacral plexopathy is less common than brachial plexopathy. Pelvic tumours for which radiation is indicated are generally associated with a poorer prognosis than breast cancer and lymphoma. The lumbosacral plexus is embedded in the substance of the psoas muscle for much of its anatomic distribution, which, together with the bulk of the adjacent vertebral column, may partially shield it from direct radiation injury. Finally, radiation doses below nerve tolerance are usually administered in this region out of respect for the vulnerability of the adjacent bowel to injury. It is seen in women who have received external and intracavity irradiation through radium implants and in patients who have undergone radiation to the para-aortic lymph nodes.

Table 22.1.   Tumour-induced reflex sympathetic dystrophy

Quality of pain
- neuralgic or dysaesthetic
- constant
- burning, numbing, tingling
- pressing, squeezing
- sharp, stabbing, shooting

Distribution of pain

Altered sensory threshold
- allodynia, hyperaesthesia, hyperpathia

Vasomotor and sudomotor abnormalities
- intermittent cyanosis, rubor or pallor
- oedema, atrophy of muscle, skin, nails
- anhydrosis, hyperhydrosis, hypohydrosis
- increased or decreased temperature

Horner's sign (upper limb)

Presenting symptoms include weakness of the legs associated with paraesthesiae and numbness. Pain occurs in only 10% of patients. Radiation necrosis of the pelvic bone commonly accompanies this disorder and can aid in diagnosis.

Techniques for pain control

Techniques for pain control can be divided into the following groups:

- sympathetic nervous system blockade;
- central nervous system blockade or destruction;
- peripheral nervous system blockade or destruction – not applicable for gynaecological cancer pain.

Sympathetic nervous system

The sympathetic nervous system has been implicated in the maintenance of cancer pain syndromes. Sympathetic blockade may be used to block either the visceral nociceptive afferent fibres or the sympathetic efferent fibres:

- blockade of the afferent visceral nociceptive fibres may reduce or eliminate visceral pain
- blockade of sympathetic efferent fibres may reduce neuropathic pain (e.g. lumbosacral plexopathy)
- destruction of sympathetic nerves is not accompanied by weakness or numbness
- neuritis and deafferentiation pain are not significant risks.

Surgical approaches have been described but are used less frequently in preference to chemical disruption as the latter techniques have been improved upon and do not require the cancer patient to be exposed to the rigours of surgery.

Anatomy of the sympathetic nervous system

The peripheral portion of the sympathetic nervous system consists of a pair of ganglionated paravertebral chains that extend from the base of the skull to the coccyx, several major prevertebral plexuses (cardiac, coeliac and hypogastric) and numerous small intermediate and terminal ganglia. The ganglia of the sympathetic chain lie on the anterolateral aspect of the vertebral column. The ganglia are inconstant in number due to fusion of adjacent components and anatomic variability. The usual arrangement consists of three paired cervical ganglia, 12 paired thoracic ganglia, four paired lumbar ganglia, four paired sacral ganglia and a single unpaired ganglion impar near the sacrococcygeal junction.

Visceral pelvic pain of lower urogenital origin may be amenable to either lumbar sympathetic, superior hypogastric plexus or ganglion impar block. Lumbosacral

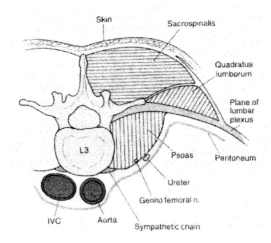

Figure 22.1. Transverse section through L3 to show position and relations of lumbar sympathetic chain; (reproduced with kind permission of Churchill Livingstone from *Principles and Practice of Regional Anaesthesia* 1987, p. 189, edited by JAW Wildsmith & EN Armitage)

plexopathy due to tumour invasion or to radiation fibrosis may be amenable to treatment with neural blockade of the lumbar sympathetic chain.

Lumbar sympathetic block

Technique

Figure 22.1 shows a transverse section through L3 to show the position of the sympathetic chains.

The patient is positioned prone with a pillow placed under the pelvis to extend the spine. Fluoroscopy is used to identify spinous processes of L2 to L4. Current practice is that only one needle is used and a skin weal is raised at the level of L3 spinous process at a distance of 8–10 cm from the midline. This distance should correspond to the lateral border of the erector spinae muscles which, in most individuals, is palpable. Infiltration of skin and deeper tissues at an angle of 45° takes place. Needle length varies from 12.5 to 17.5 cm and either a 20-gauge or 22-gauge needle is selected. The needle is introduced at 45° with the midline and advanced until the vertebral body is contacted. The depth is noted, the needle withdrawn and redirected so that its tip slides just past the lateral margin of the corresponding vertebral body to a depth of about 1 cm beyond the prior insertion. Some authors advocate attaching a glass or plastic syringe and using a loss of resistance technique to further identify the correct fascial plane.

Once the needle is placed and aspiration is negative for blood or cerebrospinal fluid, 1–3 ml of non-ionic contrast medium is injected through the needle and the spread of dye is observed. The characteristic appearance on lateral views is of a thin column of dye anterior to the vertebral bodies, with a smooth posterior contour corresponding to the anterior border of the psoas fascia. Anterior views should demonstrate contrast confined to the paramedian region with no tracking along the psoas muscle. Most commonly, either 10 ml of 0.25% bupivacaine plain as a diagnostic test or 5 ml of 6–7% aqueous phenol is injected. Alternatively, but less commonly, CT may be used to aid needle location.

Complications

Genitofemoral neuralgia, intravascular injection, backache and trauma to kidney or ureter are potential complications. Subarachnoid injection is occasionally seen but easily recognisable and should not constitute a hazard.

Superior hypogastric plexus block

Surgical interruption of the hypogastric plexus (presacral neurectomy) is a procedure that has been demonstrated to relieve a variety of painful pelvic conditions – predominantly of non-oncological origin. Presacral neurectomy for chronic pelvic pain showed success rates of 73% in relieving dysmenorrhoea, 77% in relieving dyspareunia and 63% in relieving other pelvic pains.[7] Superior hypogastric plexus block is analogous to presacral neurectomy and has emerged as an important option for intractable pelvic pain due to cancer.

Technique

The superior hypogastric plexus is a retroperitoneal structure located bilaterally at the level of the lower third of the fifth vertebral body and upper third of the first sacral vertebral body at the sacral promontory and in proximity to the bifurcation of the common iliac vessels. This plexus is in continuity with the coeliac plexus and lumbar sympathetic chains above and innervates the pelvic viscera via the hypogastric nerves (Figure 22.2).

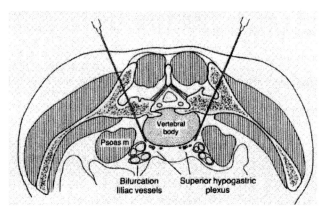

Figure 22.2.   Cross-sectional schematic view illustrating bilateral hypogastric plexus block and needles' relationship to fifth lumbar vertebrae, psoas muscle, and iliac vessels; (reproduced with kind permission of JB Lippincott Company from *Cancer Pain* 1993; p. 416, edited by RB Patt)

Superior hypogastric plexus block is performed with the patient in the prone position with a pillow placed beneath the pelvis to flatten the lumbar lordosis. The lumbosacral region is cleaned aseptically. The location of the L4–L5 interspace is approximated by palpation of the iliac crests and spinous processes and is then verified by X-ray. Skin wheels are raised 5–7 cm bilaterally to the midline at the level of the L4–L5 interspace. A 7-inch (17.5 cm) 22-gauge short bevelled needle with a depth marker placed 5–7 cm along the shaft is inserted through one of the skin weals with the needle bevel directed towards the midline. From a position perpendicular in all planes to the skin, the needle is orientated about 30° caudad and 45° medial so that its tip is directed towards the anterolateral aspect of the bottom of the L5 vertebral body. The needle is advanced until the body of the L5 vertebra is encountered or its tip is observed under X-ray to lie at its anterolateral aspect. If the vertebral body is encountered, the tip is 'walked off' the vertebral body. The needle tip is advanced about 1 cm past the depth at which contact with the vertebral body occurred and at a point at which a loss of resistance may be felt, indicating that the needle has passed the anterior fascial boundary of the ipsilateral psoas muscle and lies in the retroperitoneal space. The contralateral needle is then advanced in a similar fashion.

X-ray screening is used and anteroposterior views should demonstrate the needle tips' location at the level of the junction L5 and S1. Lateral views confirm placement of the needle tip just beyond the vertebral bodies anterolateral margin. Needle position is further verified by the injection of 3–4 ml of water-soluble contrast media through each needle. In the anteroposterior view, the contrast should be confined to the paramedian region. In the lateral view, a smooth posterior contour corresponding to the anterior psoas fascia indicates that needle depth is appropriate (Figure 22.3). Alternatively, computerised axial tomography can be used.

For a diagnostic superior hypogastric plexus block, 6–8 ml of 0.25% bupivacaine plain can be given through each needle. For neurolytic blockade, 6–8 ml of 10% aqueous phenol can be used through each needle.

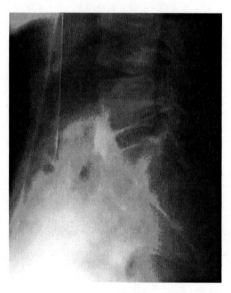

Figure 22.3.   Lateral radiograph demonstrating correct needle placement for unilateral hypogastric plexus block

Complications

Vascular puncture, with a risk of subsequent haemorrhage and haematoma formation, is possible due to the close proximity of the common iliac vessels. Intramuscular or intraperitoneal haemorrhage may result from improper estimation of depth. These and less likely complications such as subarachnoid and epidural injection, somatic nerve injury, renal or ureteral puncture can usually be avoided by careful technique.

Results

In the first published study, 28 patients with neoplastic involvement of pelvic viscera secondary to cervical cancer (20 patients), prostatic cancer (four patients), testicular cancer (one patient) and radiation injury (three patients) were treated with neurolytic superior hypogastric plexus block. Pain was significantly reduced or eliminated in all cases and no serious complications occurred. A mean reduction in pain of 70% was observed and residual pain seemed to be of somatic origin.[8]

Twenty-six patients with extensive gynaecological, colorectal or genitourinary cancer and uncontrolled pelvic pain underwent superior hypogastric plexus block. Eighteen (69%) patients achieved satisfactory lasting pain relief after one or two procedures [visual analogue scale (VAS) reduced from 10 to 3 or below] and the remaining eight patients achieved partial relief (VAS reduced from 10 to 4–7). No complications were encountered.[9]

Superior hypogastric plexus block is an effective minimally hazardous palliative block for visceral cancer pain emanating from one or more of the following organs: descending colon and rectum, vaginal fundus and bladder, prostate and prostatic urethra, testes, seminal vesicles, uterus and ovary.

Ganglion impar block

The ganglion impar is a solitary retroperitoneal structure located at the level of the sacrococcygeal junction that marks the termination of the paired paravertebral sympathetic chains.

Characteristically, sympathetic pain in the perineum is vague and poorly localised and is accompanied by sensations of burning and urgency. It is possible that the sympathetic component of this pain derives at least in part from ganglion impar.

Technique

The patient is positioned in the lateral decubitus position and a skin weal is raised in the midline at the superior aspect of the intergluteal crease just above the anus. The stylet is removed from a standard 22-gauge 8.8-cm spinal needle which is manually bent about 2.5 cm from its hub to form a 25–30° angle. This manoeuvre facilitates the positioning of the needle anterior to the concavity of the sacrum and coccyx (Figure 22.4).

The needle is inserted through the skin weal, with its concavity oriented posteriorly and under X-ray is directed anterior to the coccyx, closely approximating to the anterior surface of the bone, until its tip is observed to have reached the sacrococcygeal

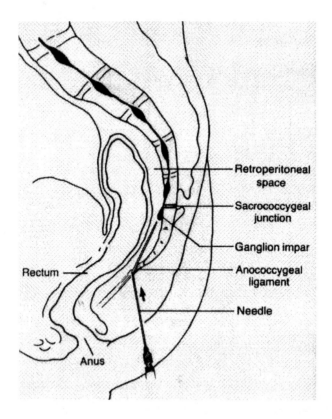

Figure 22.4. Lateral schematic view demonstrating correct needle placement for blockade of ganglion impar; (reproduced with kind permission of JB Lippincott Company from *Cancer Pain* 1993; p. 419, edited by RB Patt)

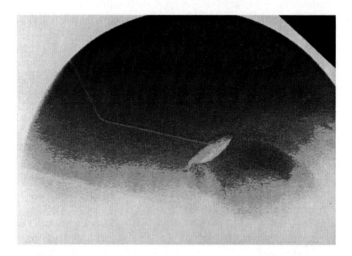

Figure 22.5. Lateral radiograph demonstrating needle placement for ganglion impar block

junction. Retroperitoneal location of the needle is verified by observing the spread of 2 ml of a water-soluble contrast solution which typically assumes a smooth margined configuration resembling an apostrophe (Figure 22.5). Four millilitres of 0.25% bupivacaine is injected for diagnostic and prognostic proposes and 4–6 ml of 10% phenol is injected for therapeutic neurolytic blockade.

Local tumour invasion may prohibit the spread of injected solutions. Observation that the spread of contrast material is restricted to the retroperitoneum is essential, as one case of epidural spread within the caudal canal has been reported. Perforation of the rectum or periosteal injection are possible. Anatomical abnormalities of the coccyx may inhibit access, in which case a further bend in the needle may be needed.

Results

The first report of the interruption of the ganglion impar for relief of perineal pain was published in 1990. Sixteen patients were studied (13 women and three men) with an age range from 24 to 87 years. All patients had advanced cancer (nine cervical, two of the colon, two of the bladder, one rectal and one endometrial) and pain had persisted in all cases despite surgery and/or chemotherapy, radiotherapy, analgesia and psychological support. Localised perineal pain was present in all cases and characterised as burning in eight cases. After preliminary local anaesthetic blockade and subsequent neurolytic block, eight patients experienced complete (100%) relief of pain. The remainder experienced significant reduction (90% for one patient, 80% for two, 70% for one and 60% for four). Blocks were repeated in two patients with further improvement. Follow-up depended on survival and was carried out for 14–120 days.[10]

Central nervous system blockade or destruction

Intraspinal opioids and local anaesthetics

Rationale for use

Oral morphine is usually used for cancer pain management because it is effective and easy to take. In some patients, high doses may cause adverse effects, such as nausea, vomiting, sedation, hallucinations and excessive sweating. Vainio and Tigerstedt[11] showed that in severe pain that requires high doses of morphine, equal pain relief using lower doses and causing fewer adverse effects can be achieved with epidural compared with oral administration. Although epidural and intrathecal morphine have been used as alternatives to oral or subcutaneous routes, results from randomised control trials are lacking.[12–14] Subcutaneous administration has also been claimed to reduce the extent of adverse effects caused by oral morphine.[15] Kalso et al.[16] reported a randomised, double-blind crossover study to compare the efficacy and acceptability of subcutaneous and epidural morphine. Subcutaneous opioid was found to be as good as epidural opioid, both in terms of efficacy and also for adverse events.

Spinal administration (either intrathecal or epidural) of a combination of both local anaesthetic and opioid has gained increasing popularity.[17–19] Neuropathic pain, intermittent visceral pain and pain on movement may not respond to spinal morphine alone and may require addition of local anaesthetic.[18,20]

In contrast to neurolytic blocks and neurosurgery, intraspinal opioid therapy produces a safe and reversible blockade that is more likely to be effective for multiple pains or for bilateral pain.

Mechanism of action

Opioid receptors are present within the spinal cord, predominantly within the dorsal horn of the spinal grey matter. The dorsal horns are the location of synapses between the primary afferent sensory neurones responsible for pain transmission (A-delta and C fibres) and the second-order spinal neurones. Opioid receptors are present pre- and post-synaptically and exert an inhibitory influence on the transmission of pain sensation across this synapse in the dorsal horn.

Intraspinal opioid therapy involves the delivery of minute quantities of drug in close proximity to the site of action in the spinal cord. The main advantage of spinal opioid analgesia is its selectivity. Motor, sensory and sympathetic systems are unaffected.

Opioids must be free of preservative and in this form morphine is available. Freeze-dried diamorphine is also suitable and easily available.

The administration of local anaesthetics into the epidural and subarachnoid space has assumed a growing role in the management of acute pain associated with obstetrics, surgery and trauma. By contrast with opioids, they are non-selective and will block motor, sensory and sympathetic fibres. However, by using dilute concentrations of local anaesthetic drugs, analgesia can be provided with no motor nor sensory loss.

Dose

For epidural administration of preservative-free morphine or diamorphine, 0.1 (1/10) of the 24-hour oral morphine dose equals the 24-hour epidural dose in milligrammes.

For intrathecal administration of preservative-free morphine or diamorphine, 0.01 (1/100) of the 24-hour oral morphine dose equals the 24-hour intrathecal dose in milligrammes.

Spinal clonidine

Clonidine is an α-2 agonist. Spinally administered clonidine has been shown to be analgesic in animals and in humans. The mechanism of analgesia is thought to be due to activation of dorsal horn α-2 adrenergic receptors, resulting in inhibition of transmission between the primary afferent nociceptive fibres and second-order dorsal horn neurones. A randomised control trial of 85 patients comparing 30 μg/hour of epidural clonidine with placebo for 14 days showed successful analgesia was more common with epidural clonidine (45%) compared with placebo (21%) and more so in neuropathic pain (56% versus 5%).[21]

Adverse effects of spinal opioids

Dose-limiting adverse effects are rare in cancer patients who have previously been exposed to oral or subcutaneous opioids. Treatment of adverse effects is usually symptomatic, but when they are severe, they can be often be treated with intravenous or intramuscular naloxone without reversal of analgesia.

Respiratory depression: Respiratory depression causes most clinical concern, although it is unlikely to happen in cancer patients who have previously been maintained on oral or subcutaneous opioids.

Factors that contribute to respiratory depression include accidental overdose, absence of severe pain, advanced age or debility, coexisting pulmonary disease, co-administration of opioids by other routes and opioid naïveté.

Constipation: Systemic opioids delay gastric emptying and decrease gastrointestinal motility by their action on the opioid receptors in the gut. Postoperative ileus persists longer when pain is treated with epidural morphine than bupivacaine. However, clinically constipation seems to be much less of a problem with spinal than oral opioids, although it may become a problem as dosage is increased.

Nausea and vomiting: Epidural morphine has been observed to reduce gastric emptying in volunteers. The incidence of nausea and vomiting may be as high as 25–30% in opioid-naïve patients, but is infrequent in patients with prior opioid use.

Urinary retention: Although acute intraspinal administration of opioids may be associated with naloxone-reversible urinary retention, it is rarely observed in opioid-tolerant cancer patients.

Pruritus: This adverse effect is extremely common and distressing in opioid naïve patients, but uncommon in cancer patients.

Infections: Serious infection has not emerged as a common sequel to intraspinal opioid therapy administered either percutaneously or via implanted catheters. Infection may occur at the catheter exit site, along superficial or deep catheter tracks, or within the epidural or intrathecal space. Undetected or untreated, an infection may lead to epidural abscess and subsequent neurological deficit.

Superficial infection at the catheter exit site may occur in as many as 6% of cases, and serves as one of the rationales for tunnelled catheters. Exit site and superficial track infections resolve with topical care and/or systemic antibiotics. Deep track infections and epidural infection require removal of the epidural catheter and antibiotic administration. Epidural infections are most commonly associated with skin flora, although haematogenous spread from systemic infection and contamination from injectate also occur.

The importance of good local skin care, observation of filtered aseptic administration and vigilant assessment cannot be overemphasised.

Misinjections: Various substances have been accidently injected through epidural and intrathecal catheters. Prevention of such incidents by affixing distinct labels to intraspinal catheters is important.

Screening

Comprehensive assessment of the patient, diagnosis of the pain problem and full efforts to optimise oral or subcutaneous therapy should always be undertaken before consideration of spinal opioids. It is important to determine whether the pain syndrome is amenable to spinal opioids. Despite a high degree of individual variability, it has been observed that continuous or intermittent somatic or visceral pain are most responsive to intraspinal opioid therapy, whereas cutaneous and neuropathic pain are most intractable (Table 22.2).[22] A proportion of patients will respond well regardless of the underlying mechanism of pain. The addition of local anaesthetic should be considered.

Epidural and intrathecal administration of opioids and local anaesthetics produce analgesia by similar modes of action and evidence is lacking for important distinctions in efficacy between routes. Each route has different advantages (Table 22.3).[23]

Mode of administration

Spinal drugs can either be given as a bolus or as an infusion. Most clinicians now favour the use of infusion. The main advantage of a continuous infusion is maintenance of stable cerebrospinal fluid levels of drug, resulting in fewer episodes of pain and

Table 22.2.   Ranking list of likelihood of cancer-related pain to respond to treatment with epidural morphine[22]

1. Continuous somatic pain
2. Continuous visceral pain
3. Intermittent somatic pain
4. Intermittent visceral pain
5. Neuropathic pain
6. Cutaneous (ulcer or fistula)

Table 22.3.   Potential advantages of epidural and intrathecal placement[23]

Placement	Advantage
Epidural	Reduced risk of post-dural puncture headache and chronic cerebrospinal fluid leak
	Dura acts as a barrier to infection
	Permits greater flexibility in drug selection
	Easier to use local anaesthetic drugs
	Side effects less common and intense
	Risk of neurological injury probably reduced
	Margin of safety increased in case of accidental overdose
Intrathecal	Technically easier to locate the intrathecal space
	Less risk of catheter obstruction from fibrosis and epidural metastases
	Less likelihood of pain on injection
	Analgesia is more intense, rapid in onset and longer duration
	Lower dose and volume of opioid and local anaesthetic required
	Absence of risk from catheter migration since catheter is already intrathecal

toxicity. Less frequent handling of the catheter system also means that there is reduced risk of infection.

A system for classifying the six basic types of implantable drug delivery systems has been suggested (Table 22.4). An understanding of each system's advantages and disadvantages is essential for optimal selection and use. However, in the UK, financial considerations mean that the least expensive option (a syringe driver and partially tunnelled epidural catheter) is often chosen other than in exceptional situations.

Ultimately the selection of the drug, the route and the mode of administration must be individualised to patient's circumstances and also to the experience of the team looking after the patient (Table 22.5).

Subarachnoid neurolytic block

Intrathecal injection of a neurolytic solution is a useful technique for the relief of intractable perineal pain related to cancer. Although the lower sacral nerve roots can be easily accessed, there is a risk that damage to the second and third sacral roots may

Table 22.4. Types of intraspinal catheters

Type I	Percutaneous epidural or intrathecal catheter
Type II	Percutaneous epidural or intrathecal catheter with a portion tunnelled subcutaneously from spinal insertion site
Type III	Totally implanted epidural or intrathecal catheter attached to subcutaneous injection port
Type IV	Totally implanted epidural or intrathecal catheter attached to implanted mechanically activated pump
Type V	Totally implanted epidural or spinal catheter attached to implanted infusion pump
Type VI	Totally implanted epidural or intrathecal catheter attached to implanted computer programmable infusion pump

Table 22.5. Spinal drugs for cancer pain

Selection	Drug
Drug	Opioid
	Opioid and local anaesthetic
	Opioid and local anaesthetic and clonidine
Route	Epidural
	Intrathecal
Catheter	Percutaneous tunnelled
	Subcutaneous port
	Totally implanted subcutaneous pump
Means of administration	Intermittent bolus
	Continuous infusion
	Continuous infusion plus PCA

result in deficits to bladder and/or bowel function. After pelvic exenteration for gynaecological cancer, when a colostomy and urinary catheter are in place, these concerns are unimportant.

Technique

The procedure is performed with the patient in the sitting position. A lumbar puncture is performed at L4–L5 or L5–S1. An injection of 1 ml of phenol in glycerol is then given with the patient tilted backwards at 45° to allow the neurolytic solution to diffuse downward in the midline to spare the motor roots. A test injection of heavy marcain is usual as a prognostic indicator before performing the neurolytic technique.

Percutaneous cordotomy

Percutaneous cordotomy is a technique that can be useful in intractable unilateral cancer pain. However, it is becoming less commonly performed due to improved non-invasive methods of pain relief. There are a few pain management and neurosurgical centres in the UK which are currently performing the procedure and it is preferable that patients are referred there for consideration of this technique.

Technique

The technique consists of introducing a Teflon™-insulated electrode with a 2-mm exposed tip through an 18-gauge lumbar puncture needle into the anterolateral aspect of the spinal cord. The needle is passed between the C1 and C2 vertebrae under image intensification. Small amounts of air and contrast material are injected intrathecally to outline the cord and the dentate ligament. The location of the tip of the needle just anterior to the dentate ligament is verified. The electrode locks into the hub of the needle so that the Teflon™ insulation projects 2 mm beyond the tip. Location of the electrode within the spinothalamic tract is confirmed with electrical stimulation. At 100 Hz, warm or cool paraesthesias occur in the contralateral part of the body, but no motor responses are seen. When the electrode is optimally located, a graded radiofrequency lesion is made with serial neurological testing in particular of ipsilateral lower limb power and contralateral analgesia.

Reported pain relief after percutaneous cordotomy is reported to be 59–96%, at the expense of a 0–6% mortality, 2.6–4.2% respiratory complications, 1–20% persistent paresis and 0–8.7% persistent bladder dysfunction. Post-cordotomy dysaesthesia has been reported in up to 20% of cases.

Conclusion

Most patients with cancer pain will have their pain successfully managed with oral or subcutaneous opioid analgesics and co-analgesic drugs. A proportion, from 10% to 30%, will need consideration of other techniques to control their pain. Anaesthetic techniques can be helpful in controlling pain and an awareness of the available techniques is important to ensure appropriate referral.

It is important that early discussion takes place between all clinicians involved in the patient's care and the patient if pain control is difficult. It is essential to ensure a comprehensive assessment of the pain and adequate discussion with the patient with regard to the benefits and risks of treatment options. This will enable the patient to play an active role in decision making about their care.

References

1.   Grond S, Zech D, Schug SA, Lynch J, Lehmann KA. Validation of World Health Organization guidelines for cancer pain relief during the last days and hours of life. *J Pain Symptom Manage* 1991;**6**:411–22.

2.   Schug SA, Zech D, Dorr U. Cancer pain management according to WHO analgesic guidelines. *J Pain Symptom Management* 1990;**5**:27–32.

3.   Kanner RM, Foley KM. Patterns of narcotic drug use in a cancer pain clinic. *Ann NY Acad Sci* 1981;**362**:161–72.

4.   Jaekle KA, Young DF, Foley KM. The natural history of lumbosacral plexopathy in cancer. *Neurology* 1985;**35**:8–15.

5.   Dalmau J, Graus F, Marco M. 'Hot and dry foot' as initial manifestation of neoplastic lumbosacral plexopathy. *Neurology* 1989;**39**:871–2.

6.   Gilchrist JM, Moore M. Lumbosacral plexopathy in cancer patients. *Neurology* 1985;**35**:1392–3.

7.   Lee RB, Stone K, Magelssen D, Belts RP, Benson WL. Presacral neurectomy for chronic pelvic pain. *Obstet Gynecol* 1986;**68**:517–21.

8.   Plancarte R, Amescua C, Patt R, Aldrete JA. Superior hypogastic plexus block for pelvic cancer pain. *Anesthesiology* 1990;**73**:236–9.

9.   Leon-Casasola OA, Kent A, Lema M. Neurolytic superior hypogastric plexus block for chronic pelvic pain associated with cancer. *Pain* 1993;**54**:145–51.

10.   Plancarte R, Amescua C, Patt RB, Allende S. Presacral blockade of the ganglion of Walther (ganglion impar). *Anaesthesiology* 1990;**73**:A751.

11.   Vainio A, Tigerstedt I. Opioid treatment in radiating cancer pain: oral administration versus epidural techniques. *Acta Anaesthiol Scand* 1988;**32**:179–85.

12.   Penn RD, Paice JA. Chronic intrathecal morphine for intractable pain. *J Neurosurg* 1987;**67**:182–6.

13.   Plummer JL, Cherry DA, Cousins MJ, Gourlay GK, Onley MM, Evans KHA. Long-term spinal administration of morphine in cancer and non-cancer pain: a retrospective study. *Pain* 1991;**44**:215–20.

14.   Ohlsson L, Rydberg T, Eden T, Persson Y, Thulin L. Cancer relief by continuous administration of epidural morphine in a hospital setting and at home. *Pain* 1992;**48**:349–59.

15.   Drexel H, Dzien A, Spiegel RW, Lang AH, Brier C. Abbrederis K, *et al.* Treatment of severe cancer pain by low-dose continuous subcutaneous morphine. *Pain* 1989;**36**:169–76.

16.   Kalso E, Heiskanen T, Rantio M, Rosenberg PH, Vainio A. Epidural and subcutaneous morphine in the management of cancer pain: a double-blind cross-over study. *Pain* 1996;**67**:443–9.

17.   Kames ES. The chronic intraspinal use of opioid and local anaesthetic mixtures for the relief of intractable pain: when all else fails! *Pain* 1993;**55**:1–4.

18.   Van Dongen RTM, Crul BJP, De Bock M. Long-term intrathecal infusion of morphine and morphine/bupivacaine mixtures in the treatment of cancer pain: a retrospective analysis of 51 cases. *Pain* 1993;**55**:119–23.

19.   Sjoberg M, Applegren L, Einarsson S, *et al.* Long term intrathecal morphine and bupivacaine in 'refractory' cancer pain. I. Results from the first series of 52 patients. *Acta Anaesthesiol Scand* 1991;**35**:30–43.

20.   Samuelsson H, Hedner T. Pain characterization in cancer pain and the analgesic response to epidural morphine. *Pain* 1991;**46**:3–8.

21.   Eisenach JC, DuPen S, Dubois M, Miguel R, Allin D. Epidural clonidine analgesia for intractable cancer pain. The Epidural Clonidine Study Group. *Pain* 1995;**61**:391–9.

22.   Arner S, Arner B. Differential effects of epidural morphine in the treatment of cancer-related pain. *Acta Anaesthesiol Scand* 1985;**29**:32–6.

23.   Waldman SD, Kennedy LD, Leak DW, Patt RB. Intraspinal opioid therapy. In Patt RB, editor. *Cancer Pain*. Philadelphia: JB Lippincott Company; 1993, p. 285–328.

Chapter 23

Postoperative pain – management options after gynaecological surgery and caesarean section

Nicholas Levy and Roshan Fernando

Introduction

In the past decade there has been an increase in awareness of postoperative pain management with the establishment of hospital acute pain teams and its entry into the undergraduate medical curriculum. This has been partly due to the joint Colleges' report *Pain after Surgery*,[1] the increased role of anaesthetists in perioperative management and also patient advocate groups. Pain is one of the more common adverse effects of surgery that patients find extremely distressing and using modern techniques it can be better controlled than a decade ago.

Physiology of acute pain

To understand how analgesic techniques work it is necessary to have a basic understanding of the physiology of acute pain.[2,3] Local tissue trauma during surgery causes the release of an inflammatory 'soup' that stimulates nociceptors, pain receptors, to produce an electrical impulse. This process is known as *transduction* and can be influenced by nonsteroidal anti-inflammatory drugs (NSAIDs). The impulse is then *transmitted* to the central nervous system via myelinated Aδ and unmyelinated C fibres. This process is known as *transmission* and can be blocked by local anaesthetic drugs such as bupivacaine. In the dorsal horn of the spinal cord, descending and also other afferent pathways *modulate* the impulse. Further *modulation* occurs within the brain stem and thalamus. Opioids, paracetamol, acetylcholine (ACh), α2-receptor agonists all effect the central modulation of pain. Transcutaneous electrical nerve stimulation (TENS) is believed to work by stimulating other afferents to the spinal cord, which in turn inhibit pain pathways. Finally the painful stimuli itself is *perceived* within the somatosensory cortex.

Applied pharmacology in the management of postoperative pain

There are essentially three reasons for the considerable advance in the pharmacological management of acute pain: first, there is a greater and more widespread understanding of the pharmacology of the drugs used in pain management; second, the development and application of reliable and inexpensive drug delivery systems such as infusion pumps; and finally the introduction of acute pain teams into a hospital setting.

The World Health Organization (WHO) analgesic ladder devised for cancer pain management can be applied to postoperative pain management. This essentially states that the first-line management is with simple analgesics (e.g. NSAIDs and paracetamol); second-line management is with weak opioids, whereas third-line management is with strong opioids. All three management options may also include adjuvant treatment.

Opioids are agonists at endogenous opioid receptors. A weak opioid is a partial agonist at these receptors whereas a strong opioid is a full agonist. Adjuvant therapy includes the use of local anaesthetics during regional blockade, other pharmacological agents and nonpharmacological techniques such as TENS, psychological techniques and acupuncture.

Comparison of analgesic efficacy

The number-needed-to-treat (NNT) is a useful statistical tool that can be used to express the analgesic efficacy of drugs. It refers to the number of patients who need to receive the active drug for one patient to achieve at least 50% pain relief compared with placebo over a 6-hour treatment period. The most effective drugs have a low NNT of about 2. This implies that for every two patients who receive the drug one patient will obtain at least 50% pain relief because of the treatment (the other patient may obtain relief but it does not reach the 50% level). For example paracetamol 1 g has a NNT of almost 5, ibuprofen a NNT of 3 and diclofenac a NNT of 2.5. These NNT comparisons are against placebo.

The simple analgesics

NSAIDs

Local tissue damage occurring during surgery causes synthesis of prostaglandins from arachidonic acid under the influence of the enzyme cyclo-oxygenase (COX). The prostaglandins permit amplification of the stimulus at the nociceptors and the local tissue trauma is transduced into an electrical impulse. There are at least two isoenzymes, COX-1 and COX-2. NSAIDs are COX inhibitors and so prevent the production of prostaglandins. Table 23.1 shows the superior efficacy of the NSAIDs on a NNT basis.

There is overwhelming evidence that:

- NSAIDs are the best performing oral analgesics after the potent opioids.

- NSAIDs have an opioid-sparing effect.

- NSAIDs enhance the quality of opioid-based analgesia.

- NSAIDs are more effective for the pain associated with movement than opioids.

- NSAID administration should be routine after surgery except where there are contraindications.

There is no evidence that NSAIDs given rectally or by injection perform better or more rapidly than the same dose given orally.[5] These other routes become appropriate when the patient cannot swallow or absorb drugs. There are many different preparations of NSAIDs available and they differ in both their adverse effect profile and also in their pharmacokinetics. Only four NSAIDs (diclofenac, flurbiprofen, ketoprofen and ketoralac) are currently licensed for postoperative use.

NSAIDs may cause adverse effects (due mainly to COX-1 inhibition) and have potential drug interactions. The more important adverse effects include gastric erosion, platelet inhibition with concurrent increased intra-operative blood loss, bronchospasm and acute on chronic renal failure.[6] In large retrospective cohort studies, short-term use of NSAIDs in those under the age of 75 years did not increase the incidence of renal failure or gastrointestinal bleeding. However, acute renal failure can be easily precipitated in at-risk patients, including those with heart disease, chronic renal failure, the elderly, those patients with impending renal failure, as in pre-eclampsia, and patients on concurrent medication such as diuretics. The newer selective COX-2 inhibitors do not appear to offer any convincing protective advantage against the traditional non-selective NSAIDs, which inhibit both COX-1 and COX-2 isoenzymes.[4,7]

Paracetamol

Paracetamol is a widely used effective analgesic with antipyretic properties. Its analgesic strength is often under appreciated but it is actually highly effective, with an NNT of 4.6 (paracetamol 1 g).[8,9] Its exact mechanism of action is unclear; however, there is evidence that it is an inhibitor of COX within the brain and affects the modulation and processing of painful stimuli. It is rapidly absorbed from the duodenum and is effective within an hour of oral administration. Its main drawback is the narrow therapeutic range with the real potential for hepatic necrosis caused by a toxic metabolite.[4]

Table 23.1. Oral analgesic league table

Drug	Number Needed to Treat (NNT)
Codeine 60 mg	16.7
Tramadol 50 mg	9.7
Tramadol 100 mg	4.8
Paracetamol 1000 mg	4.6
Paracetamol 650 mg and dextropropoxyphene 65 mg	4.4
Paracetamol 600 mg and codeine 60 mg	3.1
Tramadol 150 mg	2.9
Ibuprofen 400 mg	2.7
Diclofenac 50 mg	2.3
Paracetamol 1000 mg and codeine 60 mg	1.9

Opioid analgesics

Opioids are agonists at specific opioid receptors within the central nervous system. They inhibit the release of excitatory neurotransmitters and hyperpolarise the postsynaptic membrane so that transmission of nociceptive stimuli is reduced. Opioid analgesia has adverse effects including respiratory depression, postoperative nausea and vomiting, and gastrointestinal and bladder dysfunction, which will all restrict the patient from mobilisation and discharge. It is also clear that opioids used alone are not effective at preventing the pain associated with coughing or moving. This has led to the concept of multimodal or balanced analgesia.

Routes of administration

Opioids are routinely administered orally, intramuscularly, intravenously or centrally (epidurally or spinally) in the control of gynaecological and obstetric postoperative pain. Although novel techniques such as transdermal, inhalational and rectal administration of opioids offer certain advantages over conventional routes, their place in mainstream clinical care is unproven.

Oral

Reduced gastric emptying is often associated with severe pain, limiting the usefulness of orally administered opioids immediately postoperatively for major surgery. However by the third postoperative day following major surgery, or sooner after minor surgery, either oral morphine or codeine with paracetamol should be effective. However, the dose needs to be increased due to first-pass liver metabolism and must be given regularly due to the lag time between drug absorption and effect. It should be noted that these drugs may cause constipation and a laxative should be considered in addition.

Intramuscular

The intramuscular route is the traditional method of administration but is generally ineffective. This is because an inadequate dose is prescribed with a dosing period that has total disregard for the drug's elimination half-life. In addition, the nursing staff do not give the drugs during the regular intervals that are required. This form of inadequate pain control has been superseded by modern techniques due to the greater understanding of the relevant pharmacokinetics. However, if a ward is adequately staffed and trained to use the intramuscular technique correctly it can still be highly effective.[10,11]

Intravenous

Opioids can now be given intravenously for the control of postoperative pain using modern syringe pumps. Syringe pumps can be programmed to give a bolus on demand as in patient-controlled analgesia (PCA) or via a continuous infusion, or even a combination of both methods. A continuous infusion may potentially lead to drug accumulation and respiratory depression, and if used should be managed according to strict protocols. Every hospital should have such a protocol for the use of any intravenous infusion, as well as a multi-disciplinary pain team to ensure maximum benefit and safe practice.

A PCA system is the favoured option as it is the safest and is more effective. In the UK morphine and pethidine (meperidine) are commonly used but diamorphine may also be used according to local policy. A typical intravenous morphine PCA regimen uses a bolus of morphine 1 mg with a 5-minute lockout period and no background infusion.

Central neuraxial blockade (epidural or spinal)

Diamorphine, morphine and fentanyl are often administered epidurally for the control of postoperative pain. They have identical pharmacodynamic properties in that they all provide analgesia, but may also cause delayed respiratory depression, pruritus and urinary retention. Due to their different pharmacokinetic properties diamorphine is the most logical choice of opioid for bolus analgesia and fentanyl for continuous infusions. Opioid drugs may also be administered as a single spinal injection (q.v.) at the time of anaesthesia.

Commonly used opioids

Morphine

Morphine is the most widely used opioid. It may be administered orally, intravenously, intramuscularly, or centrally. Since it has a half-life of less than three hours, intramuscular injections should be administered three-hourly as required. It is highly emetogenic and should be avoided if possible during daycare procedures such as laparoscopy. Morphine is hydrophilic, so it has a slower onset of action and if centrally administered has a greater potential for rostral spread than the more lipid-soluble opioids (diamorphine and fentanyl) resulting in a higher incidence of postoperative nausea and vomiting and a greater potential for respiratory depression.

Diamorphine

Diamorphine's main advantage is due to its high lipid solubility. When administered centrally, it is taken up rapidly by the neural tissue of the spinal cord with minimal rostral spread. Since rostral drug migration is limited, there is less potential for nausea and vomiting and respiratory depression compared with morphine.

Fentanyl

Fentanyl is more lipid soluble than diamorphine and has a rapid onset time but also a shorter half-life. This makes it ideal for epidural infusions. Due to its high lipid solubility fentanyl has minimal rostral spread and therefore a very low incidence of nausea and vomiting and respiratory depression when given centrally.

Codeine

Codeine is a drug of low potency, which has to be metabolised to morphine to be effective. The enzyme for its metabolism is missing in approximately 10% of the population. As sole agent codeine 60 mg has an NNT of 16 (poor analgesic efficacy), however it is more effective if given together with paracetamol (Table 23.1).

Pethidine

This is an opioid with a short half-life, which should not be used routinely for postoperative pain. Its toxic metabolite, norpethidine, accumulates with repeated administration and may rarely cause fitting.

Tramadol

Tramadol is an opioid with low potency. It can be an effective analgesic in higher doses but its use is limited by adverse effects of nausea, vomiting and somnolence.

Compound analgesic preparations

These include codeine, dihydrocodeine and dextropropoxyphene with paracetamol. Review of the literature suggests that both dihydrocodeine and dextropropoxyphene are ineffective analgesics individually.[12,13] In addition, when combined with paracetamol they are of limited benefit and may be just as successful as paracetamol alone. However, a paracetamol/codeine combination is highly effective.[8]

Local anaesthetic techniques

Local anaesthetic drugs

Local anaesthetics are sodium-channel blockers, which prevent propagation of the nerve impulse. In the control of postoperative pain they may be injected into the wound during local infiltration, used for a peripheral nerve block (e.g. rectus sheath block), or as part of a central neuraxial technique such as an epidural or a spinal.

Bupivacaine is the most commonly used local anaesthetic drug and is presented in its racemic form. Its main drawbacks are the real potential for cardiac and central nervous system toxicity. If used in high concentrations it can also cause profound motor block as well as sensory block. The drive within the pharmaceutical industry to produce single isomer drugs with improved safety has resulted in the manufacture of two new drugs, ropivacaine and levobupivacaine.[14]

Ropivacaine, the S-isomer of the propyl homologue of bupivacaine, has been introduced into clinical practice with the claim by the manufacturers that it produces selective sensory blockade. However, it is now known that it is 40% less potent than racemic bupivacaine.[15,16]

Levobupivacaine, the S-isomer of bupivacaine itself, has a more favourable safety profile in laboratory testing than the racemate. Clinical trials have shown it to have similar potency to racemic bupivacaine.[17]

Local anaesthetic regional blockade

Wound infiltration

Simple infiltration of the operative site may provide useful analgesia. This is especially true for superficial operations and some laparoscopic procedures.[18]

Peripheral nerve block (e.g. rectus sheath)

A rectus sheath block may potentially be an effective technique to overcome the pain associated with the entry sites of laparoscopy.[19,20]

Epidural

The epidural space is a fat-filled space within the spinal canal. By injecting local anaesthetics into this space, nerve-root transmission of pain can be blocked. Epidural opioids can also modulate pain pathways once within the epidural space by diffusion through the dura mater into the cerebrospinal fluid and so to the opioid receptors of the spinal cord. In practice, an epidural block for gynaecological operations is normally performed using a lumbar intervertebral approach. A single-shot epidural technique is uncommon due to the limited nature of postoperative analgesia. A continuous epidural method using an indwelling epidural catheter, through which drugs are given for postoperative analgesia, is more usual. A caudal block is a single-shot epidural injection via the sacral hiatus (sacrococcygeal membrane), which can be used to provide perineal analgesia for a limited period.

An epidural or spinal (q.v.) block may be used to provide sole anaesthesia for certain gynaecological operations or more often in combination with general anaesthesia. In the latter case the epidural can naturally be used to provide prolonged postoperative analgesia. Epidurals provide excellent analgesia, however they may rarely be associated with complications, such as headache and neurological problems. A review of 141 trials has conclusively shown that central neuroaxial blockade reduces mortality and serious morbidity post surgery,[21] although the benefit to the generally healthier gynaecological patient is less clear. For this reason, before embarking on central neuroaxial pain relief it is essential that the patient is made aware of the benefits and disadvantages of this technique and gives consent for the procedure to be performed. There are only a few contraindications to central neuroaxial blockade. These include patient refusal, bleeding diathesis (the risk of developing an extradural haematoma even with low-dose subcutaneous heparin or low molecular weight heparin is rare), hypovolaemia and sepsis.

Modern epidural drug regimens use a low-dose combination of local anaesthetic and opioid by continuous infusion. A popular mixture in the UK is 0.1% bupivacaine with 2 μg/ml of fentanyl (4–12 ml/h). Using low-dose mixtures of opioids and local anaesthetic, the risk of drug adverse effects, such as motor block or systemic toxicity, is minimised, while optimal analgesia is achieved. Central blocks are rarely used alone in daycare surgery due to concerns of delayed mobility and micturition.

A relatively novel method of epidural pain relief is patient-controlled epidural analgesia (PCEA). Similarly to PCA, it allows the patient to titrate the analgesia required. The same low-dose mixture of bupivacaine and fentanyl can be used for a PCEA regimen.

Spinal

At the time of anaesthesia an opioid and a local anaesthetic may be administered intrathecally as a single-shot spinal injection. An opioid such as morphine or diamorphine may provide useful postoperative analgesia for up to 12–24 hours.

Miscellaneous centrally administered agents

Some clinicians are now administering α2-receptor agonists intrathecally or epidurally, usually in combination with local anaesthetics and opioids. In contrast to opioids, these drugs, which include epinephrine and clonidine, are not associated with respiratory depression. Spinal cholinergic receptors have also been shown to have a potent antinociceptive action, an effect that can be mimicked by spinal cholinesterase inhibitors such as neostigmine. Intrathecal injection of neostigmine inhibits the metabolism of acetylcholine released within the spinal cord and produces prolonged analgesia in both animals[22,23] and humans[24–27] without the risk of respiratory depression or pruritus, adverse effects which are normally seen with opioids. However, severe emesis limits its use.

Nonpharmacological options

TENS is a form of analgesia that is safe and devoid of major adverse effects. However, in a review of 17 randomised controlled studies, only two showed a benefit of TENS over placebo.[28] Relaxation training, procedural information, cognitive coping methods and behavioural instructions can all reduce postoperative analgesia consumption.

Multimodal analgesia

The concept of multimodal treatment has evolved since no single drug is ideal or free of adverse effects and complications. By utilising several different techniques simultaneously lower doses of individual drugs can be used: small amounts of opioids in epidural mixtures reduce the quantity of local anaesthetic required, resulting in less lower limb weakness; NSAIDs and local anaesthetics have an opioid-sparing effect and so reduce the incidence of the adverse effects of opioid analgesia, namely respiratory depression, nausea, vomiting, pruritus and intestinal and urological dysfunction.

Postoperative nausea and vomiting

Nausea and vomiting are more frequent after gynaecological surgery than general surgery. As opioid-based techniques are potent causes of nausea and vomiting, multimodal techniques must be used for this population. Regular administration of the more effective anti-emetics is required as well as avoidance of emetogenic stimuli.

Pruritus

Opioids given epidurally or spinally are associated with a high incidence of pruritus. The exact mechanism is unknown but it is presumed to be centrally mediated due to opioid μ-receptor activation. Small doses of naloxone can treat pruritus without reversing the analgesia. Other opioid antagonists, such as naltrexone and nalmefene, and even subhypnotic doses of the anaesthetic induction drug propofol have all been successfully used to treat pruritus.

Choice of analgesia

The pre-operative visit by the anaesthetist allows a pain management plan to be formulated and discussed. It is important that an appropriate history is obtained since other factors apart from the type of surgery influence the amount of pain perceived by the patient and the techniques that may be used in the management of the postoperative pain.

Practical management of postoperative analgesia

Gynaecological procedures

Because of wide personal variations, pain may not be predicted by the type of operation and must be assessed individually, however certain principles can be used as a guide. The Office of Population Censuses and Surveys classification of operations and surgical procedures can be used as a basis for analgesic strategies. The system divides operations into five broad categories: minor, intermediate, major, major plus and complex major.

Minor procedures

These include suction termination of pregnancy, cervical dilatation and curettage, laser ablation of cervical lesions and superficial vulval surgery. Patients should all receive paracetamol and NSAIDs provided there are no contraindications.[29-31] For the shorter procedures it must be remembered that paracetamol and enteral NSAIDs are not going to be effective for at least one hour, so should be given as premedication. If appropriate local anaesthetic infiltration by the surgeon should be performed.

Intermediate procedures

These include diagnostic laparoscopy, laparoscopic tubal ligation, cone biopsy (including laser) and hysteroscopy. It is unusual to experience major discomfort following hysteroscopy and a combination of NSAIDs and paracetamol can be used as above. However, contrary to popular belief laparoscopic procedures can cause pain. There are several strategies that can be used to reduce the pain. As always, simple analgesics are used for initial management. NSAIDs can be used together with paracetamol as premedication and short-acting opioids, such as fentanyl, can be given intraoperatively. Long-acting opioids such as morphine should be avoided since they are associated with a high incidence of nausea and vomiting. Local anaesthetic block may also be appropriate for laparoscopy.[32] A rectus sheath block[19] or simple entry site infiltration is effective for the superficial pain. Injecting the mesosalpinx,[19,33] irrigating the fallopian tubes[34] or pouch of Douglas,[35] using lidocaine gel on the sterilisation clips[36-38] can reduce the pain associated with laparoscopic sterilisation. Shoulder-tip pain is a frequent complaint after laparoscopic surgery and irrigating the intraperitoneal cavity or the hemidiaphragm with large volumes of diluted local anaesthetic can reduce its incidence.[39,40] Other analgesic strategies include leaving catheters in the pouch of Douglas or intraperitoneally for postoperative local anaesthetic infusions.

Day-case surgery considerations

Day-case surgery[41,42] provides a particular challenge to both the surgeon and anaesthetist; the patient must be pain free with no nausea and vomiting before discharge. This can only be achieved by a meticulous surgical and anaesthetic technique. It is important not to forget the lag time between administration and effect of drugs, especially of the simple analgesics. Another important issue is the emetic effect of the longer-acting opioids, so that drugs such as morphine should only be given as a last resort. Incremental boluses of the short-acting opioid fentanyl are more appropriate. If the pain is severe, longer-acting opioids must be administered and it must be accepted that some of these patients will be admitted to hospital overnight.

Surgical factors are also important in reducing pain after laparoscopy. A gentle surgical technique, using clips rather than rings for laparoscopic sterilisation,[43] limiting the volume of distending gas[44] and expelling as much residual gas as possible at the end of the procedure can all help to reduce postoperative pain.[45-47]

It is important that an acceptable level of analgesia is achieved prior to discharge and that advice is given on the administration of the postoperative analgesics at home.[48] A combination of a NSAID and paracetamol with or without codeine is probably the ideal combination. It is important that the patient takes them regularly, and is made aware of possible interactions and the adverse effects, and should be advised not to take any other paracetamol-containing drugs or operate machinery.

Major procedures

These include more complex laparoscopic procedures such as laser ablation of endometriosis, tubal surgery, removal of ovarian cysts and laparoscopically assisted vaginal hysterectomy. Other major procedures include both abdominal and vaginal hysterectomy, myomectomy, bladder-neck suspension and anterior colporrhaphy.

Apart from simple analgesics it is highly likely that long-acting opioids, for example in the form of an intravenous morphine PCA, will need to be used in the postoperative period. It is good practice to prescribe paracetamol and NSAIDs at regular intervals on the drug prescription chart and not as required. An epidural (placed at the time of operation) infusion of low-dose bupivacaine and fentanyl is another option instead of intravenous morphine PCA. Coexisting medical problems (e.g. severe pulmonary or cardiovascular dysfunction) may make an epidural a more attractive option. Since a patient's pain requirements normally decrease over subsequent postoperative days, an epidural or PCA regimen can gradually be reduced and eventually discontinued. Oral therapy, such as oral morphine preparations, NSAIDs and other simple analgesics, can then be substituted. The day-to-day management of such decisions is usually delegated to the hospital's acute pain team.

Many anaesthetists will perform a single-shot epidural or spinal at induction of general anaesthesia using a long-acting opioid such as diamorphine in combination with bupivacaine. However, this strategy may be inadequate for procedures when major postoperative pain is anticipated for a few days. The use of intravenous morphine PCA or indeed any systemic opioid following such single-shot techniques should only be used if adequate agreed protocols are in place.

Complex major procedures

These include Wertheim's hysterectomy, pelvic exenteration and radical vulvectomy, all of which may be associated with significant morbidity. It is this group of patients that may benefit the most from effective epidural analgesia. If an epidural is contraindicated, morphine PCA should be available. The PCA or epidural can as before generally be removed by the third postoperative day and oral opioid analgesia can be substituted.

Caesarean section

A caesarean section is classified as major surgery and the resultant postoperative pain can be severe.

Regional analgesia

Today, caesarean sections are usually performed under regional anaesthesia. A single-shot spinal, an epidural or a combined spinal epidural (CSE) can be used to provide anaesthesia for surgery as well as postoperative analgesia using long-acting opioids.[49,50] Various strategies can be used to extend the analgesia into the postoperative phase, the most effective being the use of morphine or diamorphine either in the intrathecal injection or epidural injection. Diamorphine compares favourably with morphine when both are administered intrathecally to provide analgesia for caesarean section, producing analgesia of similar duration to morphine (15–20 h) but of faster onset, with fewer adverse effects.[51,52] For an elective procedure the intrathecal route may cause less nausea and vomiting compared with the epidural route; 250 μg of diamorphine intrathecally caused six times less nausea and vomiting than 5 mg epidural diamorphine for elective caesarean section.[53] This is thought to be due to a greater systemic absorption of drug from the epidural space. Due to its high lipid solubility, diamorphine is rarely associated with respiratory depression and using a popular intrathecal-dosing regimen of between 250 and 300 μg this complication has not been reported in the obstetric population. If fentanyl is substituted for a long-acting opioid, the duration of postoperative analgesia is short. A dose of 100 μg of epidural fentanyl combined with bupivacaine may only provide two hours of analgesia after caesarean section.[54]

Occasionally, if an epidural only or a CSE technique is used for surgery, there may be indications to leave the epidural catheter in place and administer low-dose local anaesthetic/opioid mixtures (e.g. bupivacaine and fentanyl) either as intermittent boluses, continuous infusion or even PCEA. This is an excellent method of providing prolonged postoperative analgesia providing the patient remains in a designated high-dependency area or on the labour ward. In an obstetric setting within the UK, often due to midwifery staffing concerns, this is usually performed for high-risk patients such as those with pre-eclampsia.

General anaesthesia

Although in some units intramuscular opioids remain popular following caesarean section under general anaesthesia they compare poorly with epidural/spinal opioids and intravenous PCA.[55,56] Morphine is the most popular drug for PCA. It provides better postoperative analgesia than fentanyl PCA[57] and is the PCA drug of choice for post-caesarean section analgesia in women who breastfeed.[58] Local anaesthesia skin infiltration to the wound at the end of the operation or bilateral ilio-inguinal blocks to provide postoperative analgesia are of uncertain benefit.[59]

NSAIDs

The use of NSAIDs and opioids has been shown to reduce opioid requirements following caesarean section. Rectal diclofenac prolongs the time to first analgesic request when used with intrathecal morphine.[60] Many obstetric units now prescribe regular diclofenac orally or rectally in the postoperative period together with paracetamol or paracetamol/opioid combinations.

Control of pain in recovery

Recovery personnel within a theatre complex are usually in the ideal position to optimise a patient's immediate postoperative analgesia requirements. If they are permitted to administer intravenous opioids, for example as agreed through local protocols, superior, more rapid and safer pain control can be achieved compared with intramuscular injections. This can also be useful when an intravenous PCA regimen is in progress, when several loading doses of opioid may be needed before a patient can obtain satisfactory pain relief using the PCA demand button.

The recovery personnel will also check to ensure any regional blockade, such as an epidural, is working and if not, notify the anaesthetist to give a further epidural bolus. Other forms of pain control can be initiated as necessary if the regional block is inadequate.

The acute pain team, audit and monitoring pain

Every hospital should have a multidisciplinary acute pain team, whose primary role is to review the management of all the patients with moderate to severe pain.[61,62] They also have important secondary roles. Firstly, in educating the junior medical and nursing staff in best practice, secondly in publishing protocols for the management of postoperative pain and the techniques employed with their safety features, and finally in auditing the pain levels in postoperative patients to ensure best practice is actually occurring.

The effects of interventions can only be assessed and improved if some form of measurement is made. Since objective assessment techniques are not available and pain cannot be assessed accurately and consistently by observers, pain severity scoring must be made by the patient. The visual analogue scale and verbal rating scale are two such reliable techniques that are widely used.

Summary

In the last decade, no new class of analgesic has been licensed for the control of postoperative pain, however it is universally agreed that our management has improved. This improvement is multi-factorial but is essentially due to a wider understanding of the relevant pharmacology, improved drug delivery techniques, the introduction of acute pain teams but moreover, the realisation that good pain management matters and may actually influence patient morbidity and mortality as well as satisfaction.

References

1.   The Royal College of Surgeons of England and the College of Anaesthetists. *Report of the Working Party on Pain after Surgery*. London: The Royal College of Surgeons of England and the College of

Anaesthetists; 1990.

2. Dickenson AH. Spinal cord pharmacology of pain. *Br J Anaesth* 1995;**75**:193–200.

3. Ekblom A, Rydh-Rinder M. Pain mechanisms: anatomy and physiology. In: Rawal N, editor. *Management of Acute and Chronic Pain*. London: BMJ Books; 1998. p. 1–22.

4. Dahl V, Raeder JC. Non-opioid postoperative analgesia. *Acta Anaesthesiol Scand* 2000;**44**:1191–1203.

5. McQuay HJ, Moore RA. Comparing analgesic efficacy of NSAIDs given by different routes in acute and chronic pain. In: McQuay HJ, Moore RA, editors. *An Evidence-Based Resource for Pain Relief*. Oxford: Oxford University Press; 1998. p. 94–101.

6. The Royal College of Anaesthetists. *Guidelines for the Use of Non-steroidal Anti-inflammatory Drugs in the Perioperative Period*. London: RCA; 1998.

7. Jackson LM, Hawkey CJ. COX-2 selective nonsteroidal anti-inflammatory drugs: do they really offer any advantages? *Drugs* 2000;**59**:1207–16.

8. McQuay HJ, Moore RA. Paracetamol with and without codeine in acute pain. In: McQuay HJ, Moore RA, editors. *An Evidence-Based Resource for Pain Relief*. Oxford: Oxford University Press; 1998. p. 58–77.

9. McQuay HJ, Moore RA. Oral ibuprofen and diclofenac in postoperative pain. In: McQuay HJ, Moore RA, editors. *An Evidence-Based Resource for Pain Relief*. Oxford: Oxford University Press; 1998. p. 94–101.

10. Gould TH, Crosby DL, Harmer M, Lloyd SM, Lunn JN, Rees GA, Roberts DE, Webster JA. Policy for controlling pain after surgery: effect of sequential changes in management. *BMJ* 1992;**305**:1187–93.

11. McQuay HJ, Moore RA. Injected morphine in postoperative pain. In: McQuay HJ, Moore RA, editors. *An Evidence-Based Resource for Pain Relief*. Oxford: Oxford University Press; 1998. p. 118–26.

12. McQuay HJ, Moore RA. Dextropropoxyphene in postoperative pain. In: McQuay HJ, Moore RA, editors. *An Evidence-Based Resource for Pain Relief*. Oxford: Oxford University Press; 1998. p. 132–7.

13. McQuay HJ, Moore RA. Dihydrocodeine in postoperative pain. In: McQuay HJ, Moore RA, editors. *An Evidence-Based Resource for Pain Relief*. Oxford: Oxford University Press; 1998. p. 127–31.

14. Reynolds F. Does the left hand know what the right hand is doing? An appraisal of single enantiomer local anaesthetics. *Int J Obstet Anesth* 1997;**6**:257–69.

15. Polley LS, Columb MO, Naughton NN, Wagner DS, van de Ven CJ. Relative analgesic potencies of ropivacaine and bupivacaine for epidural analgesia in labor: implications for therapeutic indexes. *Anesthesiology* 1999;**90**:944–50.

16. Capogna G, Celleno D, Fusco P, Lyons G, Columb M. Relative potencies of bupivacaine and ropivacaine for analgesia in labour. *Br J Anaesth* 1999;**82**:371–3.

17. Lyons G, Columb M, Wilson RC, Johnson RV. Epidural pain relief in labour: potencies of levobupivacaine and racemic bupivacaine. *Br J Anaesth* 1998;**81**:899–901.

18. Alexander JI. Pain after laparoscopy. *Br J Anaesth* 1997;**79**:369–78.

19. Smith BE, MacPherson GH, de Jonge M, Griffiths JM. Rectus sheath and mesosalpinx block for laparoscopic sterilization. *Anaesthesia* 1991;**46**:875–7.

20. Yentis SM, Hills-Wright P, Potparic O. Development and evaluation of combined rectus sheath and ilioinguinal blocks for abdominal gynaecological surgery. *Anaesthesia* 1999;**54**:475–9.

21. Rodgers A, Walker N, Schug S, McKee A, Kehlet H, van Zundert A, *et al*. Reduction of postoperative mortality and morbidity with epidural or spinal anaesthesia: results from overview of randomised trials. *BMJ* 2000;**321**:1493–1505.

22. Detweiler DJ, Eisenach JC, Tong C, Jackson C. A cholinergic interaction in alpha 2 adrenoceptor-mediated antinociception in sheep. *J Pharmacol Exp Ther* 1993;**265**:536–42.

23. Bouaziz H, Tong C, Eisenach JC. Postoperative analgesia from intrathecal neostigmine in sheep. *Anesth Analg* 1995;**80**:1140–44.

24. Mercier FJ, Benhamou D. Promising non-narcotic analgesic techniques for labour. *Baillieres Clin Obstet Gynaecol* 1998;**12**:397–407.

25. Liu SS, Hodgson PS, Moore JM, Trautman WJ, Burkhead DL. Dose-response effects of spinal neostigmine added to bupivacaine spinal anesthesia in volunteers. *Anesthesiology* 1999;**90**:710–17.

26. Lauretti GR, Hood DD, Eisenach JC, Pfeifer BL. A multi-center study of intrathecal neostigmine for analgesia following vaginal hysterectomy. *Anesthesiology* 1998;**89**:913–18.

27. Chung CJ, Kim JS, Park HS, Chin YJ. The efficacy of intrathecal neostigmine, intrathecal morphine, and their combination for post-cesarean section analgesia. *Anesth Analg* 1998;**87**:341–6.

28. McQuay HJ, Moore RA. Transcutaneous electrical nerve stimulation (TENS) in acute postoperative

pain. In: McQuay HJ, Moore RA, editors. *An Evidence-Based Resource for Pain Relief.* Oxford: Oxford University Press; 1998. p. 172–8.

29. Green CR, Pandit SK, Levy L, Kothary SP, Tait AR, Schork MA. Intraoperative ketorolac has an opioid-sparing effect in women after diagnostic laparoscopy but not after laparoscopic tubal ligation. *Anesth Analg* 1996;**82**:732–7.

30. Liu J, Ding Y, White PF, Feinstein R, Shear JM. Effects of ketorolac on postoperative analgesia and ventilatory function after laparoscopic cholecystectomy. *Anesth Analg* 1993;**76**:1061–66.

31. Rosenblum M, Weller RS, Conard PL, Falvey EA, Gross JB. Ibuprofen provides longer lasting analgesia than fentanyl after laparoscopic surgery. *Anesth Analg* 1991;**73**:255–9.

32. Moiniche S, Jorgensen H, Wetterslev J, Dahl JB. Local anesthetic infiltration for postoperative pain relief after laparoscopy: a qualitative and quantitative systematic review of intraperitoneal, port-site infiltration and mesosalpinx block. *Anesth Analg* 2000;**90**:899–912.

33. Alexander CD, Wetchler BV, Thompson RE. Bupivacaine infiltration of the mesosalpinx in ambulatory surgical laparoscopic tubal sterilization. *Can J Anaesth* 1987;**34**:362–5.

34. Koetsawang S, Srisupandit S, Apimas SJ, Champion CB. A comparative study of topical anesthesia for laparoscopic sterilization with the use of the tubal ring. *Am J Obstet Gynecol* 1984;**150**:931–3.

35. Haldane G, Stott S, McMenemin I. Pouch of Douglas block for laparoscopic sterilisation. *Anaesthesia* 1998;**53**:598–603.

36. Ezeh UO, Shoulder VS, Martin JL, Breeson AJ, Lamb MD, Vellacott ID. Local anaesthetic on Filshie clips for pain relief after tubal sterilisation: a randomised double-blind controlled trial. *Lancet* 1995;**346**:82–5.

37. Eriksson H, Tenhunen A, Korttila K. Balanced analgesia improves recovery and outcome after outpatient tubal ligation. *Acta Anaesthesiol Scand* 1996;**40**:151–5.

38. Tool AL, Kammerer-Doak DN, Nguyen CM, Cousin MO, Charsley M. Postoperative pain relief following laparoscopic tubal sterilization with silastic bands. *Obstet Gynecol* 1997;**90**:731–44.

39. Narchi P, Benhamou D, Fernandez H. Intraperitoneal local anaesthetic for shoulder pain after day-case laparoscopy. *Lancet* 1991;**338**:1569–70.

40. Cunniffe MG, McAnena OJ, Dar MA, Calleary J, Flynn N. A prospective randomized trial of intraoperative bupivacaine irrigation for management of shoulder-tip pain following laparoscopy. *Am J Surg* 1998;**176**:258–61.

41. Millar JM. Gynaecological procedures in day surgery. In: Millar JM, Rudkin GE, Hitchcock M, editors. *Practical Anaesthesia and Analgesia for Day Surgery.* Oxford: BIOS Scientific Publishers Ltd; 1997. p. 168–91.

42. Millar JM. Laparoscopy. In: Millar JM, Rudkin GE, Hitchcock M, editors. *Practical Anaesthesia and Analgesia for Day Surgery.* Oxford: BIOS Scientific Publishers Ltd; 1997. p. 153–66.

43. Chi IC, Cole LP. Incidence of pain among women undergoing laparoscopic sterilization by electrocoagulation, the spring-loaded clip, and the tubal ring. *Am J Obstet Gynecol* 1979;**135**:397–401.

44. Lindgren L, Koivusalo AM, Kellokumpu I. Conventional pneumoperitoneum compared with abdominal wall lift for laparoscopic cholecystectomy. *Br J Anaesth* 1995;**75**:567–72.

45. Fredman B, Jedeikin R, Olsfanger D, Flor P, Gruzman A. Residual pneumoperitoneum: a cause of postoperative pain after laparoscopic cholecystectomy. *Anesth Analg* 1994;**79**:152–4.

46. Jackson SA, Laurence AS, Hill JC. Does post-laparoscopy pain relate to residual carbon dioxide? *Anaesthesia* 1996;**51**:485–7.

47. Alexander JI, Hull MG. Abdominal pain after laparoscopy: the value of a gas drain. *Br J Obstet Gynaecol* 1987;**94**:267–9.

48. Codd C. Are analgesics necessary for women at home following laparoscopic gynaecological day surgery? *Nurs Pract* 1991;**5**:8–12.

49. Dahl JB, Jeppesen IS, Jorgensen H, Wetterslev J, Moiniche S. Intraoperative and postoperative analgesic efficacy and adverse effects of intrathecal opioids in patients undergoing cesarean section with spinal anesthesia: a qualitative and quantitative systematic review of randomized controlled trials. *Anesthesiology* 1999;**91**:1919–27.

50. Westmore MD. Epidural opioids in obstetrics – a review. *Anaesth Intensive Care* 1990;**18**:292–300.

51. Husaini SW, Russell IF. Intrathecal diamorphine compared with morphine for postoperative analgesia after caesarean section under spinal anaesthesia. *Br J Anaesth* 1998;**81**:135–9.

52. Roulson C, Chan A, Albin M, Carli F. Intrathecal morphine or diamorphine for caesarean section? Preliminary findings. *Int J Obstet Anesth* 1994;**3**:181.

53. Hallworth SP, Fernando R, Bell R, Parry MG, Lim GH. Comparison of intrathecal and epidural diamorphine for elective caesarean section using a combined spinal-epidural technique. *Br J Anaesth* 1999;**82**:228–32.

54.   Grass JA, Sakima NT, Schmidt R, Michitsch R, Zuckerman RL, Harris AP. A randomized, double-blind, dose-response comparison of epidural fentanyl versus sufentanil analgesia after cesarean section. *Anesth Analg* 1997;**85**:365–71.
55.   Macrae DJ, Munishankrappa S, Burrow LM, Milne MK, Grant IS. Double-blind comparison of the efficacy of extradural diamorphine, extradural phenoperidine and i. m. diamorphine following caesarean section. *Br J Anaesth* 1987;**59**:354–9.
56.   Eisenach JC, Grice SC, Dewan DM. Patient-controlled analgesia following cesarean section: a comparison with epidural and intramuscular narcotics. *Anesthesiology* 1988;**68**:444–8.
57.   Howell PR, Gambling DR, Pavy T, McMorland G, Douglas MJ. Patient-controlled analgesia following caesarean section under general anaesthesia: a comparison of fentanyl with morphine. *Can J Anaesth* 1995;**42**:41–5.
58.   Wittels B, Glosten B, Faure EA, Moawad AH, Ismail M, Hibbard J, *et al.* Postcesarean analgesia with both epidural morphine and intravenous patient-controlled analgesia: neurobehavioral outcomes among nursing neonates. *Anesth Analg* 1997;**85**:600–606.
59.   Huffnagle HJ, Norris MC, Leighton BL, Arkoosh VA. Ilioinguinal iliohypogastric nerve blocks–before or after cesarean delivery under spinal anesthesia? *Anesth Analg* 1996;**82**:8–12.
60.   Dennis AR, Leeson-Payne CG, Hobbs GJ. Analgesia after caesarean section. The use of rectal diclofenac as an adjunct to spinal morphine. *Anaesthesia* 1995;**50**:297–9.
61.   Black AM. Taking pains to take away pain. *BMJ* 1991;**302**:1165–6.
62.   Rawal N, Berggren L. Organization of acute pain services: a low-cost model. *Pain* 1994;**57**:117–23.

Chapter 24

Pain in cancer and postoperative pain

Discussion

___

Discussion following the papers of Mr Tookman, Dr Collett and Dr Fernando

Steege: Is anybody on this side of the pond using warmed CO_2 for a laparoscopy? It has been touted as a pain reducer in the USA – warming the gas through the insufflator. They are trying to sell us the gear.

Stones: On a related note, what about nitrous oxide rather than carbon dioxide? Is anybody advocating that?

Crowhurst: The embolism risk is too great. If there is any left behind or if it gets into the lesser sac and so on, it will stay there for a while, you get expansion and it is just too much of a problem, too insoluble.

Berkley: I was interested in Dr Tookman's comments about the ever-expanding palliative care in this country. In the USA, I believe that in order to be referred to palliative care a physician has to diagnose less than six months of life, so you are ahead of us.

Tookman: Palliative care in the UK is very different from palliative care in the USA. You are right, there is the six-month entry condition. I believe it is MediCare that has said it has to be six months, and there have been all sorts of criteria to try to assess patients' prognosis that have mainly been driven by the Americans, none of which have been very successful – which is what we all know when we try to assess prognosis. In the UK palliative care is diversifying greatly, which is good on one level and bad on another. We are diversifying into non-malignant work and we see a lot of patients with chronic problems such as chronic renal problems, chronic rheumatological problems, we see a lot of vascular patients. A good deal of that is chronic pain work, using opioids.

   The other thing is the changing nature of cancer care. There is a lot of pressure for cancer rehabilitation. At the end of the year 2001, in December, there is to be a government launch of something called the Supportive Care Strategy, which is all about supporting patients with advanced cancer through their cancer journey, and palliative care has nominated itself to be responsible for a big proportion of that supportive care. As I said, that comes with an up-side and a down-side which are obvious. But palliative care is certainly a growing specialty.

Fernando: In obstetrics we have recommendations from our association – they are rather old-fashioned now – about 500 deliveries per consultant session. Do you have any recommendations for that?

Tookman: Yes, there are recommendations. There is one consultant per 150 000 population. It is one consultant per teaching hospital, two consultants for each hospice unit. I would advise you not to do the figures because you know which way they are going to go. That has been published.

Fernando: From our point of view we regard our figures from the 1960s as very old-fashioned, and with Calman training we go for at least ten sessions. In other words, all week is covered by a consultant anaesthetist.

Crowhurst: I want to mention the question of thrombo-embolic problems after major surgery in cancer patients and gynaecology and a lot of other cancer surgery. I draw your attention to something that Dr Fernando has in his chapter although he did not mention it today. In the *British Medical Journal* before Christmas was published a very definitive review of trials of regional anaesthesia[1] and their benefit with respect to postoperative morbidity after major surgery, known as the CORTRA study. There is no doubt that regional anaesthesia, central neuraxial anaesthesia, is of enormous benefit when you have major surgery, abdominal and pelvic surgery as well as cardiac and so on. The reduced pain and reduced thrombotic problems and other morbidities are quite astounding on this study that took in over 10 000 mixed surgical patients, a lot of them orthopaedic but nevertheless in the age group of the patients we are talking about here.

Thrombosis and prophylaxis are described later in this volume but regional anaesthesia in this sort of patient is very important and I believe we will see its growth come on enormously. Having said all that, can I ask the Americans here whether regional, neuraxial anaesthesia is used a lot after major gynaecological surgery in the USA?

Steege: To some degree, especially in cancer patients with lengthier procedures and larger incisions. In the routine, benign procedures, relatively seldom, and zero in the laparoscopic procedures. One major difficulty in our hospital – and it is true of many – is that we do not have an anaesthesia work room aside from the operating room, so if there is a regional anaesthetic to be placed it takes up another half an hour of operating room time, which is precious, so it tends to be discouraged by the surgeons – strongly.

Stones: I should like to ask Dr Collett about superior hypogastric plexus block. We are aware with presacral neurectomy that there are serious problems with adverse post-surgical effects on bowel function. Is that something that you would expect to see after a local anaesthetic block for a neurolytic procedure?

Collett: I have performed only five superior hypoglastric plexus blocks. Four were with local anaesthetic for pelvic pain, so that was benign and we just used the block to see whether it would take the pain away, in a way seeing whether presacral neurectomy as a surgical approach might be something that the surgeons might want to consider. This was some years ago when we were looking to see whether this was a route that we should go down and whether we should be using diagnostic local anaesthetic blocks. We did not see it in that. In the other two patients who had a malignancy we did it with phenol and we did not see any bowel problems afterwards at all. That was a male patient with carcinoma of the bladder and a patient with cervical cancer.

Sutton: Did it help the pelvic pain in the four cases?

Collett: The patients who were non-malignant – no, it did not. I have just done one on a patient who has testicular pain and it has removed his testicular pain but we are only about two weeks post-block, so I don't know whether the effect will be long-lasting.

Stones: Was that with phenol?

Collett: No, that was with local anaesthetic.

Steege: We did a randomised control trial of a presacral block as a pre-hysterectomy procedure in both laparoscopic and abdominal hysterectomies, attempting a pre-emptive analgesic technique. We had an open trial of presacral block (manuscript in preparation) and 25 or more patients showed about a 50% reduction in post-operative narcotic use. The randomised control trial, however, showed no difference between the active drug and placebo, so it is a beautiful theory spoiled by an ugly fact. In that group there was no impact on bladder or bowel function postoperatively.

Foster: I was wondering whether any of the UK anaesthetists have had any experience with conscious pain mapping and any secrets of how you do it here? As gynaecologists we find the anaesthesia techniques are probably more important than anything we can do with a probe.

Stones: We use fentanyl and midazolam. I used to use a rectus block but now I find that it is simpler to infiltrate only the puncture site. It does not seem to add anything to do a rectus block.

Crowhurst: In a few chronic pain patients – the chronic pain syndromes and other neuropathies that are beyond the scope of what we are dealing with here – I have had a little bit of experience. I trained with Professor Michael Cousins and I keep up with that sort of work, and it is developing greatly. I was rather puzzled when you said earlier that you raise your eyes to heaven when you get a one-sided vulvodynia. That is the sort of patient that I would approach with some prospect of cure, because one would be able to do, say, a selective L1 block on that side or whatever and attack it. They might have a neuroma somewhere – that sort of thing. So that sort of thing is developing.

There is a technique that is just starting to be researched of a way of getting drugs specifically to areas of the lower cord without endangering it. There is some exciting stuff for the future.

Foster: We have been using conscious pain mapping for a fair amount of time – similar to midazolam and fentanyl type therapy – but it requires a lot of counselling of the patient beforehand and getting them very prepared for what to expect. There is quite a variation in how people respond to that type of anaesthesia.

Steege: Our experience has been similar. For the more anxious patient we use fentanyl, midazolam and some propofol on top of it. They are fairly well sedated, so you can do your complete survey scope first and then shut the propofol off as the patient emerges; then you can begin to question. Even with the best of preparation, there is about one-third of the time where you do not get usable information.

Regarding unilateral penile or vulval neuropathy, we have had a number of patients do quite well using the xylocaine ointment preparation overnight, poultice fashion, much along the lines of post-herpetic neuropathy. We had a few remissions. Don't ask me why.

Foster: That is a great way to go. Our use of a steroid lanacane cream that is applied four to six times a day probably has a similar effect. You want to keep this lidocaine continuously in place similar to the lidocaine patch and it has a very beneficial additive effect if you are using a tricyclic or something else in addition. Even in our early vulvodynia patients, purely topical lidocaine repeatedly can be very effective, along with behavioural changes.

Berkley: I want to change the subject back to the palliative care expansion. I was a member of a study when Cathy Fowler first started her movement within the States to do some cross-hospital clinical trials devoted to cancer pain management. Part of the rationale during that entire study section meeting was, because of the possibility of using the information from cancer patients to whom physicians could more freely prescribe opiates, to use that information then to spread out into the 'benign' community. In other words, it was what is happening now in the UK. That was one reason that studies were funded because that rationale sounded wonderful as a way to help a specific population that may be in need of specialised care and at the same time to use them to mine that information experimentally for expansion. If that is happening here, it sounds like a wonderful opportunity to use what is happening in the UK to go after all the issues, both financial and applying to non-cancer patients and so forth. Coming from over the sea, I see this as a wonderful situation.

Tookman: The use of opioids in non-cancer chronic pain management is well established, accepted by many, but there are still a few who feel uncomfortable with that – sometimes for a justifiable reason, and I would be interested to hear what Dr Collett has to say about it. I have attended many meetings where there is now an established use of strong analgesics in chronic non-cancer pain. Clearly there are devotees to that approach because, in essence, the drugs are safe. There are more deaths on non-steroidals than there are on opioids. But I know that there are some people who feel that that may not be the correct approach. The opportunities offered by opioid rotations may be a way forward in using opioids chronically.

Collett: It is difficult to talk about opioids in non-malignant pain. If we are talking about gynaecological pain the people that I see in the gynaecology pain clinic who are on opioids have usually called up the GP at two o'clock in the morning on a Saturday night with really bad pain and have been given oral pethidine and they have gone on using that. Or they have come into hospital with an acute exacerbation of pain. They have been sitting in a hospital bed and have been given intramuscular pethidine; then have gone on to oral pethidine, and nobody can get them off. The patients that we see who are on opioids tend to be the ones who are most distressed. They may be distressed because the opioids are not working. There may be various other reasons for distress such as being out of control or not being in charge of the situation or feeling they are not believed.

In a pelvic pain population it is a very complex problem and from our point of view we feel that before we put patients with pelvic pain on opioids we need to do a better assessment of all the issues that are involved in their pain from a multidisciplinary aspect, and then to see whether they are the best drugs, whether they have any features that might make you cautious about prescribing opioids in that group of patients. Do they have previous addictions? Many of these women have previously used alcohol or recreational drugs or are using opiates that they have bought off the street as well.

We have to look at that person as a whole and look at the various issues that are going on before we can make the right decision. I don't think it is contraindicated, but we need to be extremely careful before we start this young population, who may have other factors that are important, on opiates.

Whorwell: I also run an abdominal pain service and some years ago tried to involve palliative care people in this service. They found it quite a problem because they found that visceral pain was harder to control. They also said that they had great difficulty with patients not dying. They had this problem of a patient going on and on and on, and it was quite a problem for them. Eventually I had to employ my own Macmillan nurse, because then she did what I told her and she could cope with these people going on and on and on. We have quite a few of these patients now on opiates and I believe we are doing quite well with them. We have had problems with GPs, particularly after the Harold Shipman case. The GPs get very nervous about giving opiates to benign patients, and I often have to write a letter saying I will take responsibility and it is my idea.

The other thing that the palliative team had difficulty with was the bowel problems. Obviously, the patients with chronic abdominal pain are often constipated, and we have to educate them that regular laxatives are not harmful, and are perfectly reasonable to use in non-palliative situations. The only thing we burnt our fingers with badly in the first place was injectable opiates. We never use those. It was a disaster, and we have two patients who are stuck, and that was a problem.

As a gastroenterologist who hates NSAIDs, 4000 people a year die in this country from the use of NSAIDs. Not many people die of morphine.

Tookman: I am sorry about your bad experience with your palliative care service. You are absolutely right – collaborative working and negotiation about difficult cases is all-important. We have an established practice of patients who are on long-term opioids and I do not believe they come to too much harm. They are a very difficult group of patients. They present to you as a very difficult, complex patient and I have sat in many meetings and discussed the long-term use of opioids. People seem to be either on one side of the camp or the other. You need to take a very balanced, rational view. You are right – people die of NSAIDs, and in primary care no one has a problem prescribing NSAIDs for life. Also, people die with chronic pain – they get depressed and they kill themselves – and there is a morbidity with chronic pain. Therefore, if someone has an opioid-sensitive pain, one has to consider that as one of the strategies that can be used. What I am not saying is give opioids to everyone; it has to be carefully thought through. The pain has to be opioid sensitive. You have to use long-acting preparations. You must not use injectable preparations. And there are other rules. But I feel they have a role.

Berkley: What do you think of the concept – I tried this at our local hospital with physicians in our town who were very resistant to prescribing opioids – of bringing the palliative care people into the hospital as part of the internal quality management mechanism, as a way of starting a dialogue? It started something in our local hospital that has proven very helpful across the hospital because some people listened. This is what I mean about spreading out the information that has come from palliative care into the acute community.

Tookman: Dialogue is very important, but there is a great difference between practice in the UK and the States in that most hospitals now – I would say all of them – have palliative care teams who operate within the hospital. There are community teams who cover the community and there are inpatient units. It is a big service and it is rapidly expanding.

The other thing to say – and I am not sure that palliative care has to have this role – is that if people are prescribed opioids there is a commitment to monitor those patients. I strongly believe that. Whether that lies with primary care or not is something to debate. Personally, I believe that people on opioids long term should be monitored by specialists who have some knowledge about using opioids. That is my personal view.

MacLean: Dr Whorwell, can I ask about the use of non-steroidals? Does your rather alarming mortality apply to the use of the drugs as Dr Fernando described in the peri-operative or postoperative period, or does it relate mainly to long-term use? I have seen one patient who a week after a vaginal hysterectomy was readmitted with a perforated duodenal ulcer from what I am sure was postoperative use of diclofenac sodium. However, my impression is that the majority of patients who use it postoperatively do not run into problems. Earlier, Mrs Barnard talked about the use of mefenamic acid and that it was ineffective for many patients. One of the problems is that many people take mefenamic acid in ineffective doses; they need to increase it until they get almost to the point of developing indigestion before they can say whether or not it works. Is it gynaecologists or postoperative pain people who are killing off all these patients with gastrointestinal tract haemorrhages, or is it rheumatologists who are doing it?

Whorwell: The most common groups are the elderly and rheumatology patients. The trouble is that they need analgesics, and they may develop an ulcer but get no pain from it, no symptoms; they are silent ulcers and result in big bleeds. I am worried about this because you see women who have just taken a short course of non-steroidals. Is that a risk? Yes, you do occasionally have a significant bleed from one dose of aspirin or a non-steroidal, but the majority of these 4000 deaths are in the elderly and in people taking them chronically. It is interesting that gynaecologists always use mefenamic acid, because mefenamic acid can give very substantial diarrhoea. I don't like NSAIDs but I don't like mefenamic acid at all. I saw recently a lady who had intractable diarrhoea from this drug. Her GP had put her on salazopyrin because he thought she had colitis, and then loperamide, and then she got sick from the salazopyrin, so she was on prochlorperazine. She was on four drugs, and all she had to do was stop the mefenamic acid.

MacLean: Unfortunately, Professor Li Wan Po has left, but he talked about the efficacy of treatment for dysmenorrhoea in the Study Group we had 12 months ago. His chapter compared the use of different non-steroidals for the management of dysmenorrhoea. If you are suggesting that mefenamic acid is not the best choice, should we actually document, certainly for this Study Group, what the better options are?

Whorwell: I just never prescribe these drugs.

Stones: There is a very good review on the Bandolier website of NSAIDs for dysmenorrhoea (http://www.jr2.ox.ac.uk/bandolier/band57/b57-2.html). The main point is that most of the studies are not mefenamic acid, and if I remember rightly, the conclusion is that ibuprofen is probably as good as anything.

Whorwell: I have always wondered why people use mefenamic acid. I don't want to stop you using a drug if it is the best NSAID for dysmenorrhoea, but if it is not it can cause even more trouble. As an aside, NSAIDs make irritable bowel syndrome worse as well. One more therapeutic thing – a lot of people are afraid of using laxatives in people with constipation, and there is absolutely no evidence that laxatives damage the bowel. It is a complete fallacy. You can give laxatives, particularly the osmotic ones, willy-nilly and they will not upset the bowel. It was based on one paper many years ago which was a totally flawed paper, because the patients already had an enteric neuropathy before they had the laxatives.

Crowhurst: Is that true for things like phenolphthalein and senna?

Whorwell: Don't give phenolphthalein. Senna is OK – it just makes you get a black colon, a melanosis. The best ones are polyethylene glycol, picosulphate. Most gastroenerologists in my area would give those. We have people taking picosulphate every day of their life – no problem. But certainly phenolphthalein, liquid paraffin – the old-fashioned laxatives – no.

Crowhurst: You are recommending those normal practices that you have for the opioid-induced constipation.

Whorwell: I am sure you use Laxoberal® (sodium picosulphate elixir; Boehringer) straightaway, or polyethylene glycol.

Tookman: We use polyethylene glycol quite a lot now. As you know we have been sold co-danthrusate as the laxative of choice. It is widely prescribed. It is also very expensive, and it gives certain animals bowel cancer, so it is very limited to our practice. Picosulphate and polyethylene glycol are drugs that we are using a lot now. The problem with the sugars is that it gives our patients abdominal distension and griping pain and wind, so we tend to lay off the lactulose.

Whorwell: He has taken the wind out of my sails. Lactulose is an awful laxative. It blows them up and if they have irritable bowel syndrome they get bloated, they are farting all day, and it is terrible stuff. We don't use lactulose.

Steege: I have one question for Dr Tookman perhaps, and others who use opiates chronically. We are also burdened with a population of patients that never die, so we have more and more people on maintenance opiates. We have more recently been aggressive in trying to wean them back down after a period of time. Usually we congratulate ourselves if we stay at a steady dose, but we have had a number of people who on their own have gradually weaned down. Is there something to be learned about the unwinding of wind-up in a person with a chronic pain disorder, from your experience?

Tookman: This is a personal opinion. There is dogma spoken about opiates that is, in my own experience, untrue. I believe that what you are saying is certainly a possibility. Patients do have problems with tolerance in the long term – and that is almost heresy from a palliative medicine physician. Opioids in the long term can 'run out of effect' and therefore you have to switch to an alternative opioid. In addition, opioids are commonly prescribed but we do not know the full detail of their pharmacological actions and their long-term effects. There are lots of other issues about opioids that are poorly understood. We know about the constipation, but we know little about erectile dysfunction that can occur, the dry mouth that nearly always occurs – we do not understand these drugs very well. In conclusion, yes, I have seen many patients who have been on opioids for a long time and they seem to have just run out of effect and they can come off them.

Barnard: Perhaps I could make a comment and throw it open to the floor to see if there is any comeback. I sense that there is a strong issue here about consent and about including patients in this decision. As I mentioned earlier, it is a strong case among women that we need something stronger when the pain is bad. Gynaecologists will give us mefenamic acid as though it were sweets and, frankly, I am opposed to the proposition that you just keep increasing the dose of that until your digestive tract goes into rebellion. I get anxious also hearing that 'we would withhold any category of drug until we have assessed the patient'. As a patient, I would like to be included in that assessment, I would like to be told what the risks of various drugs are, and I would like to be given the choice of having a slightly risky drug and no pain or, if I like to, of carrying on with a lot of pain but without the risk of horrible drugs. If we are going to make recommendations, please can we make one that includes proper consent from patients rather than being perennially prescriptive about it?

Collett: When we prescribe opioids in the pain clinic, we always tell the patient about the potential problems: that they will probably get physically addicted; they may become psychologically dependent on that drug. We split the physical addiction and psychological dependency. What we do not do is, like many pain clinics in the USA, get them to sign a consent form to say that the patient has agreed to that.

Talking about coming off opioids, if you look at the data from pain management programmes, there are quite a lot of people who have been on pain management programmes in whom the opiate can be withdrawn. Whether they have come to the end of that period of their life whereby they no longer need that and they can come off it, or whether there are other methods of controlling the pain and therefore they do not need the opioid, we probably don't know. We see patients who come off the drug in the pain management programme with other techniques, yet you see patients who just stop it one day and phone up and say 'Well, actually, I'm much better and I don't need that opioid any more.' We don't know. Certainly, if we use drugs for neuropathic pain I tend to give people gabapentin or amitriptyline, if it helps, for six or nine months and then tell them to try to come off it to see whether the pain comes back, on the assumption that you are switching off central sensitisation and can then reduce the dose. But I have not the faintest idea whether that is valid.

Crowhurst: Dr Tookman might like to comment on this. In the non-terminal patient this problem is often helped by using methadone. In many pain units – certainly many in Australia – methadone is a very popular drug in this group of patients, perhaps not initially but they are switched to it, just as it is used in substitution therapy in the addicts. It is a very good drug, as Dr Tookman implied before. It has a long half-life, it is a once-a-day dose, and some of the side effects in my experience are much less with it as well.

Tookman: I would agree with that. Methadone is very useful drug. Having said that, as you get older I don't know if you become more stupid or you become more wise. You speak to other people who use these drugs and we have recently been involved with the drug dependency service, the academic service, talking things through in general. It is said that methadone blocks the NMDA (N methyl-D-aspartate) receptors, and NMDA receptors are receptors for memory in the brain. Therefore the effects that methadone may have on cognitive function, short-term memory, are not understood. I am just adding my own personal note of 'I wonder what is going to happen in the future'. I believe that methadone is a very useful agent if used in low doses. It gets stored in the fat as well, which can make it a difficult drug to use because it can leach out and you can get side effects many days, if not weeks, after stabilising the dose.

Stones: I should like to raise a different topic. Probably a significant proportion of the readership of this Study Group's proceedings is likely to be from parts of the developing world and I would appreciate some comment from the anaesthetists regarding anaesthesia for caesarean section in the developing world. Do you see any new technical developments which might have an impact on the developing world? It is probably true to say that in large parts of the world most people are stuck with spinal anaesthetic or intravenous agents and that is probably it. Do you see any technologies that might be useable by mid-level service providers rather than highly trained physicians?

Fernando: For the foreseeable future I believe spinal anaesthetics will continue to be used. It is a simple technique. I don't think combined spinal techniques are necessarily suitable to be used. It is a lot more expensive – two needles – compared with a straight spinal technique. In the developing world I just see one-shot spinals being used to provide fairly good analgesia.

Crowhurst: I agree with that. I go to Bangladesh and India and the Middle East to teach, often a couple of times a year. In many countries in the Far East many of the anaesthetists are not trained in the way that anaesthesiologists are here or in North America. They are extremely slick with regional techniques for all sorts of surgery. It is very cheap for them. The drugs are cheap – the local anaesthetics and so on – and many of them will re-use needles and do things that we would never do here, but they are very slick and regional anaesthesia will continue to prosper. I have learned many things from people in those parts of the world.

Sutton: I worked for three years on Overseas Aid in Fiji as a consultant obstetrician and gynaecologist and there we almost exclusively used ketamine, which is a terrible drug for Caucasians – gives them dreadful hallucinations – but the Fijians and the Indians did not have that problem and it was very safe and easy to use.

Crowhurst: If you went there now, many of my colleagues have been to Fiji in the last few years and they do a lot more regional anaesthsia. Ketamine has been mentioned a couple of times and I mention it briefly in my chapter. It is a most interesting drug but it is like a lot of other drugs in that its history is chequered with great over-use and misunderstanding. Like methadone we still don't know a lot about it, but the doses in which it has been used in the past have been grossly excessive. I use very low-dose ketamine in *in vitro* fertilisation, for example, for monitored sedation of people having eggs collected and things like that. I know some intensivists who use it in preference to opiates in the short term and so on, but in low doses that are not in the textbooks. Low dose is something that we are coming round to, as Dr Fernando intimated with regional blocks for postoperative analgesia. We are just getting better and better at it, especially with combinations of things. Ketamine is a drug that is going to come into some prominence in the future, I believe – revisited, as it were.

Whorwell: May I just respond to Mrs Barnard's point? The way we take on a pain patient is that we discuss all the options open to them from TENS to opiates. I also run a hypnotherapy service, so they have that offered. It is quite interesting – you then say to them, 'Which of these treatments do you feel like having first?' – having explained the pros and cons – and they often go for the lowest form first and leave the morphine until last. They certainly usually plump for the hypnotherapy before the morphine. It is interesting that they usually adopt the route that I would have imposed on them if I had imposed one on them.

Reference

1.   Rodgers A, Walker N, Schug S, McKee A, Kehlet H, van Zundert A, *et al*. Reduction of postoperative mortality and morbidity with epidural or spinal anaesthesia: results from overview of randomised trials. *BMJ* 2000;**321**:1493.

SECTION 7

PAIN DURING PREGNANCY

Chapter 25

Musculoskeletal considerations and the role of physiotherapy in the management of peripartum spinal and pelvic pain

Yvonne Coldron and Kathleen Vits

Introduction

Musculoskeletal pain, particularly back pain, is a common occurrence in pregnancy, so much so that women themselves and medical staff involved in their care often regard it as 'a normal part of pregnancy'. This can lead to what could have been a minor treatable acute episode developing into a chronic long-term problem due to lack of appropriate physiotherapy treatment.

During pregnancy, the female body undergoes significant hormonal, postural, musculoskeletal and biomechanical changes. Increases in oestrogen and progesterone concentrations produce visceral and smooth muscle changes.[1] An increase in serum relaxin increases collagen synthesis.[2] Changes in connective tissue of the pubic symphysis during pregnancy in animal studies have been described by MacLennan and include an increase in total collagen, increased water uptake and a decrease in viscosity of the ground substance.[3] This remodelled collagen has greater pliability and extensibility and predisposes ligaments of the musculoskeletal system to laxity, so compromising joint stability.

Incidence of peripartum spinal and pelvic pain

The incidence of low back pain during pregnancy has been reported to range from 50% to 70%. Studies from the UK and Scandinavia report an incidence of 48–59%.[4-9] The varying methods used for determining the degree and nature of the pain may well explain the wide variation. Fast *et al.* in the USA showed that ethnic origin appeared to be a factor in personal perception of pain and is therefore worth considering in epidemiological studies.[5]

One-third of women report that their back pain is severe, interfering with daily life and compromising their ability to work.[7] From a survey in Sweden, it was noted that pain continued for 18 months postnatally in over one-third of women who had backache in pregnancy.[10] Russell and Reynolds reported that most backache resolves in the first few weeks postpartum but for some may continue for many months or may present postpartum for the first time.[11]

Mens *et al.* concluded that peripartum pelvic pain seriously interfered with activities of daily living and most patients experienced a relapse around menstruation and in a subsequent pregnancy.[12]

Distribution and origin of spinal and pelvic pain

The terminology for the different types of peripartum pain varies across the literature – for the purposes of this paper the terms peripartum spinal and pelvic pain (encompassing sacro-iliac and symphysis pubis pain) will be used.

The structural origins of spinal and pelvic pain during pregnancy are difficult to determine. Women describe pain occurring in the low back, sacral areas, posterior thigh and leg, pubic, groin and hip areas, and this pain may occur simultaneously or separately, antenatally, during delivery or postnatally.[13] There is often associated cervical, thoracic and coccygeal pain.

Attempts at localisation of the origin of spinopelvic pain in pregnancy have been studied using pain drawings[7,12] or clinical examination (for example use of sacro-iliac pain provocation tests and functional tests).[6]

Nilsson-Wikmar and Harms-Ringdahl used ten passive manual tests of the spinal and pelvic joints on postnatal women to determine whether provoked pain from these tests could be localised to the hips, sacro-iliac joints, lumbar spine and symphysis pubis.[14] They distinguished four different localisation groups – posterior pelvic pain (27%), lumbar pain (18%), mixed pain (39%) and no pain (16%). They concluded that back pain can be provoked from different structures in postpartum women, and hence back pain postpartum is not a unitary concept. It follows that, for women with peripartum spinal and pelvic pain, individual examination and assessment of the spine and pelvis by a specialist physiotherapist is vital to determining the probable cause. This allows a pain management and rehabilitation programme to be designed for the individual woman.

Spinal and pelvic stability

It is normal for there to be an increased laxity of the musculoskeletal system during pregnancy and there is potential for decreased stability of the spine and pelvis. In some women this decreased stability may be sufficient to cause abnormal joint movements, poor muscular control and pain.

The stability of the neuromusculoskeletal system is dependent on the interaction of the nervous system, the muscular system and the inert connective tissue system. Panjabi discussed these systems in relation to the lumbar spine and categorised them into control, active and passive subsystems.[15] The systems are interdependent to achieve optimal function, and faults in one subsystem affect one or both of the others.

The bony configuration of the spine renders it inherently unstable. Clinical instability is defined as a significant decrease in the capacity of the stabilising system of the spine to maintain the intervertebral neutral zone within the physiological limits. Clinical instability may result from a passive subsystem failure and/or failure of the active and control subsystems to maintain dynamic control (via prime stability muscles) of a lumbar motion segment.[15]

Pelvic stability also requires the interdependent functioning of the three subsystems. The pelvic ring (two sacro-iliac joints and the pubic symphysis) is inherently stable due to the bony configuration and ligamentous support of the sacro-iliac joints. However, Vleeming *et al.* determined that both the ligamentous and bony system (form closure) and the muscular system (force closure) are necessary to provide passive and dynamic stability of the pelvis.[16]

During pregnancy, the inherent bony and ligamentous stability of both the spine and pelvis may be compromised due to altered collagen synthesis. It is hypothesised that in order to maintain stability of these joints, correct muscular activity is a necessity.

Dynamic function of muscles stabilising the spine and pelvis

Most abdominal and spinal muscles contribute to the stability of the spine and pelvis either via a local function of individual joint stability or a global function to maintain the body's equilibrium in response to trunk perturbation. The global stabilisers also have a torque-producing function.

Joint stiffness and maintenance of a steady joint angle are dependent upon the ratio of tension generated by the agonist and antagonist muscles at a given muscle length[17] as well as the integrity of the passive ligamentous system. Muscle stiffness is determined by the intrinsic elastic stiffness and viscoelastic properties of the muscle itself. Total muscle tension depends on the basic viscoelastic properties (passive tension) and the degree of activation of the contractile elements of the muscle (active tension).[18] For optimal joint stability, muscles need to be recruited appropriately and to have normal intrinsic contractile properties. Hence, stability dysfunction of the spine and pelvis may be due to inefficient motor control[19] plus changes to muscle structure leading to weakness and increased fatigability.

The local stabilising muscles of the spine are believed to be transversus abdominis, lumbar multifidus, the pelvic floor muscles and diaphragm.[19,20] They use intra-abdominal pressure and attachments to the thoracolumbar and abdominal fascia to form a corset around the spine and give external stability. The global stabilisers linking the thoracic cage to the pelvis are the internal and external oblique muscles, thoracic erector spinae and latissimus dorsi.

In studies on subjects with acute low back pain it has been shown that there is altered function of transversus abdominis and lumbar multifidus. Transversus abdominis demonstrated a delayed action in response to trunk perturbation when compared with normal subjects. The authors concluded that the mechanism for preparatory spinal control was altered in people with low back pain.[19] In subjects with acute, first episode unilateral back pain, unilateral segmental inhibition of the multifidus muscle was demonstrated, and spontaneous recovery was not found when the painful symptoms disappeared.[21]

Dynamic stability of the sacro-iliac joint is thought to be maintained by the gluteus maximus working with the contralateral latissimus dorsi.[22] The symphysis pubis is stabilised through the oblique abdominals of one side working with the contralateral adductors, and the hip is stabilised through the actions of the gluteus medius and the contralateral adductors.[23]

The function of some or all of these muscles may be affected by musculoskeletal changes in pregnancy.

Musculoskeletal changes during pregnancy

Postural changes

Evidence of backache due to postural changes is inconclusive and inconsistent.[24,26] A significant relationship between altered posture and back pain during pregnancy was not found critically but in a later study Bullock-Saxton determined that the adaptive changes to thoracic and lumbar curves were maintained 12 weeks postnatally.[24-26] She hypothesised that muscle imbalances would result and could lead to alteration in the stresses imposed on joint structures.

The overall equilibrium of the spine and pelvis alters as pregnancy progresses. With increased weight gain, increased blood volume and ventral growth of the fetus the centre of gravity no longer falls over the feet and the woman may need to lean backwards to gain equilibrium.[27] This leads to a disorganisation of spinal curves so that the lumbar curve may move dorsally or may be accentuated.[28] Alteration in posture in the lumbar curve causes a compensatory alteration in the thoracic and cervical curves as the woman tries to maintain equilibrium in an upright posture.

Sandler theorised that 75% of women have a posterior posture where the weight of the gravid uterus is carried posterior to the centre of gravity and the woman leans backwards to compensate,[29] and the remaining 25% have an anterior posture. It could be concluded, therefore, that those with an exaggerated posterior posture may take more weight on the lumbo-sacral junction and pelvic joints, while those with an anterior posture may take more weight on the lumbar spinal zygapophyseal joints and intervertebral discs. This could be one reason for some women having predominantly pelvic problems and others having predominantly spinal problems.

Muscular changes in pregnancy

During pregnancy, the enlarged uterus stretches and elongation of the abdominal muscles results, together with some separation of the linea alba.[30] There is a paucity of research related to abdominal muscle changes during pregnancy and research has concentrated on the rectus abdominis alone.

Rectus abdominis

As pregnancy progresses, the rectus abdominis has been shown to separate, elongate (by 115%) and widen.[31] Gilleard and Brown found a decreased ability to stabilise the pelvis in late pregnancy and discovered that poor stability persisted at eight weeks postpartum.[31] The strength of gross muscle flexion has been shown to be impaired at

24 weeks postpartum. It was concluded that a state of imbalance exists between flexors and extensors which may lead to postpartum low back pain.[32]

In most females there is divarication of the linea alba during pregnancy which varies from 2–3 cm wide and 2–5 cm long, to 2–20 cm wide and extending the whole length of the rectus abdominis.[1,33] This is probably due to tissue creep and relaxation of the recti fascia. A gap of more than 2 cm between the bellies of rectus abdominis postpartum is defined as a diastasis.[30] There is little information on the prevalence of divarication/diastasis, or on rehabilitation of the recti.[33]

There has been a reported incidence of 66% of diastasis during the third trimester that may persist in 30–60% of cases in the postpartum period.[30] A study of two single cases found nonreduction of diastasis at 12 weeks postpartum.[34] However, this is contrary to the findings of Gilleard and Brown, who reported that the diastasis had resolved to the 22-week level at eight weeks postpartum.[31] Lo *et al.* identified the risk factors as age, multiparity, large fetus, multiple pregnancy, increased weight gain and caesarean section.[33] It is not established whether diastasis of the recti is a factor in low back or pelvic pain.

Lateral abdominal muscles

The three lateral (deep) muscles (transversus abdominis, internal oblique and external oblique) insert into the aponeurosis which forms the linea alba. There is little information on the effect of pregnancy on these muscles and no study has been made of the effect of divarication/diastasis of the recti on them. However, research (on normal subjects) has identified the importance of transversus abdominis as a prime stabiliser of the trunk.[35]

It is thought that women may present with structural alterations in the lateral abdominal muscles as well as in the rectus abdominis, resulting in stretch weakness. Stretch weakness is defined as weakness in a muscle that has remained elongated beyond its neutral physiological rest position for a period of time but not beyond the normal range of muscle length.[36]

Gluteus medius

If the trunk is in a posterior posture, the gluteus medius tends to lose its abductor function, resulting in a wobbling gait.[27] This in turn may lead to decreased stability in the pelvic joints. This waddling gait is seen classically in peripartum women with pelvic problems. This may be caused by painful compression of the superior aspect of the symphysis pubis during normal nutation of the sacrum while walking. The result is that the ilia rotate anteriorly with counternutation of the sacrum that leaves the pelvis in an unstable position. This will inhibit the function of the glutei and lead to further pelvic instability. The effect of this pelvic instability will have an effect on the lumbar spine and further alter the articular and muscular biomechanics and function of the whole spinopelvic system.

Pelvic floor muscles

During pregnancy and vaginal delivery there is stretching of the pelvic floor and trauma/tearing during labour and delivery.[27] It is now thought that the function and recruitment of transversus abdominis and the pelvic floor musculature is closely associated, which implies that inhibition of the correct action of the pelvic floor muscles will affect the function of transversus abdominis and vice versa.[21] Favery and O'Sullivan have shown evidence of pelvic floor muscle dysfunction in patients with sacro-iliac joint syndrome.[37] Thus re-education of the pelvic floor musculature plays an important part in rehabilitation. It has been shown by Bump *et al.* that women require individual instruction and vaginal assessment to allow effective rehabilitation of the pelvic floor musculature thus reinforcing the recommendation of individual assessment for peripartum women.[38]

Articular changes

The complicated ligamentous structures of the spine and pelvis play a key role in the self-locking mechanism of the pelvis, which functions to maintain the integrity of the low back and pelvis during transfer of energy from the spine to the lower extremities during gait.[39] Several major muscle groups influence the ligamentous support mechanism, and active tension in certain muscles exerts influence on the passive ligamentous and fascial stability structures. The main cause of reduced pelvic stability during pregnancy is the effect on collagen metabolism and connective tissue extensibility from altered levels of relaxin, oestrogen and progesterone.[2] These altered hormonal levels may result in a disturbance of ligamentous co-ordination and result in a small but important decrease in the stability of the passive system of the pelvis.[2] This instability may be inconsistent with normal body movement. Ostgaard argues that this instability increases muscle tension in the posterior pelvis to re-establish stability; this may then lead to pain and fatigue and a secondary muscle insufficiency. This ligamentous laxity may continue for many months postpartum.

Biomechanical changes of the joints of the spine and pelvis during pregnancy may involve an increase in sacral promontory, increase in the lumbosacral angle, laxity in one or both sacro-iliac joints and/or pubic symphysis joints. These mechanical changes predispose a woman to back pain during pregnancy, particularly if the woman has an antepartum history of low back pain and decreased fitness.[2]

Golightly noted that during pregnancy there is a forward rotatory movement of the innominate bones at the sacro-iliac joints that carries the pubes downwards and forwards.[40] As body weight is transmitted through the pelvis, increased laxity makes joints more vulnerable putting increased stress on the lumbosacral junction and the sacro-iliac joints. This may or may not be accompanied by an increase in lumbar lordosis.

Asymmetry in the pelvic joints from trauma (which may be minor during pregnancy) may result in one sacro-iliac joint being hypermobile and one being hypomobile. Rost *et al.* described asymmetry of the pelvis as causing pelvic pain in pregnancy. They described a forward rotation and oblique slip of the ilia that is caused by overactivity in the adductor muscles of the thigh. Displacement of the ilium can cause a secondary problem in the symphysis pubis by placing upon it added torsion. Thus, poor use of the glutei ensues with lack of force closure of the pelvis leading to disruption of the self-locking mechanism.[41]

Symphysis pubis dysfunction

Historically, symphysis pubis dysfunction was thought to be rare but research in the 1990s has shown it to be a relatively common complaint with reported figures of 1:300 to 1:800.[42-44] The severity of the problem varies considerably, but at its most severe pain and lack of mobility causes severe social difficulties.[45,46]

The normal gap of 4–5 mm of the symphysis may increase during pregnancy and the level of separation may cause severe pain. Scriven demonstrated that the width of the gap postpartum could vary from 10 mm to 35 mm in a symptomatic group of patients but the width was less important than the reduction of the gap over time in determining the likely outcome of the condition.[43]

The interaction between the symphysis pubis and the sacro-iliac joints give the bony pelvis its stability; therefore when assessing the symphysis an assessment of the sacro-iliac joints is equally important. Dalastra showed that the symphysis has its maximum load at the beginning of the swing phase of gait, which may explain why many of the patients find walking extremely difficult and tend to shuffle without lifting the feet.[47]

In summary, therefore, changed load, lax ligaments and weak muscles will alter spinopelvic stability and affect load transfer between the trunk and leg that may lead to spinal and/or pelvic pain and trunk and pelvic muscle inhibition. When examining and treating these patients therefore, attention must be paid to both the spine and the pelvis and their articular and muscular systems.

Other factors contributing to spinal and pelvic pain are:

- high relaxin concentrations in women with the onset of pelvic pain during pregnancy[48] or a susceptibility to relaxin and the other hormones of pregnancy[46]

- physically strenuous work during pregnancy[13]

- fatigue with poor posture, clumsiness, carelessness and weight gain[8]

- work involving bending, twisting, lifting and sitting[13]

- large abdominal sagittal and transverse diameters[49]

- naturally large lumbar lordosis[49]

- multiparous mothers and increased maternal age[50]

- posterior pelvic pain associated with parity, weight of the newborn and smoking[2]

- low back pain associated with pre-pregnancy lower back pain and decreased fitness levels[2]

- younger physical age.[7]

Epidural anaesthesia

The role of epidural analgesia is controversial. The groups of both MacArthur and Russell implicated epidural anaesthesia in the development of chronic backache in retrospective studies, which could also have been due to mothers adopting unsuitable positions in labour.[51,52] However Russell et al., in a later prospective study, did not find epidural anaesthesia to be associated with the development of chronic backache.[9] Other prospective studies did not demonstrate an association between new onset postpartum backache and epidural analgesia.[53,54]

The conclusion is that the factors contributing to peripartum musculoskeletal pain are multifactorial and involve joint laxity and abdominal muscle changes; these may not fully resolve post partum.

Management and treatment of spinopelvic pain

Advice, education and general exercise

Advice and education to prevent back and pelvic pain early in pregnancy should be available to women. Treatment of back pain with physiotherapy and patient education has been shown to reduce sick leave during pregnancy.[55] It has also been shown that individual assessment and treatment was more effective than group treatment and that following initial individual assessment, advice and exercise, further management could be continued in a group setting with other women with similar pain distribution.[2,55]

From these studies it has been shown that early education, advice and exercise intervention given by a specialist physiotherapist help to reduce back and pelvic pain in pregnant women and to reduce sick leave and that the benefits continue into the postnatal period. The conclusion of the above studies was that the costs of the physiotherapists' time could be balanced with improved healthcare outcome for the women and an earlier return to work.

Muscle re-education

It has long been recognised that re-education and restoration of abdominal muscle function is essential in the rehabilitation of pregnant and postpartum women. Until recently, re-education has been via the use of general abdominal strengthening exercises such as curl-ups and posterior pelvic tilting. However, non-obstetric research on abdominal re-education has shown that active trunk stabilisation programmes benefit patients with spinal instability problems and low back pain rather than general abdominal strengthening programmes.[56-59] Concurrently, research into postpartum spinal pelvic pain and pelvic instability has concentrated on the role of re-education of the active stabilisation system of pelvic musculature as well as the trunk musculature.[60]

The purpose of rehabilitation of the trunk and pelvis in antenatal and postnatal women is to increase active stability of potentially unstable passive systems of the trunk and pelvis, to assist in pain reduction and increase functional activities by increasing overall muscle performance. Training of the prime stability muscles of the spine has reduced the amount of rectus abdominis diastasis in postpartum women who had a chronic diastasis. This area requires further research to be undertaken.

In studies on non-pregnant patients with low back pain, success has been recorded in the use of specific stabilisation exercises.[61] O'Sullivan argues that an individual spinal segmental stability exercise programme for patients with instability and low back pain is the optimum treatment strategy.[62] Lee also uses prime and global stability exercises with patients who have pelvic instability.[63,64]

With rehabilitation of peripartum women, attention needs to be paid to rehabilitation of both pelvic stability muscles and spinal stability muscles. Rehabilitation needs to be concise, as many women cannot regularly attend physiotherapy department, due to family commitments.

Manipulative therapy joint treatments

Peripartum spinopelvic pain often responds to manual therapy, although the evidence for manipulative (manual) techniques in pregnancy is limited. However, manipulative and mobilisation techniques applied to the pelvis and spine have been used successfully by many practitioners.[8,29] Reported effects of manual therapy include unlocking a locked joint, improving the tensile strength of ligaments, inhibition of chemically mediated pain, reduction of oedema, reduction of extra-articular muscle spasm and increased joint and disc nutrition. Zusman reviewed these theories and concluded that evidence for efficacy was limited and that further research is urgently needed.[65]

Other authors advocate the use of muscle energy techniques to treat spinal and pelvic joint dysfunction.[66] The aim is to restore mobility, reduce joint oedema, stretch fibrotic tissue and retrain the stabilising function of intersegmental muscles.

Practioners such as Rost advocate a combined manual therapy and muscle re-education approach to restore optimal mobility and improve muscle function.[41]

Management of chronic pain and general fitness

The problems of chronic pain are two-fold. One aspect is fear that movement will cause re-injury or increase the pain, and the second aspect is the resulting physical deconditioning.[67] From experience, it has been noted that many women who present with peripartum pain and/or low back pain who have had pain throughout pregnancy are generally unfit and have low exercise tolerance. It is important, therefore, that once core stability has been gained that the patient is encouraged to increase her strength and general aerobic and cardiovascular fitness. Encouragement to undertake general fitness will aid behavioural rehabilitation with the aim of decreasing disability levels by learning and practising skills to cope better with pain. Pain management strategies may be used concurrently with the above suggestions for treatment.

Orthoses

With pelvic instability, the use of a sacro-iliac belt both antenatally and postnatally may decrease pain and allow the woman to recruit disused muscles more easily and improve general mobility. Snijders et al. suggested that a pelvic belt is a substitution for the work of the internal oblique muscle.[68] Mens et al. applied a pelvic belt to women with peripartum pelvic pain women and found that their active straight leg raise improved.[12] Women should be advised to re-educate the internal oblique and transversus abdominis muscles concurrently with wearing the pelvic belt.

Special consideration for the management/treatment of symphysis pubis dysfunction

As well as the preceding methods there are the following additional guidelines to be considered when dealing with symphysis pubis dysfunction.

An individual assessment and exercise programme is essential. Pelvic support, trochanteric belt or tubigrip may be indicated.[69,70] Advice regarding activities that involve unilateral weight bearing and hip abduction should be given. Crutches, or in the most severe cases a wheelchair, may be required. Rost advocates an active regimen ignoring the pain involved and records encouraging results. However, there is no research comparing the efficacy of working within the limits of pain to a more aggressive regimen.[41]

During labour and delivery, present guidelines produced by the Association of Chartered Physiotherapists in Women's Health stress awareness of the masking effect of epidural and spinal anaesthesia in relation to excessive abduction of hips. It is advised that women should adopt the most comfortable position for them during labour. Delivery positions of left lateral or kneeling upright with support are suggested and women should be discouraged from placing their feet on attendants' hips because of the excessive forced hip abduction and strain on the pelvis. Care should be taken if lithotomy is required and suturing should take place in the most comfortable position for the mother.[71] To date, there is no evidence to suggest that caesarean section is indicated.

Other methods

It is recommended that other pain control methods using electrotherapy modalities (including TENS) should be confined to the postnatal period as their effects on the developing fetus remain to be researched. The use of drug therapy should be discussed with the medical team involved.

Conclusions and recommendations

Peripartum spinal and pelvic pain is a common multifactorial problem, but with correct treatment and advice, research has shown that the longstanding sequelae can be reduced.

Education in back care and activities of daily living, and instruction in appropriate exercises (aimed at optimising spinal and pelvic stability) by a physiotherapist should be available to all pregnant women.

Women presenting with spinal or pelvic pain in pregnancy should be referred to a specialist physiotherapist for individual examination, assessment and treatment.

Collaborative multidisciplinary research projects into the causes and management of musculoskeletal spinal and pelvic pain (including symphysis pubis dysfunction) should be undertaken by the obstetric team. Current research is being undertaken by the first author of this paper to investigate changes in size and electrical function of abdominal muscles and lumbar multifidus in postpartum women, together with the relationship to spinal and pelvic pain.

References

1. Polden M, Mantle J. *Physiotherapy in Obstetrics and Gynaecology*. Oxford: Butterworth Heinemann; 1990.
2. Ostgaard HC. Lumbar back and posterior pelvic pain in pregnancy. In: Vleeming A, Mooney V, Dorman T, Snidjers C, Stoeckart R, editors. *Movement, Stability and Low Back Pain*. Edinburgh: Churchill Livingstone; 1997. p. 411–20.
3. MacLennan AH. Relaxin – A review. *Aust NZ J Obstet Gynaecol* 1981;**21**:195–201.
4. Mantle MJ, Greenwood RM, Currey HLF. Backache in pregnancy. *Rheumatol Rehab* 1977;**16**:95–101.
5. Fast A, Shapiro D, Ducommun EJ. Low back pain in pregnancy. *Spine* 1987;**12**:368–71.
6. Berg G, Hammar M, Moller-Nielsen J. Low back pain during pregnancy. *Obstet Gynecol* 1988;**71**:71–5.
7. Ostgaard HC, Andersson GB, Karlsson K. Prevalence of back pain in pregnancy. *Spine* 1991;**16**:549–52.
8. Mantle J. Back pain in the childbearing year. In: Boyling JD, Palastanga N, editors. *Grieve's Modern Manual Therapy*. Edinburgh: Churchill Livingstone; 1994. p. 799–808.
9. Russell R, Dundas R, Reynolds F. Long term backache after childbirth: prospective search for causative factors. *BMJ* 1996;**312**:1384–8.
10. Ostgaard HC, Andersson GBJ. Postpartum low-back pain. *Spine* 1992;**17**:53–5.
11. Russell R, Reynolds F. Back pain, pregnancy and childbirth. *BMJ* 1997;**314**:1062.
12. Mens MA, Vleeming A, Stoeckart R, Stam HJ, Snijders CJ. Understanding peripartum pelvic pain. *Spine* 1996;**21**:1363–70.
13. Heiberg E, Aarseth SP. Epidemiology of pelvic pain and low back pain in pregnant women. In: Vleeming A, Mooney V, Dorman T, Snidjers C, Stockart R, editors. *Movement, Stability and Low back Pain*. Edinburgh: Churchill Livingstone; 1997. p. 405–10.
14. Nilsson-Wikmar L, Harms-Ringdahl K. Back pain in women post-partum is not a unitary concept. *Physiother Res Int* 1999;**4**:201–13.
15. Panjabi MM. The stabilising system of the spine. Part 1. Function, dysfunction, adaption and enhancement. *J Spinal Disord* 1992;**5**:383–96.
16. Vleeming A, Snidjers CJ, Stoeckart R, Mens JMA. A new light on low back pain. In: Vleeming A, Mooney V Dorman T, Snidjers C, editors. *Proceedings of 2nd Interdisciplinary World Congress on Low Back Pain*. San Diego, CA, 9–11 November 1995, p. 149–67.
17. Brooks VB. *The Neural Basis of Motor Control*. New York: Oxford University Press; 1986.
18. Simons DG, Mense S. Understanding and measurement of muscle tone a related to clinical muscle pain. *Pain* 1998;**75**:1–17.
19. Hodges PW, Richardson CA. Inefficient muscular stabilisation of the lumbar spine associated with low back pain. *Spine* 1996;**21**:2640–50.
20. Richardson CA, Jull G. Muscle control – pain control. What exercises would you prescribe? *Manual Ther* 1996;**1**: 2–10.
21. Hides JA, Richardson CA, Jull GA. Multifidus muscle recovery is not automatic after resolution of acute, first-episode low back pain. *Spine* 1996;**21**:2763–9.
22. Mooney V, Prozos R, Vleeming A, Gulick J, Swenski D. Coupled motion of contralateral latissimus dorsi and gluteus maximus: its role in sacroiliac stabilisation. In: Vleeming A, Mooney V Dorman T, Snidjers C, Stoeckart R, editors. *Movement, Stability and Low Back Pain*. Edinburgh: Churchill Livingstone; 1997. p. 115–22.
23. Lee D. Instability of the sacroiliac joint and the consequences to gait. In: Vleeming A, Mooney V Dorman T, Snidjers C, editors. *Proceedings of the 2nd Interdisciplinary World Congress on Low Back Pain*. San Diego, CA, 9–11 November 1995, p. 473–84.
24. Bullock JE, Jull GA, Bullock MI. The relationship of low back pain to postural changes during pregnancy. *Aust J Physiother* 1987;**33**:10–17.
25. Bullock-Saxton JE. Changes in posture associated with pregnancy and the early post-natal period measured in standing. *Physiother Theory and Practice* 1991;**7**:103–9.
26. Snidjers CJ, Snidjers JG, Hoest HT. Change in form of the spine as a consequence of pregnancy. In: *Digest of 11th International Conference on Medical and Biological Engineering, Ottawa, 1976*, p. 670–71.
27. Abitbol MM. Quadrupedalism, bipedalism, and human pregnancy. In: Vleeming A, Mooney V, Dorman T, Snidjers C, Stoekart R, editors. *Movement, Stability and Low Back Pain*. Edinburgh: Churchill Livingstone; 1997. p. 395–404.

28. Snijders CJ, Vleeming A, Stoeckart R, Kleinrensink GJ, Mens JMA. Biomechanics of sacro-iliac joint stability: validation experiments on the concept of self-locking. In: Vleeming A, Mooney V, Dorman T, Snidjers C, editors. *Proceedings of the 2nd Interdisciplinary World Congress on Low Back Pain.* San Diego, CA, 9–11 November, 1995. p. 75–91.

29. Sandler SE. The management of low back pain in pregnancy. *Manual Ther* 1996;**1**:178–85.

30. Boissonnault JS, Blaschak MJ. Incidence of diastasis recti abdominus during the childbearing year. *Physical Ther* 1988;**86**:1082–6.

31. Gilleard WL, Brown JMM. Structure and function of the abdominal muscles during pregnancy and the immediate post birth period *Physical Ther* 1996;**7**:750–62.

32. Potter HM Effect of an intense training programme for the deep antero-lateral muscles on rectus abdominis diastasis: a single case study. In: *10th Biennial Conference Proceedings of the Manipulative Physiotherapists Association of Australia, 'Clinical Solutions'.* Victoria: Manipulative Physiotherapists Association of Australia, 1997.

33. Lo CG, Janssen P. Diastasis of the Recti Abdominis in pregnancy: risk factors and treatment. *Physiotherapy Canada.* 1999;**44**:32–7.

34. Hsia M, Jones S. Natural resolution of rectus abdominis diastasis. Two single case studies. *J Physiother* 2000;**46**:301–7.

35. Hodges PW. Is there a role for transversus abdominis in lumbo-pelvic stability? *Manual Ther* 1999;**4**:74–86.

36. Gossman MR, Sahrmann SA, Rose SJ. Review of length-associated changes on muscle. *Physical Ther* 1982;**62**:1799–1807.

37. Favery A, O'Sullivan PB. Evidence of pelvic floor muscle dysfunction in subjects with chronic sacro-iliac pain syndrome. In: Singer K, editor. *Proceedings of the 7th Scientific Conference of the International Federation of Orthopaedic Manipulative Therapists.* Perth: University of Western Australia. 2000, p. 35–8.

38. Bump RC, Hurt W, Fantl JA,Wyman JF. Assessment of Kegel pelvic muscle exercise performance after brief verbal instruction. *Am J Obstet Gynecol* 1991;**165**:322–9.

39. Vleeming A, Snidjers CJ, Stoeckart R, Mens JMA. The role of the sacroiliac joints in coupling between spine, pelvis and arms In: Vleeming A, Mooney V, Dorman T, Snidjers C, Stoeckart R, editors. *Movement Stability and Low Back Pain.* Edinburgh: Churchill Livingstone; 1997. p. 53–72.

40. Golighty R. Pelvic arthropathy in pregnancy and the puerperium. *Physiotherapy* 1982:**68**:216–20.

41. Rost C. *Bekkenpijn Tijden En Na De Zwangerschap: Een Programma ter Voorkoming van Chronische Bekkeninstabiliteit.* Maarssen: Elsevier/De Tijdstroom; 1999.

42. Snow RE, Neubert AG. Peripartum Pubic Symphysis separation: a case series and review of the literature. *Obstet Gynecol Surv* 1997;**52**:438–43.

43. Scriven MW, Jones DA, McKnight L. The importance of pubic pain following childbirth: a clinical and ultrasonographic study of diastasis of the pubic symphysis. *J R Soc Med* 1995, **88**:26–30.

44. Kubitz RL, Goodlin RC. Symptomatic separation of the pubic symphysis. *Southern Med J* 1986;**79**:578–80.

45. Fry D. Perinatal symphysis pubis dysfunction: a review of the literature. *Journal of the Association of Chartered Physiotherapists in Women's Health* 1997;**85**:11–18.

46. MacLennan AH, MacLennan SC. Symptom-giving pelvic girdle relaxation of pregnancy, postnatal pelvic joint syndrome and dysplasia of the hip. *Acta Obstet Gynecol Scand* 1997;**76**:760–64.

47. Dalastra M. Biomechanics of the human pelvic bone. In: Vleeming A, Mooney V, Dorman T, Snidjers C, Stoeckart R, editors. *Movement Stability and Low Back Pain.* Edinburgh: Churchill Livingstone; 1997. p. 91–102.

48. Kristiansson P. S-Relaxin and pelvic pain in pregnant women. In: Vleeming A, Mooney V, Dorman T, Snidjers C, Stoeckart R, editors. *Movement Stability and Low Back Pain.* Edinburgh: Churchill Livingstone; 1997, p. 421–4.

49. Ostgaard HC, Andersson GBJ, Schuttz AB, Miller JA. Influence of some biomechanical factors on low-back pain in pregnancy. *Spine* 1993;**18**:61–5.

50. Heckman JD, Sassard R. Musculoskeletal considerations in pregnancy. *J Bone Joint Surg* 1994;**76**:1720–26.

51. MacArthur C, Lewis M, Knox BJ, Crawford JS. Epidural anaesthesia and long-term backache after childbirth. *BMJ* 1990;**301**:9–12.

52. Russell R, Groves P, Taub N, O'Dowd J, Reynolds F. Assessing long term backache after childbirth. *BMJ* 1993;**306**(6888):1299–1303.

53. Breen TW, Ransil BJ, Groves PA, Oriol NE. Factors associated with back pain after childbirth. *Anesthesiology* 1996;**81**:29–34.

54. Macarthur C, Weeks S. Epidural anaesthesia and low back pain after delivery: Prospective cohort

study. *BMJ* 1995;**311**:1336–9.

55.   Noren L, Ostgaard S, Nielson TF, Ostgaard HC. Reduction of sick leave for lumbar back and posterior pain in pregnancy. *Spine* 1997;**22**:2157–60.

56.   Richardson C, Toppenburg R, Jull G. An initial evaluation of eight abdominal exercises for their ability to provide stability for the lumbar spine. *Aust J Physiother* 1990;**36**:6–11.

57.   Richardson C, Jull G, Toppenburg R, Commerford M. Techniques for active stabilisation for spinal protection: a pilot study. *Austral J Physiother* 1993;**38**:105–11.

58.   Jull G, Richardson C, Toppenberg R, Comerford M, Bui B. Towards a measurement of active muscle control for lumbar stabilisation. *Austral J Physiother* 1993;**39**:187–93.

59.   O'Sullivan PB, Twomey L, Allison G. Evaluation of specific stabilising exercises in the treatment of chronic low back pain with radiological diagnosis of spondylosis or spondylolisthesis. In: *Proceedings of the Manipulative Physiotherapists Association of Australia Ninth Biennial Conference.* 1995, p. 113–4.

60.   Vleeming A, Buyruk HM, Stoeckart R, Karamursel S, Snijders CJ. Towards an integrated therapy for peripartum pelvic instability. *Am J Obstet Gynecol* 1992;**166**:1243–7.

61.   O'Sullivan PB, Twomey L, Allison GT. Evaluation of specific stabilising exercises in the treatment of chronic low back pain with radiological diagnosis of spondylosis or spondylolisthesis. *Spine* 1997;**22**:2959–67.

62.   O'Sullivan PB. Lumbar segmental 'instability'. Clinical presentation and specific stabilising exercises management. *Manual Ther* 2000;**51**:2–12.

63.   Lee D. Treatment of pelvic instability. In: Vleeming A, Mooney V, Dorman T, Snidjers C, Stoeckart R, editors. *Movement Stability and Low Back Pain.* Edinburgh: Churchill Livingstone; 1997. p. 445–60.

64.   Lee D. Muscles posture and ergonomics. In: Lee D, editor. *The Pelvic Girdle,* 2nd edn. Edinburgh: Churchill Livingstone; 1999. p. 153–69.

65.   Zusman M. What does manipulation do? The need for basic research. In: Boyling JD, Palastanga N, editors. *Grieve's Modern Manual Therapy.* Edinburgh: Churchill Livingstone; 1994. p. 651–9.

66.   Fowler C. Muscle energy techniques for pelvic dysfunction. In: Boyling JD, Palastanga N, editors. *Grieve's Modern Manual Therapy.* Edinburgh: Churchill Livingstone; 1994. p. 781–91.

67.   Vlaeyen JWS, Cole-Snidjers AMJ, Heuts PHTG, van Eek H. Behavioural analysis of fear of movement/(re)injury and behavioural rehabilitation in chronic low back pain. In: Vleeming A, Mooney V, Dorman T, Snidjers C, Stoeckart R, editors. *Movement, Stability and Low Back Pain.* Edinburgh: Churchill Livingstone; 1997. p. 433–44.

68.   Snijders CJ, Ribbers MTLM, de Bakker HV, Stoeckart, R, Stam HJ. EMG recordings of abdominal and back muscles in various standing postures: validation of a biomechanical model on sacroiliac joint. *J Electromyogr Kinesiol* 1998;**8**:205–14.

69.   Fry D, Tudor A. Pelvic support belt. *Journal of the Association of Chartered Physiotherapists in Womens' Health* 1997;**81**:40.

70.   McIntosh JM. Treatment note: Alternative pelvic support. *Journal of the Association of Chartered Physiotherapists in Womens' Health* 1995;**76**:28.

71.   Association of Chartered Physiotherapists in Women's Health. *Symphysis Pubis Dysfunction – Guidelines* 1996. Available from the Chartered Society of Physiotherapy, 14 Bedford Row, London WC1R 4ED.

Chapter 26

Abdominal pain in pregnancy

Timothy G. Overton, Manu Vatish and Steven Thornton

Acute abdominal pain in pregnancy is caused by pathological conditions either related or unrelated to the pregnancy. Non-obstetric causes can be difficult to recognise because the anatomical and physiological state is altered by pregnancy confounding the investigation and findings. Management of the acute abdomen requires careful assessment to reduce the chance of unnecessary surgical intervention while not increasing the risk of miscarriage or preterm labour by undue delay. This chapter outlines the anatomical changes which occur during pregnancy. There follows a discussion of the numerous causes, classified depending on the organ principally involved.

Anatomical and physiological changes in pregnancy

The uterus increases in weight from approximately 70 g to 1100 g and in volume by 5 litres or more.[1] After 12 weeks of gestation the uterus rises out of the pelvis. The adnexa become abdominal organs, making the ovaries more difficult to palpate. With continued enlargement of the uterus, the intestines and omentum are displaced superiorly and laterally. The appendix progressively moves upwards and laterally away from McBurney's point to the level of the iliac crest by the sixth month. The presence of the uterus makes it more difficult for the omentum to restrict localised peritonitis and elevation of the anterior abdominal wall may mask the symptoms of parietal peritoneal irritation. Even after delivery, the relaxed abdominal wall musculature does not demonstrate the characteristic guarding or rebound associated with underlying inflammation. The enlarging uterus compacts the bowel, making the intestine more vulnerable to penetrating injury. Uterine expansion places the supporting ligaments under increasing tension, which can produce discomfort in the lower abdomen. Part of this pain is caused by smooth muscle contraction within the round ligaments, an event more common in multigravid women.[2]

Interpretation of physical signs also becomes more difficult in pregnancy. Nausea and vomiting are frequent in the first trimester and a physiological tachycardia develops. The general hyperadrenocortical state of pregnancy can diminish the evidence of the toxicity which occurs during acute surgical conditions such as appendicitis. Changes in standard laboratory reference ranges also occur. There is a progressive leucocytosis in pregnancy with an elevation of the normal range to $12\,000-16\,000 \times 10^9/l$, which overlaps with values in acute intra-abdominal conditions. The expansion of plasma volume exceeds the increase in the red cell mass, resulting in a 3–4% fall in the haematocrit and a relative anaemia that can hamper the prompt diagnosis of intra-abdominal bleeding. There is also a 30% decrease in the albumin concentration[3] increasing the likelihood of pulmonary oedema if care is not taken with crystalloid fluid replacement. The alkaline phosphatase is progressively elevated in pregnancy and hepatic amniotransferases need to be interpreted according to the gestational age.[4]

There is a general reluctance, sometimes inappropriately, to subject pregnant woman to radiological investigations and to rely on newer imaging modalities such as ultrasound. Unfortunately, the expertise needed for these tests is not always available in an emergency situation and the input of senior clinicians is important at an early stage to avoid unnecessary delay in diagnosis.

Uterine causes of abdominal pain

Miscarriage

Vaginal bleeding, lower abdominal pain and a positive pregnancy test are indicative of a compromised pregnancy. In the first trimester the differential diagnosis is essentially miscarriage (threatened, complete, or incomplete) or ectopic pregnancy. Pain due to miscarriage is usually intermittent and often associated with cervical changes on vaginal examination. Increasingly sensitive ultrasound imaging coupled with serum β-human chorionic gonadotrophin (βhCG) usually enables the accurate diagnosis of miscarriage, enabling the option of surgical or conservative management.

Septic abortion with peritonitis is rarely seen in the UK but remains an important cause of death worldwide. Amenorrhoea associated with shock (due to blood loss and sepsis) may give the clue to the diagnosis. Interference is often denied. The abdomen is usually slightly distended, with tenderness and guarding more marked in the lower abdomen.[5] On pelvic examination, the cervix is open and soft. There is usually an offensive bloodstained discharge and possibly signs of trauma. There may be pyrexia, leucocytosis and tachycardia but in severe cases the temperature may be low. Prompt treatment with antibiotics is required but surgical exploration of the uterus should be deferred for 24 hours if possible.

Acute retention of urine

This usually presents between 12 and 14 weeks of gestation and is caused by impaction of the retroverted gravid uterus beneath the sacral promontory. The patient presents with symptoms of severe abdominal pain and urinary frequency. A cystic swelling arising out of the pelvis is palpable on abdominal examination. The diagnosis is confirmed by catheterisation, which allows spontaneous anteversion of the uterus.

Uterine torsion

Uterine torsion is defined as rotation more than 45° around the long axis of the uterus.[6] It is rare, and a review of the literature in 1992 revealed only 212 reported cases.[6] While it usually occurs in the third trimester, it has been reported as early as 6 weeks.[7] Most cases that occur at term do so in the first stage of labour. The aetiology is unclear. Predisposing factors are congenital abnormalities of the uterus, pelvic tumours and adhesions. Symptoms are usually related to the degree of torsion. Torsion needs to be considered in cases of long-lasting and obstructed labour or unremitting, intense abdominal pain in pregnancy. The severity of abdominal pain is variable and associated with shock (19%), intestinal symptoms (nausea, vomiting, diarrhoea and abdominal distension in 16%), urinary symptoms (frequency, urgency, nocturia, oliguria or haematuria in 8%), vaginal bleeding (10%) and obstructed labour (12%).[6] On examination the presence of a spiral running urethra or rectum, twisted vagina or pulsating uterine artery in either the anterior or posterior fornix are pathognomonic signs. Although there is often difficulty in diagnosis between uterine torsion and other surgical conditions, laparotomy is usually required. Nevertheless, if confused with a non-surgical cause or a complication of labour managed without laporotomy the consequences may prove disastrous. At caesarean section, the baby may need to be delivered through an incision in the posterior wall of the uterus which spontaneously returns to its normal position after closing the wound.

Uterine fibroids

Uterine fibroids are common and occasionally complicate pregnancy. Studies indicate that the majority of fibroids do not enlarge greatly during pregnancy.[8] Approximately 10% undergo red degeneration causing pain. This is thought to be due to haemorrhagic infarction caused by an acute inadequacy of blood supply. The abdominal pain, mild pyrexia and leucocytosis are usually self-limiting. The importance of the diagnosis is that treatment is predominantly nonsurgical, with bed rest, analgesia and hydration. Occasionally conservative management fails and surgery is required. Although there are many reports to support the safety of myomectomy in pregnancy these often relate to pedunculated tumours[9–11] and conservative management remains the treatment of choice.[8]

Preterm labour

Although an obvious cause of abdominal pain in pregnancy, it is surprising how often it is overlooked, especially in the second trimester. Its characteristic nature should usually alert the clinician to assess the cervix. It is especially important to consider the possibility of preterm labour during the postoperative period following laparotomy for the other causes of abdominal pain discussed in this article. It is prudent to undertake external tocodynamometry during the initial 24-hour postoperative period when the routine use of analgesics may well mask the symptoms of preterm labour.[2]

Placental abruption

When significant placental separation occurs, there is usually severe, acute abdominal pain. Vaginal bleeding may not be evident. Abruption is associated with maternal hypertension, cigarette smoking, multiple pregnancy and fibroids. The pain is unrelenting and often described as sharp, tearing or burning. The patient may be hypotensive, anaemic and can rapidly develop a coagulopathy. With a large separation, fetal death is likely and the uterus is characteristically 'woody hard' on palpation. Fetal parts are difficult to distinguish. Such findings of major abruption should prompt a rapid search for the fetal heart and if present, urgent caesarean section should be considered because of the likelihood of imminent fetal demise.

Acute polyhydramnios

Polyhydramnios presenting as acute abdominal pain is relatively uncommon. However, the twin–twin transfusion syndrome complicates 15–20% of monochorionic twin pregnancies and can cause severe polyhydramnios and abdominal pain. The abdomen is tense and the diagnosis is easily made following ultrasound examination. Acute hydramnios can also be associated with fetal anomalies, such as oesophageal atresia and neural tube defects.

Chorioamnionitis

Chorioamnionitis usually follows prelabour rupture of the membranes. Occasionally, however, infection can cause uterine inflammation and abdominal pain in the absence of membrane rupture.

Problems with the adnexa

Ectopic pregnancy

Ectopic pregnancy occurs in approximately 2% of pregnancies[12] and remains an important cause of maternal mortality in the first trimester. Its frequency is increasing, possibly due to an increase in the prevalence of sexually transmitted diseases, sterilisation and delay in childbearing until later in life. In addition, with better imaging techniques and more sensitive biochemical assays, ectopic pregnancies are diagnosed earlier and may hitherto have resolved spontaneously, remaining undiagnosed. Abdominal pain with amenorrhoea are the most common presenting complaints. Vaginal bleeding is present in only 40–50%[13] of cases and can be mistaken for a normal period. Abdominal tenderness occurs in 75%, which may or may not be accompanied by rebound, guarding, or shoulder tip pain. Cervical excitation is elicited in two-thirds of ectopic pregnancies and there is a palpable adnexal mass in approximately 50%.[12] Prior to the routine use of first-trimester ultrasound with biochemical screening, more than 80% of ectopic pregnancies presented after rupture whereas the figure is now less than 20%.

The diagnosis of ectopic pregnancy must be considered with abdominal pain and irregular vaginal bleeding. A pregnancy test is important for diagnosis. Blood and urine tests for the β subunit of hCG are now so sensitive that they are nearly always positive in the presence of an ectopic pregnancy. Although there are reported cases of ruptured tubal pregnancies with negative tests, these are extremely rare. The main diagnostic difficulty occurs when the pregnancy test is positive and differentiation from a viable intrauterine pregnancy or threatened miscarriage is required. Serial measurements of βhCG levels can help the diagnosis. In a viable intrauterine pregnancy, the βhCG level doubles approximately every 1.5 days in early pregnancy and every 3.5 days at 7 weeks of gestation.[12] Ectopic pregnancies and failing intrauterine pregnancies show a suboptimal rise in βhCG (usually increasing less than 66% every 48 hours) or a fall. Unfortunately, biochemical testing does not allow the distinction between ectopic pregnancy and a failing intrauterine pregnancy. Transvaginal ultrasound is then required. The sensitivity of modern transvaginal ultrasound equipment should enable the visualisation of a viable intrauterine pregnancy with a βhCG level of >2000 miu/ml and in many cases a sac can be visualised with levels >1000 miu/ml.[14] While a combination of serial βhCG measurements and transvaginal ultrasound usually allows diagnosis, laparoscopy is required for atypical presentations. Rarely a heterotopic pregnancy occurs where an intrauterine pregnancy coexists with an ectopic pregnancy. The incidence of this is very low (1 in 15 000 to 1 in 30 000) but should be considered if there are unusual presentations of pain and bleeding in the first trimester.

Adnexal torsion

Twisting of the adnexa on the infundibulopelvic ligament is usually secondary to enlargement of the ovary from a functional ovarian cyst or neoplasm, or, more rarely, from an enlarged fallopian tube due to hydrosalpinx or tubo-ovarian abscess. The presenting complaint is usually pain, which is abrupt in onset and severe. It is often localised to the right or left iliac fossa, and associated with nausea and vomiting. It is slightly more common on the right, possibly because of the position of the sigmoid colon.[15] The pain may be intermittent if there is incomplete torsion. Initially there will be little in the way of a fever but if the torsion leads to necrosis, pyrexia develops with leucocytosis. A tender mass may be felt on pelvic examination. This is a surgical emergency which, if untreated, can lead to infarction of the fallopian tube, ovary and peritonitis.

Haemorrhage and rupture of ovarian cysts

Ovarian cysts do not usually cause pain unless they tort, bleed or rupture. Ovarian tumours most commonly seen in pregnancy are dermoid, pseudomucinous cysts, serous cystadenoma, corpus luteum cysts of pregnancy, paraovarian cysts and fibromas.[16] Haemorrhagic cysts in the first trimester present in a similar way to a ruptured ectopic pregnancy and require similar prompt action, as life-threatening haemorrhage can result.

Genitourinary causes of abdominal pain

Pyelonephritis

This usually occurs in the second or third trimester, complicating approximately 1–2% of pregnancies.[17] It is generally the result of untreated, asymptomatic bacteriuria and is predisposed by obstructive uropathy or urinary stasis. Loin pain is variable in severity but can be intense if infection causes ureteric spasm. Nausea, fever, rigors and dysuria are often present. A negative urine examination does not rule out pyelonephritis. Aggressive treatment with intravenous antibiotics and hydration is needed to prevent progression to septicaemia.

Cystitis

This is relatively common in pregnancy and is usually easily diagnosed in the presence of suprapubic pain, dysuria, frequency and haematuria.

Gastrointestinal causes of abdominal pain

Acute intestinal obstruction

Intestinal obstruction is a rare but significant complication of pregnancy, with a reported incidence of 1 in 5000 to 1 in 60000 deliveries. Higher incidence is reported in more recent reviews due to an increase in abdominal surgery in young women. A review of 66 patients presenting with obstruction between 1966 and 1991[18] demonstrated that a minority occur following delivery ($n = 13$). The causes found at laparotomy were adhesions (59%), volvulus (23%), intussusception (5%), hernia (3%), carcinoma (1%), appendicitis (1%) and idiopathic (8%). Volvulus, particularly of the caecum, has a much higher incidence in pregnancy, presumably because the enlarging uterus displaces the mobile caecum out of the pelvis to the right upper quadrant.

The symptoms of intestinal obstruction remain similar to those in nonpregnant women, with abdominal pain occurring in 98%, vomiting in 82% and constipation in 30%. Accurate diagnosis is hampered by the pregnancy-associated changes. Although colicky abdominal pain radiating to the back is invariable, there is often no abdominal tenderness unless there is underlying peritoneal irritation.[15] Abdominal tenderness in association with obstruction is often an indication of intestinal ischaemia, which requires urgent surgical intervention. Faeculent vomiting occurs if obstruction persists for longer than 24 hours, when prolonged stasis allows bacterial colonisation of the intraluminal contents. The white cell count is usually raised in obstruction but can be normal. It is prudent to assess baseline renal function and electrolyte balance. A plain erect abdominal radiograph will often show evidence of obstruction but a barium enema may also be useful. The significant morbidity and mortality of this condition outweighs the small potential risk of radiation exposure to the fetus. A dose of 1 rad (equivalent to ten times the dose from two abdominal films or one barium enema) is associated with a risk of congenital fetal malformation of less than 1 per 1000 compared with the normal background malformation rate of approximately 3%.[15] Nevertheless, care should be taken with appropriate shielding if possible because of the potential for oncogenesis.

Once a diagnosis of obstruction has been made, there is general agreement that surgery is required.[15,18,19] Conservative management, with fluid replacement and nasogastric decompression, should only be used while the patient is being prepared for theatre. Electrolyte and acid–base balance disturbances should be corrected, and urine output should be monitored. Aggressive intravenous fluid therapy may contribute to an increased risk of pulmonary oedema.[20] Tocolytic therapy for an irritable uterus is controversial. Magnesium sulphate tocolysis may contribute to a paralytic ileus.[21]

Undue delay in the length of time between admission to hospital and laparotomy contributes to an increased mortality rate.[18] A midline incision is preferred. The bowel must be carefully inspected for necrosis; 15 of 66 patients in one series required resection of nonviable bowel.[18] Hypotension and hypoxia, common causes of fetal morbidity and mortality, must be avoided.

Mortality and morbidity from intestinal obstruction remains high. In 1966, maternal mortality rates of 12% and fetal mortality rates of 20% were reported.[22] In a more recent series the figures are similar (6% and 26% respectively).[18] The fetal mortality rates increase as gestation advances and may be as high as 64% by the third trimester.[23]

Acute appendicitis

Appendicitis is the most common acute abdominal condition requiring surgery in pregnancy.[24] Its incidence, approximately one in 1700 pregnancies, about the same as in nonpregnant women.[25] It can occur at any time in pregnancy but there is an increased incidence in the second (45%) compared with the first (30%) and third (25%) trimesters.[26] With improved surgical techniques and antibiotics, maternal mortality has decreased significantly from 25% in the early 20th century[2] to 0.5% in 1977[27] and is rarely encountered today. However, the diagnosis is important as there is considerable fetal loss, especially in the presence of perforation and peritonitis. In one series, first-trimester appendicectomy for appendicitis was associated with miscarriage in 30% (3/10 cases) and in the second trimester premature delivery occurred in 11% (2/18 cases).[24]

Diagnosis can be difficult, since symptoms of appendicitis are similar to those normally encountered in pregnancy. Signs and symptoms common to both include anorexia, nausea and vomiting, mild to moderate elevation in the white cell count and pain. Nevertheless, a clinical diagnostic accuracy of between 60% and 80% has been reported by several authors.[24,28]

The pain of appendicitis is reported to move upward as the uterus enlarges and displaces the appendix cephalad. This should change the position of the perceived pain towards the right flank or right upper quadrant. However, some reports dispute this and suggest the majority of patients present with pain in the lower right quadrant irrespective of the gestation.[24,26] Rebound tenderness and guarding are found less frequently due to increased laxity of the abdominal wall in pregnancy.

Maternal temperature is not reliably elevated in pregnant patients with appendicitis. In one study, only one-third of patients with or without perforation, had a temperature greater than 37.5°C,[24] and in another the mean maximal temperature for proven appendicitis was 37.6°C compared with 37.8°C in those with normal histology.[26]

Laboratory investigations are also unreliable. The white cell count was greater than 16 × 10⁹/l in only around 40% of cases in these two reviews. While the C-reactive protein is not reliably raised in appendicitis, it is more likely if perforation has occurred.[24]

The type of incision for treatment depends on the gestation. In the first trimester, a paramedian incision is generally appropriate given the false-positive rates.[5] In the second and third trimesters, a muscle-splitting incision over the point of maximal tenderness may give the best access. Prophylactic treatment with antibiotics prior to surgery is recommended.[24] There are thus no reliable symptoms or signs with which to diagnose appendicitis in pregnancy but a high clinical suspicion combined with good clinical judgement will make the diagnosis in the majority.

Hepatobiliary and pancreatic causes of abdominal pain

Acute cholecystitis and cholelithiasis

Cholelithiasis is more common than acute cholecystitis in pregnancy.[5] Cholelithiasis occurs in approximately 3.5% of pregnant women[29] whereas the incidence of acute cholecystitis is 0.01–0.06%.[30] The increased incidence of cholelithiasis in pregnancy is due to an increase in serum cholesterol and lipids in combination with decreased gallbladder motility. The increase in progesterone during pregnancy (a smooth muscle relaxant and inhibitor of cholecystokinin) decreases gallbladder emptying and increases residual volume. Both oestrogen and progesterone lead to biliary cholesterol hypersaturation and virtually all gall stones in pregnancy are made of cholesterol. While gallstone formation is particularly common in pregnancy, most stones remain asymptomatic until the puerperium, when normal gall bladder contractions resume and the potential for obstruction of the cystic or common bile duct increases.

Biliary colic, which is pain in the right upper quadrant associated with documented cholelithiasis, is usually of sudden onset and radiates to the back, right scapula or shoulder blade. Acute cholecystitis occurs with the obstruction of the cystic duct and also causes sudden onset right upper quadrant pain. This can be constant, colicky, or stabbing in nature. The symptoms may be associated with nausea, vomiting, fever (>38.5°C), abdominal tenderness, and non-specific laboratory findings such as a leucocytosis, elevation of serum amylase and bilirubin. Tenderness under the right costal margin on deep inspiration (Murphy's sign) is less common in pregnancy. Progression to gall stone pancreatitis is associated with an elevation in amylase, lipase, direct bilirubin and transaminases. Alkaline phosphatase estimations are less useful as these are normally raised in pregnancy. Diagnosis is reliably made by ultrasound,[31] which demonstrates the presence of stones, thickening of the gallbladder wall and dilatation in the diameter of the common bile duct.

Management has traditionally been conservative, especially in the first and early second trimester, comprising adequate intravenous hydration, analgesia, restricted oral intake, nasogastric aspiration, and antibiotics where necessary. Cholecystectomy has traditionally been reserved for cases where there have been recurrent attacks or suspected perforation, sepsis or peritonitis. However, with increasing recognition that morbidity is the consequence of the disease rather than of the surgery, a more aggressive approach is being recommended by some.[32-34] While pregnancy has generally been regarded as a contraindication to laparoscopic cholecystectomy, recent experience suggests that this may be a safe alternative to open surgery, especially in the second trimester.[35]

Pre-eclampsia and acute fatty liver of pregnancy

Liver disease associated with pregnancy must always be considered in the differential diagnosis of a pregnant woman presenting with right upper quadrant pain, especially in the second or third trimester. Significant liver involvement complicates about 10% of cases of pre-eclampsia[2] and typically presents with sudden onset of nausea and vomiting, right upper quadrant and epigastric pain and the characteristic features of hypertension and proteinuria. The abdomen is tender and the liver edge may be palpable. Blood tests will usually reveal a falling platelet count, elevated serum transaminases and uric acid levels, and as the disease progresses, a deranged clotting screen with disseminated intravascular coagulation. Hyperbilirubinaemia is found in approximately 10% of cases[36] and is usually indicative of microangiopathic haemolytic anaemia. In extreme cases, subcapsular haematoma formation can occur with subsequent liver rupture and carries a high risk of maternal mortality. These patients present with shock due to a rapidly developing haemoperitoneum.

Acute fatty liver of pregnancy is a rare condition complicating approximately one in 10 000 pregnancies.[37] It usually occurs in the third trimester. Hepatic encephalopathy, haemorrhage secondary to disseminated intravascular coagulation, pancreatitis and sepsis contribute to the high maternal mortality. Early diagnosis is essential and should be considered when vomiting in the third trimester is associated with tiredness, upper abdominal pain (often for days or weeks), jaundice, drowsiness or confusion. Blood tests resemble those seen in pre-eclampsia,[38] although the serum uric acid is often extremely elevated. Hypoglycaemia occurs as hepatic failure supervenes.

The treatment of severe pre-eclampsia and acute fatty liver of pregnancy is prompt delivery once the maternal condition has been stabilised. Delay can result in a worsening of the condition with higher perinatal and maternal mortality rates.

Hepatitis

Acute hepatitis is an inflammation of the liver which results in pain due to stretching of the liver capsule. The most common cause is viral infection (hepatitis A, B, C, E or G, Epstein–Barr, herpes simplex viruses, or cytomegalovirus). Other causes include alcoholic and autoimmune hepatitis.

Clinically the symptoms and signs are anorexia, abdominal pain, malaise (fever is uncommon), dark urine, light stools and scleral icterus. The liver edge is commonly palpable and occasionally tender but marked hepatomegaly is uncommon. The clinical course of acute hepatitis varies from mild symptoms requiring no treatment to fulminant liver failure requiring transplantation.

Of diagnostic importance is a history of exposure to infected contacts, recent intravenous drug use or transfusions, sexual orientation, travel history and drug or toxin exposure. Laboratory evaluation will help to confirm the presence of acute liver injury, distinguish the cause and monitor the course of the disease. An increase in bilirubin and transaminases are to be expected. A low albumin and raised INR are poor prognostic features, reflecting diminished hepatic protein synthetic capacity.

Initial serologic testing should include hepatitis A immunoglobulin M antibody (HAV-IgM), hepatitis B surface antigen (HB$_s$Ag), anti-hepatitis C virus antibody (anti-HCV), other hepatotrophic viruses and an autoimmune screen. Abdominal ultrasound may help to exclude biliary tract disease but liver biopsy is rarely indicated.

Most cases of acute viral hepatitis resolve spontaneously and the treatment is supportive. In cases of infectious hepatitis, the disease must be notified and contact tracing instituted. The natural course of acute hepatitis may not be altered in pregnancy, although hepatitis E virus and herpes simplex virus infections can be more complicated.[39] Both cause fulminant hepatic failure and have a high maternal mortality, particularly during the third trimester.[40,41] Herpes simplex virus infection can be treated with acyclovir.[42] In women with hepatitis B in the second or third trimester, maternal immunoprophylaxis with hyperimmune globulin may be indicated and the neonate will require immunisation after delivery.[43] Vertical transmission of hepatitis B, C, E[44] and G have been reported. The possibility is increased in hepatitis C if there is co-infection with human immunodeficiency virus[45] but clarification of interventions which may be helpful is awaited.[46] Caesarean section reduces vertical transmission of some hepatotrophic viruses.[47]

Inflammatory bowel disease

There has been considerable debate regarding the effect of inflammatory bowel disease on pregnancy. The general consensus is that the chance of a full-term normal delivery is the same as for unaffected women with the proviso that ulcerative colitis or Crohn's disease active at conception doubles the miscarriage rate.[48] The risk of worsening the disease is not affected by pregnancy, although active disease in the first trimester is associated with a tendency to relapse in the puerperium. Patients usually present with diarrhoea, anaemia, weight loss and abdominal pain. Diagnostic confirmation by sigmoidoscopy and biopsy need not be avoided in pregnancy. Inflammatory bowel disease is usually responsive to medical treatment and surgery is reserved for major complications such as toxic megacolon.

Reflux oesophagitis and peptic ulceration

Mild to moderate acid reflux, described as 'heartburn', complicates approximately 40% of pregnancies and is often associated with nausea and vomiting.[49] The frequency is caused by a decrease in lower oesophageal sphincter tone due to a rise in progesterone and intra-abdominal pressure created by the enlarging uterus. Peptic ulceration is, by contrast, rare and pregnancy seems to confer a protective effect. Peptic ulceration needs to be considered when symptoms persist in a dramatic fashion or do not respond to conventional treatment. Endoscopy remains the confirmatory diagnostic test but is rarely necessary. Severe epigastric pain in the third trimester should lead to consideration of the other causes of abdominal pain discussed, in particular, pre-eclampsia.

Acute pancreatitis

Acute pancreatitis in pregnancy complicates between 1 in 1000 and 1 in 12000 deliveries.[50] Although pregnancy was once regarded as a predisposing factor, especially in primiparous women, this has now been contested.[50,51] Pancreatitis tends to be more common with advancing gestation.[50] In nonpregnant patients, gallstones or alcohol abuse are contributors to over 80% of cases but alcohol is rarely implicated in pregnancy and cholelithiasis is by far the most common cause. The clinical significance of the disease lies in the fetal loss rate of 10–20% and the maternal mortality rate of up to 15%.[49]

Symptoms of pancreatitis are similar in pregnancy to those in nonpregnant women and include mid-epigastric or left upper quadrant pain with characteristic radiation through to the back. Pain, is not however, consistently present and the diagnosis needs consideration when there are any upper abdominal symptoms or signs. Nausea, vomiting, ileus and a low-grade fever are seen in a proportion of women. Haemorrhagic pancreatitis should be considered when there is hypovolaemic shock. Serum amylase and lipase are usually raised and remain the key diagnostic tests for confirmatory diagnosis, although hyperamylasaemia can also occur with bowel obstruction, perforated viscus, or cholecystitis.[2] It has been reported that amylase levels rise in normal pregnancy, further complicating the diagnosis[52] but this has been disputed.[53,54] Ultrasound examination may be useful to diagnose pancreatic oedema and will identify gallstones. Pancreatic oedema may also be diagnosed by magnetic resonance imaging.[50]

Treatment is usually conservative with intravenous fluids, restricted oral intake, nasogastric suction (if vomiting is excessive) and analgesia. Although cholecystectomy if required, can usually be delayed until after delivery, there are reports on its safety, especially in the second trimester. When there is significant hypertriglyceridaemia, specific metabolic manipulation may be required, including dietary restriction and parenteral nutrition. Triglyceride levels usually fall after delivery and delivery may be required in unusually severe disease.

Musculoskeletal causes of abdominal pain

Rupture of the rectus abdominus muscle

This is a rare complication of pregnancy usually seen in multigravid women. It is often precipitated by coughing which causes bleeding from the deep epigastric vessels behind the muscle.[5] If the bleeding occurs below the linea semilunaris, where there is no posterior sheath, blood will irritate the peritoneum causing peritonism. This may be difficult to distinguish from other causes of acute abdominal pain in pregnancy. Careful inspection of the abdomen may reveal a unilateral, elongated, tender swelling. Smaller haematomas can usually be managed conservatively, whereas more profuse bleeding can present with shock necessitating surgery.

Haematological causes of abdominal pain

Sickle cell disease

Sickle cell disease is caused by a structural abnormality of the haemoglobin (Hb) chain resulting in an abnormal variant (HbS). The abnormality is a single base mutation in the gene coding for β-globin. In the homozygous state, both genes are abnormal, resulting in sickle cell disease, whereas the heterozygous form results in sickle cell trait. In sickle cell disease the red blood cells deform (sickle) under various conditions such as cold, dehydration, infection, acidosis, hypoxia and pregnancy.

Three types of acute episodes, or crises, may occur. These are termed infarctive, sequestrative and haemolytic. By far the most common are infarctive crises, characterised by severe pain, which may persist for several days or weeks. Abdominal pain may be caused by infarction of the kidneys, spleen or liver. Fever is common but anaemia rare, in contrast to sequestrative or haemolytic crises where anaemia may be marked. Sickle trait is generally asymptomatic but sickling can occur under conditions of severe hypoxia.

The diagnosis is made by haemoglobin electrophoresis. Stable sickle cell anaemia and sickle cell trait require no acute clinical intervention although care should be taken to avoid dehydration and precipitating events during pregnancy and delivery. Acute painful infarctive crises in sickle cell disease should be treated supportively ensuring adequate analgesia, hydration and oxygenation.[55] Any underlying precipitant causes should be investigated and treated.

Pregnancy can exacerbate the frequency and intensity of sickling crises[56] and repeated transfusions may be used to reduce the proportion of circulating HbS.[57] Sickle cell disease is associated with an increased risk of intrauterine growth restriction, antepartum hospital admissions, pre-eclampsia,[58] preterm labour and postpartum infection. It is thus particularly important that the patient is aware of the precipitants for sickling and the importance of seeking early medical attention during pregnancy. Sickle cell patients and their partners should be offered specific genetic counselling and testing.[59]

Porphyria

This heterogeneous group of inborn errors of metabolism are caused by abnormalities of enzymes involved in the biosynthesis of haem, resulting in overproduction of intermediate compounds called porphyrins. Porphyrias are classified as acute or nonacute. Acute porphyrias (in contrast to nonacute) are characterised by an increase in delta-aminolevulinic acid (δ-ALA).[60] All forms of acute porphyria are associated with abdominal pain,[61] nausea and vomiting. The pain may be severe enough to mimic an acute abdomen. Polyneuropathy and psychiatric manifestations are also common. The symptoms may be precipitated by pregnancy,[62–65] infection, dieting, alcohol or drugs (sulphonamides, barbiturates, anticonvulsants).[60] The diagnosis should be considered whenever there is a combination of the clinical features or a family history of porphyria. Investigations may demonstrate elevated bilirubin, transferase enzymes and urea with a low serum sodium.[66] The type of porphyria may be distinguished by the analysis of faecal and urinary porphyrins.

Management is largely supportive.[66] A high carbohydrate intake is given by dextrose infusion during the acute phase since this has an indirect effect on porphyrin production. It is also prudent to administer dextrose during labour, even in asymptomatic individuals. Narcotics should be given for the pain due to acute porphyria.

Other causes of abdominal pain

Diabetic ketoacidosis

Diabetic ketoacidosis (DKA) is a state of uncontrolled catabolism associated with insulin deficiency. It is usually caused by reducing or omitting insulin in diabetics, often due to the anorexia caused by nausea or vomiting in pregnancy.[67] It may also be precipitated by the stress of intercurrent illness, sometimes in hitherto unrecognised diabetes mellitus.[68] The pathophysiological mechanism is an absence of insulin which increases hepatic glucose production and reduces peripheral uptake. The high plasma glucose levels lead to osmotic diuresis, loss of fluid and electrolytes and dehydration. Progressive dehydration impairs renal excretion of hydrogen ions and ketones, aggravating the acidosis. Respiratory compensation leads to hyperventilation, described as 'air hunger'. The reduced insulin is also associated with lipolysis, which produces ketone bodies, identified by a characteristic fetor on the breath.

The clinical features of ketoacidosis are prostration, hyperventilation (Kussmaul respiration), nausea, vomiting and abdominal pain. The latter may cause confusion with a surgical acute abdomen. The diagnosis is made by demonstrating hyperglycaemia and acidosis with ketonaemia or heavy ketonuria. Untreated, severe ketoacidosis can be fatal for mother and/or fetus.[69] Treatment should therefore be started urgently[70] with aggressive hydration (including potassium supplementation), replacement of electrolytes and sliding scale insulin.[69,70]

Malaria

Malaria is a protozoal disease transmitted by the bite of the infected *Anopheles* mosquito. Four species of the genus *Plasmodium* cause nearly all infections in humans. Of these *Plasmodium falciparum* is the most serious. Malaria should be considered in patients who are from, or who have travelled to, regions where malaria is endemic. Administration of an antimalarial medication and preventing mosquito bites reduces but does not eliminate the risk of developing malaria.[71]

The classical features of malaria include fever, abdominal pain, malaise, splenic enlargement, hypoglycaemia and secondary anaemia. Malaria is often more severe in pregnancy and therefore has a higher risk of morbidity and mortality.[72] The fever of malaria in pregnancy can be continuous low-grade or periodic hyperpyrexia although in the second half of pregnancy, fever may not be a feature. Destruction of red cells and removal by the spleen in conjunction with ineffective erythropoeisis may lead to marked anaemia and its associated symptoms. An important and common complication of malaria in pregnancy is hypoglycaemia, which is associated with a poor prognosis. In severe disease, the clinical signs of hypoglycaemia may be masked and the neurological impairment can then (mistakenly) be attributed to the underlying infection.

Abdominal pain is relatively common when malaria occurs in pregnancy[73,74] and may be accompanied by guarding and rigidity. Diagnosis requires demonstration of the asexual forms of the parasite in peripheral blood. Fever, hypoglycaemia and anaemia are all detrimental to fetal wellbeing. Furthermore, the malarial parasite is sequestered and can develop in the placenta leading to insufficiency. The perinatal mortality rate is 15–70% ,[72,75] dependent upon the malarial species. Spontaneous abortion, preterm labour, stillbirth, intrauterine growth restriction and fetal distress are all commonly associated with malarial infection.[72]

Treatment consists of antimalarials, depending upon the strain of plasmodium.[71] Most forms are choloroquine-resistant and therefore quinine or intravenous quinidine is often used in the first instance. These are relatively safe during pregnancy. Correction of hydration with dextrose and anaemia with blood transfusion may be required.

Intraperitoneal haemorrhage

Such bleeding may occur around the time of childbirth. In some instances, laparotomy fails to reveal the source of the bleeding. In pregnancy, the ovarian and broad ligament veins significantly increase in size with a doubling of the venous pressure.[5] Spontaneous rupture has been reported in labour, giving rise to acute lower abdominal pain and shock. Urgent laparotomy is required with opening of the peritoneal space to secure the bleeding.

Splenic artery aneurysm rupture in pregnancy deserves special consideration. The precise incidence is unknown but relatively high incidences have been reported.[76,77] Interestingly, arterial aneurysms usually occur more frequently in men but splenic artery aneurysms are four times more common in women.[77] Unfortunately, very few women present with any symptoms before rupture. Warning signs include epigastric or left upper quadrant pain that may radiate to the back. There may be pain in the left shoulder (Kehr's sign) as the aneurysm enlarges. Splenomegaly is present in approximately 44% and a bruit may be heard in the left upper quadrant.[77] It may be diagnosed incidentally on plain abdominal radiography since the majority are calcified. The diagnosis can often be made with ultrasound but arteriography remains the gold standard. In the majority of cases, the aneurysm ruptures directly into the peritoneal cavity and the presence of symptoms and signs should prompt an urgent laparotomy. Sometimes the aneurysm will initially rupture into the lesser sac causing syncope, hypotension and pain in the flank. As the lesser sac fills with blood and clot, partial tamponade may allow some recovery. The haematoma eventually ruptures into the peritoneal cavity causing severe pain, hypotension, tachycardia and cyanosis. There may be associated fetal bradycardia as the uteroplacental perfusion pressure decreases. This sequence is described as the 'double-rupture' syndrome.

When a splenic artery aneurysm is discovered in pregnancy, surgery is required to ligate the vessel on either side of the aneurysm. Occasionally splenectomy is needed. After rupture, resuscitation followed by laparotomy to clamp the splenic hilum is recommended.

Summary and conclusions

Abdominal pain in pregnancy can present a difficult diagnostic challenge. Delays in diagnosis and treatment represent the most significant risks for poor outcome in mother and fetus. Delays occur because of the tendency to attribute many of the early symptoms to those routinely experienced in pregnancy, the masking of symptoms due to the anatomical and physiological changes of pregnancy, and caution in investigating pregnant women. As diagnostic techniques become safer, the use of these at an earlier stage may avoid unnecessary delay and improve fetal and maternal outcome.

References

1.   Hytten FE, Weight changes in pregnancy. In: Hytten F, Chamberlain G, editors. *Clinical Physiology in Obstetrics*. London: Blackwell Scientific; 1991. p. 171–203.
2.   Nathan L, Huddleston JF, Acute abdominal pain in pregnancy. *Obstet Gynecol Clin N Am* 1995;**22**:55–68.
3.   Mendenhall HW. Serum protein concentrations in pregnancy. I. Concentrations in maternal serum. *Am J Obstet Gynecol* 1970;**106**:388–99.
4.   Girling JC, Dow E, Smith JH. Liver function tests in pre-eclampsia: importance of comparison with a reference range derived for normal pregnancy. *Br J Obstet Gynaecol* 1997;**104**:246–50.
5.   Sivanesaratnam V. The acute abdomen and the obstetrician. *Baillieres Best Pract Res Clin Obstet Gynaecol* 2000;**14**:89–102.
6.   Jensen JG. Uterine torsion in pregnancy. *Acta Obstet Gynecol Scand* 1992;**71**:260–65.
7.   Carter TD. A further case of torsion of the pregnant uterus. *Centr Afr J Med* 1961;**7**:258.
8.   Lumsden MA, Wallace EM. Clinical presentation of uterine fibroids. *Baillieres Clin Obstet Gynaecol* 1998;**12**:177–95.
9.   Burton CA, Grimes DA, March CM. Surgical management of leiomyomata during pregnancy. *Obstet Gynecol* 1989;**74**:707–9.
10. Glavind K, Palvio DH, Lauritsen JG. Uterine myoma in pregnancy. *Acta Obstet Gynecol Scand* 1990;**69**: 617–19.
11. Mollica G, Pittini L, Minganti E, Perri G, Pansini F. Elective uterine myomectomy in pregnant women. *Clin Exp Obstet Gynecol* 1996;**23**:168–72.
12. Carr RJ, Evans P. Ectopic pregnancy. *Prim Care* 2000;**27**:169–83.
13. Fylstra DL. Tubal pregnancy: a review of current diagnosis and treatment. *Obstet Gynecol Surv* 1998;**53**:320–28.
14. Bree RL, Edwards M, Bohm-Velez M, Beyler S, Roberts J, Mendelson EB. Transvaginal sonography in the evaluation of normal early pregnancy: correlation with HCG level. *Am J Roentgenol* 1989;**153**:75–9.
15. Tarraza HM, Moore RD. Gynecologic causes of the acute abdomen and the acute abdomen in pregnancy. *Surg Clin North Am* 1997;**77**:1371–94.
16. Klufio CA, Amoa AB, Rageau O. Abdominal pain in pregnancy. *P N G Med J* 1993;**36**:342–52.
17. Gilstrap LC, Cunningham FG, Whalley PJ. Acute pyelonephritis in pregnancy: an anterospective study. *Obstet Gynecol* 1981;**57**:409–13.
18. Perdue PW, Johnson HW Jr, Stafford PW. Intestinal obstruction complicating pregnancy. *Am J Surg* 1992;**164**:384–8.
19. Meyerson S, Holtz T, Ehrinpreis M, Dhar R. Small bowel obstruction in pregnancy. *Am J Gastroenterol* 1995;**90**:299–302.
20. Pisani RJ, Rosenow EC. Pulmonary edema associated with tocolytic therapy. *Ann Intern Med* 1989;**110**:714–18.
21. Hill WC, Gill PJ, Katz M. Maternal paralytic ileus as a complication of magnesium sulfate tocolysis. *Am J Perinatol* 1985;**2**:47–8.
22. Goldthorp WO. Intestinal obstruction during pregnancy and the puerperium. *Br J Clin Pract* 1966;**20**:367–76.
23. Fallon WF, Newman JS, Fallon GL, Malangoni MA. The surgical management of intra-abdominal

inflammatory conditions during pregnancy. *Surg Clin North Am* 1995;**75**:15–31.

24. Andersen B, Nielsen TF. Appendicitis in pregnancy: diagnosis, management and complications. *Acta Obstet Gynecol Scand* 1999;**78**:758–62.
25. Mahmoodian S. Appendicitis complicating pregnancy. *South Med J* 1992;**85**:19–24.
26. Mourad J, Elliott JP, Erickson L, Lisboa L. Appendicitis in pregnancy: new information that contradicts long-held clinical beliefs. *Am J Obstet Gynecol* 2000;**182**:1027–9.
27. Babaknia A, Parsa H, Woodruff JD. Appendicitis during pregnancy. *Obstet Gynecol* 1977;**50**:40–44.
28. Weingold AB. Appendicitis in pregnancy. *Clin Obstet Gynecol* 1983;**26**:801–9.
29. Stauffer RA, Adams A, Wygal J, Lavery JP. Gallbladder disease in pregnancy. *Am J Obstet Gynecol* 1982;**144**:661–4.
30. Lanzafame RJ. Laparoscopic cholecystectomy during pregnancy. *Surgery* 1995; **118**:627–31; 631–3.
31. Sharp HT. Gastrointestinal surgical conditions during pregnancy. *Clin Obstet Gynecol* 1994;**37**:306–15.
32. Davis A, Katz VL, Cox R. Gallbladder disease in pregnancy. *J Reprod Med* 1995;**40**:759–62.
33. Dixon NP, Faddis DM, Silberman H. Aggressive management of cholecystitis during pregnancy. *Am J Surg* 1987;**154**:292–4.
34. Swisher SG, Schmit PJ, Hunt KK, Hiyama DT, Bennion RS, Swisher EM. Biliary disease during pregnancy. *Am J Surg* 1994;**168**:576–9; 580–81.
35. Reedy MB, Galan HL, Richards WE, Preece CK, Wetter PA, Kuehl TJ. Laparoscopy during pregnancy. A survey of laparoendoscopic surgeons. *J Reprod Med* 1997;**42**:33–8.
36. Simon JA. Biliary tract disease and related surgical disorders during pregnancy. *Clin Obstet Gynecol* 1983;**26**:810–21.
37. Kaplan MM. Acute fatty liver of pregnancy. *N Engl J Med* 1985;**313**:367–70.
38. Purdie JM, Walters BN. Acute fatty liver of pregnancy: clinical features and diagnosis. *Aust N Z J Obstet Gynaecol* 1988;**28**:62–7.
39. Hunt CM, Sharara AI. Liver disease in pregnancy. *Am Fam Physician* 1999;**59**:829–36.
40. Kang AH, Graves CR. Herpes simplex hepatitis in pregnancy: a case report and review of the literature. *Obstet Gynecol Surv* 1999;**54**:463–8.
41. Aggarwal R, Krawczynski K. Hepatitis E: an overview and recent advances in clinical and laboratory research. *J Gastroenterol Hepatol* 2000;**15**:9–20.
42. Johnson LG, Saldana LR. Herpes simplex virus hepatitis in pregnancy. A case report. *J Reprod Med* 1994;**39**:544–6.
43. Michielsen PP, Van Damme P. Viral hepatitis and pregnancy. *Acta Gastroenterol Belg* 1999;**62**:21–9.
44. Irshad M. Hepatitis E virus: a global view of its seroepidemiology and transmission pattern. *Trop Gastroenterol* 1997;**18**:45–9.
45. Hunt CM, Carson KL, Sharara AI. Hepatitis C in pregnancy. *Obstet Gynecol* 1997;**89**:883–90.
46. Zanetti AR, Tanzi E, Newell ML. Mother-to-infant transmission of hepatitis C virus. *J Hepatol* 1999;**31**(suppl. 1):96–100.
47. Ohto H, Ujiie N, Sato A, Okamoto H, Mayumi M. Mother-to-infant transmission of GB virus type C/HGV. *Transfusion* 2000;**40**:725–30.
48. Walters BNJ. Hepatic and gastrointestinal disease. In: James DK, Steer PJ, Weiner CP, Gonik B, editors. *High Risk Pregnancy; Management Options*. London: W. B. Saunders; 1999. p. 787–802.
49. Epstein FB. Acute abdominal pain in pregnancy. *Emerg Med Clin North Am* 1994;**12**:151–65.
50. Ramin KD, Ramin SM, Richey SD, Cunningham FG. Acute pancreatitis in pregnancy. *Am J Obstet Gynecol* 1995;**173**: 187–91.
51. Scott LD. Gallstone disease and pancreatitis in pregnancy. *Gastroenterol Clin North Am* 1992;**21**:803–15.
52. Kaiser R, Berk JE, Fridhandler L. Serum amylase changes during pregnancy. *Am J Obstet Gynecol* 1975;**122**: 283–6.
53. Strickland DM, Hauth JC, Widish J, Strickland K, Perez R. Amylase and isoamylase activities in serum of pregnant women. *Obstet Gynecol* 1984;**63**:389–91.
54. Ordorica SA, Frieden FJ, Marks F, Hoskins IA, Young BK. Pancreatic enzyme activity in pregnancy. *J Reprod Med* 1991;**36**:359–62.
55. Steinberg MH. Management of sickle cell disease. *N Engl J Med* 1999;**340**:1021–30.
56. Berkane N, Nizard J, Dreux B, Uzan S, Girot R. Sickle cell anemia and pregnancy. Complications and management. *Pathol Biol (Paris)* 1999;**47**:46–54.
57. Howard RJ, Tuck SM, Pearson TC. Pregnancy in sickle cell disease in the UK: results of a multicentre survey of the effect of prophylactic blood transfusion on maternal and fetal outcome. *Br J Obstet Gynaecol* 1995;**102**:947–51.
58. Larrabee KD, Monga M. Women with sickle cell trait are at increased risk for preeclampsia. *Am J*

Obstet Gynecol 1997;**177**:425–8.

59.   Xu K, Shi ZM, Veeck LL, Hughes MR, Rosenwaks Z. First unaffected pregnancy using preimplantation genetic diagnosis for sickle cell anemia. *JAMA* 1999;**281**:1701–6.

60.   Gordon N. The acute porphyrias. *Brain Dev* 1999;21:373–7.

61.   Thadani H, Deacon A, Peters T. Diagnosis and management of porphyria. *Br Med J* 2000;**320**:1647–51.

62.   Kanaan C, Veille JC, Lakin M. Pregnancy and acute intermittent porphyria. *Obstet Gynecol Surv* 1989;44: 244–9.

63.   Keung YK, Chuahirun T, Cobos E. Acute intermittent porphyria with seizure and paralysis in the puerperium. *J Am Board Fam Pract* 2000;**13**:76–9.

64.   Soriano D, Seidman DS, Mashiach S, Sela BA, Blonder J. Acute intermittent porphyria first diagnosed in the third trimester of pregnancy. Case report. *J Perinat Med* 1996;**24**:185–9.

65.   Shenhav S, Gemer O, Sassoon E, Segal S. Acute intermittent porphyria precipitated by hyperemesis and metoclopramide treatment in pregnancy. *Acta Obstet Gynecol Scand* 1997;76:484–5.

66.   Morales Ortega X, Wolff Fernandez C, Leal Ibarra T, Montana Navarro N, Armas-Merino R. Porphyric crisis: experience of 30 episodes. *Medicina* 1999;**59**:23–7.

67.   Cullen MT, Reece EA, Homko CJ, Sivan E. The changing presentations of diabetic ketoacidosis during pregnancy. *Am J Perinatol* 1996;**13**:449–51.

68.   Sills IN, Rappaport R. New-onset IDDM presenting with diabetic ketoacidosis in a pregnant adolescent. *Diabetes Care* 1994;**17**:904–5.

69.   Steel JM, Johnstone FD. Guidelines for the management of insulin-dependent diabetes mellitus in pregnancy. *Drugs* 1996;**52**:60–70.

70.   Ramin KD. Diabetic ketoacidosis in pregnancy. *Obstet Gynecol Clin North Am* 1999;**26**:481–8;viii.

71.   Winstanley P. Malaria: treatment. *J R Coll Physicians Lond* 1998;**32**:203–7.

72.   Carles G, Bousquet F, Raynal P, Peneau C, Mignot V, Arbeille P. Pregnancy and malaria. Study of 143 cases in French Guyana. *J Gynecol Obstet Biol Reprod (Paris)* 1998;**27**:798–805.

73.   Sarma PS, Kumar RS. Abdominal pain in a patient with falciparum malaria. *Postgrad Med J* 1998;**74**:425–7.

74.   Prien-Larsen JC, Stjernquist M. Malaria in pregnancy: a master of masquerade. *Acta Obstet Gynecol Scand* 1993;**72**:496–7.

75.   Nyirjesy P, Kavasya T, Axelrod P, Fischer PR. Malaria during pregnancy: neonatal morbidity and mortality and the efficacy of chloroquine chemoprophylaxis. *Clin Infect Dis* 1993;**16**:127–32.

76.   Stanley JC, Fry WJ. Pathogenesis and clinical significance of splenic artery aneurysms. *Surgery* 1974;**76**:898–909.

77.   Angelakis EJ, Bair WE, Barone JE, Lincer RM. Splenic artery aneurysm rupture during pregnancy. *Obstet Gynecol Surv* 1993;**48**:145–8.

Chapter 27

Pain during pregnancy

Discussion

Discussion following the papers of Mrs Coldron and Dr Vits and of Mr Overton and Professor Thornton

Fernando: I have a question for Mrs Coldron. You said TENS was recommended postnatally but it is very commonly used antenatally. It is even sold over the counter, and is widely available.

Coldron: That is a point of controversy. We do not know the effects of TENS on the fetus and whether it leads to premature labour, so our recommendation is not to use it – apart from during labour, and also perhaps in the last three weeks, from 37 weeks of gestation. Perhaps it needs more study to see what effect electrical stimulation around the abdomen and the back has on the developing fetus.

Fernando: Are you saying it should not be used in labour?

Coldron: It should be used in labour but not used antenatally.

Fernando: Are there any guidelines?

Coldron: We have not written them down. It is a point of debate at the moment within the committee of the women's health group, but we recommend that up to 37 weeks' gestation TENS is not used.

Fernando: One last thing was about symphysis pubic dysfunction. You said that an epidural may be contraindicated in some situations.

Coldron: No, I said that it is controversial. It is just to be aware of the fact that if somebody presents with symphysis pubis dysfunction or pain antenatally, it should be written in their antenatal notes. The amount of abduction the woman can achieve needs consideration since an epidural can mask that. If the woman only has 10–20 degrees of abduction and her thighs are forcibly abducted during labour because she cannot feel it, these women can get huge problems postnatally with their symphysis pubis.

Fernando: I thought that in some situations an epidural may be of advantage if they were opting for a normal delivery. They would get better pain relief and be able to adopt a better position, in conjuction with the physiotherapist.

Coldron: That is the point, is it not? The best position for the woman needs to be determined antenatally and then perhaps an epidural may help.

Fernando: It is rare that we have women like these unless they have an elective caesarean section, but I remember that from time to time we have had physiotherapists within the labour ward room with the women with epidural delivery. That is fairly unusual and needs highly motivated physiotherapists.

Coldron: It is, and that is why it needs to be discussed with the midwife, because they are more likely to be with the woman, as to what positions will be best for the woman, if possible. Sometimes in an emergency we know that they have to be up in stirrups, and that is that. But if the woman cannot abduct, being up in stirrups – or particularly putting her feet on the attendant's hips and pushing unilaterally with one foot – is rather dangerous for someone who already has an unstable symphysis pubis. So one has to be aware of that and be aware of the masking effects of an epidural.

Fernando: Old-fashioned epidurals were much worse because a lot of the muscle tone was lost – with 0.25% ropivacaine, for example. These days, with more modern epidurals, with preservation of muscle tone, that risk is far less. That is just a personal opinion.

Crowhurst: That is true. We had a case recently where a woman was on crutches for most of the pregnancy, and she needed an epidural for her labour. But we were careful about doing a very low-dose block for her, and she had normal movements and abduction and could get into the lithotomy position without damaging anything.

Something should perhaps be said about backache in relation to epidurals. It is a very topical subject that comes up all the time. The best evidence to date that I know of is based on a study done at St Thomas's Hospital about three years ago – a prospective study of about 600 women.[1] They showed that with the modern, low-dose neuraxial blocks that we are using, there is no significant change in the incidence of backache postpartum for up to 12 months. I notice it was said that the backache could go on for 18 months in the population, but this was a definitive study and it put to rest a good deal of the earlier work, which did show back problems because of the higher dose and the motor block and so on.

Thornton: Thank you, that is a very important point. Have you included that in your chapter?

Coldron: I have put it in my chapter, and said that it is controversial. As you say, the early studies have said that epidural was associated with back pain, but the later studies are saying that it is not, and clinically it often is not. Because the pain has come on during pregnancy and there is new onset back pain during labour, the women believe that it is due to the epidural when it may well be due to the musculoskeletal problems or to differences during labour itself.

MacLean: Mrs Coldron, can I ask you to comment about the role of caesarean section in people with symphysis pubis dysfunction? There is an increasing trend to use this, as Dr Fernando described. Some of these patients spend a long time hobbling around on crutches and there is a feeling that an easy way out is elective caesarean section, but clearly that interrupts your anterior abdominal wall. I wonder whether there is any evidence to show that caesarean section has any benefit? I imagine it could possibly be harmful.

Vits: There is no evidence at all that caesarean section is helpful. Certainly in our unit we do not use section electively, but we have a problem in that the symphysis pubis dysfunction support group feels that caesarean section for some of its members is the way to go. Unfortunately, you cannot delivery a lady twice. You cannot take the baby out by caesarean section and say how did you get on with that, then deliver it vaginally and say was that better? However, there is absolutely no clinical data that supports caesarean section for symphysis pubis dysfunction.

MacLean: Could we include that as one of the recommendations? There is an increasing move towards that and if one of your recommendations is that there is no evidence to support this, it would be a very important comment.

Vits: One of the problems is that there is no evidence either way. We only have one single paper, a very small study done quite a long time ago, to say that it does not make any difference. What you really need to do is look for the evidence and go forward. Now that women with this condition are being identified more, you could do a prospective study and look at them in a unit where maybe caesarean section has been used to see whether the outcomes were different from another unit where it was not being used. I don't think you would find decent data to back that up as a recommendation *per se*. You need to produce the data.

Stones: I want to ask about the sacro-iliac joint, which you have only briefly talked about.

Coldron: I used the word 'articular changes' which was predominantly sacro-iliac and symphysis pubis. Also lumbar spine, because with these women it may be lumbar spine or sacro-iliac or it may be both; the problem is sorting the wood from the trees. We prefer to use the word 'pelvic' pain because the pelvic ring is an entity with the sacrum and the two innominate bones, but if you want to look at the sacro-iliac *per se*, there is often associated pubic pain, and *vice versa* the symphysis pubis has associated sacro-iliac pain. It has to be because of the dysfunction. Yes, we do see an acute sacro-iliitis in some women, and we also see sacro-iliac dysfunctions that are perhaps more pronounced in the pregnant population than the normal population because of the associated joint laxity. We would approach them in the way that I have suggested – reduce any manual displacement and then work the muscles over the top to retain the correct positioning of the pelvis.

Berkley: I have a question about referred hyperalgesia in muscles from the uterus. In the three talks this morning I did not hear much discussion about back pain. We heard about dealing with back pain, but some of the source of that back pain may be referred from uterine contractions or the residual of uterine contractions in the back. And abdominal pain.

Coldron: That is the important thing, and this is why we recommend that if you are concerned about back pain the patient should be referred to us because we will do a musculoskeletal examination. It will not be a gynaecological or obstetric examination but musculoskeletal, and therefore we would expect to pick up musculo-skeletal signs if there was a musculoskeletal cause. We take a subjective history and we listen, and sometimes it is quite obvious if the pain is not coming from the musculoskeletal system but from the organic or visceral system, and in this case we refer back.

Berkley: The reason I bring this up is the referred pains during breastfeeding in the week or two after birth. These pains increase with parity. We have just finished a study with Anita Holdcroft on this. It is like a dose–response – each child further increases the pain during lactation.

Vits: That is true. Having two children myself, I would agree. But it is a very different pain and it is quite easy then to bring them in. We can screen for this pain and we can discount musculoskeletal involvement. If you are having a problem with breastfeeding pain and you do not know what it is, it will take us 20 minutes to discount completely the fact that it is a back problem.

Thornton: Just picking up on that, do you think that it is the perception of that pain that is different or do you think that the actual uterine contraction is stronger in the multiparas?

Berkley: That is a good question. We also had tocographic data, which did indeed show an increase with parity in the duration and frequency of uterine contractions during breastfeeding.[2]

Crowhurst: Mr Overton was talking about using radiographs in the acute abdomen. These days I find myself having to request radiology of perhaps ten or so women a year, usually with kyphoscoliosis or they have had previous spinal surgery and we want to avoid giving them general anaesthesia. I have had many discussions with radiologists over the past several years about this, and a good rule of thumb that I have been told is that one plain film of the lumbar spine, which is what I am usually looking at, is equivalent in radiation dose to somebody flying from here to the Costa del Sol or somewhere that they go for their holidays – about an hour and a half at 35 000 feet – in the daytime, I might add, there is more radiation in the daytime. A plain abdominal film, which is a little less than that, is probably only like a flight from London to Paris or from New York to Chicago. It is a good analogy to use to tell patients.

I don't know whether this is true of the acute abdomen and such conditions but I put this question to you. More recently, our radiology department at Hammersmith have been using something called a spiral computerised tomography (CT) scan, which gives a much lower dose even than a couple of plain films, and it is ideal for what I look for in a back X-ray in a pregnant woman. I don't know whether the spiral CT is of any benefit in your conditions?

Overton: The only contact I have with spiral CT is for investigation of possible pulmonary emboli. I certainly did not come across that when I was reviewing the literature for this chapter on the use of spiral imaging for acute abdominal conditions. Are you aware of any uses of it for abdominal imaging, Professor Thornton?

Thornton: Presumably it is only equivalent to a flight to Skegness! I would probably go to Paris. In answer to your question, no, I have not used spiral CT.

Fernando: Just a word on backache. All the data that suggested that epidurals caused backache many years ago spanning over at least ten years were all retrospective studies, and at least three prospective studies have now shown that early backache is not due to epidurals. It does not seem to matter whether you use a low-dose epidural or high-dose.

At the Royal Free Hospital, London, we often get patients who come complaining of anything to do with the back, and the epidural gets blamed. We often refer them to our physiotherapy colleagues. Do you have any sort of referral mechanism or recommendations if we get problems like this?

Coldron: Each hospital has its own referral system, which is the problem. There is a debate at the moment in the wider profession about this business of medical referral. In the private sector we do not need medical referral; patients can walk in off the street. But in the hospital system patients have the gate-keeping of the medical referral. That is why they come to us from all sorts of medical sources. Within the obstetric-physio world we broaden that referral to midwives. Community midwives in the first ten days postpartum will often refer, and antenatally as well. We get a lot of patients through the midwifery service.

You need to look at the policy for referral within each hospital – how do you refer to your physiotherapy department? I don't work at the Royal Free, so I don't know. I would imagine that consultant or registrar referral is straightforward – you just send a referral form down to the department for the attention of the physiotherapist in women's health.

Fernando: Is there any objection to mothers referring themselves to you, for example?

Coldron: On the whole, no. Again, you need to check the policy of the hospital but there is often a blanket referral system whereby the mother can self-refer during the antenatal period. It is a way of giving the patients their own responsibility for the management of their condition.

Foster: In the urogynaecological area there is a suggestion that early physical therapy rehabilitation after delivery may improve pelvic floor functioning, perhaps even improving the re-innervation of the pelvic floor from the pudendal nerve. Is there any evidence in other parts of the body where early rehabilitation might reduce a long-standing diastasis or other types of muscular dysfunction?

Coldron: I will not venture to speak on the pelvic floor because that is Miss Vits' area. Yes, there are recent studies – one from Australia, one by Sally Sheppard at the Royal Free – where they have looked at diastasis of the recti.[3-4] By using the stabilisation programme that we have looked at, i.e. using the lateral abdominals to contract the anterior abdominal fascia, this seems in these single case studies to have reduced the incidence and the amount of diastasis of the recti in early postpartum rehabilitation.

Foster: Have you tried that in somebody who, say, is five or ten years out, and do you get a similar response, or we do we know anything about that?

Coldron: There are no data on that.

Whorwell: Just a predictable comment – I am surprised you did not mention irritable bowel pain in these patients. When I get asked to see abdominal pain in pregnant patients, very often I can reassure them that it is irritable bowel. Critically, that is based on the prepregnant history obviously of the typical symptoms.

The only other comment is anecdotal. It is my experience, but I do not know whether it is has been written up, that inflammatory bowel disease usually gets worse after delivery of the child, which would go along with what has been said.

A diagnostic comment on tuberculosis (TB) – extra-pulmonary TB is nearly always in non-Caucasians – very unusual in the other groupings.

Stones: On malaria, I was not quite clear why somebody with malaria in pregnancy would be presenting with abdominal pain.

Thornton: As far as malaria is concerned, you are right, the presentation can be one of a number of symptoms. What I probably did not get across very well was that in those patients with infection where you are thinking about malaria, one of the presenting features is anorexia, abdominal pain, generally feeling unwell and bowel disturbance. It was one of the causes of abdominal pain that perhaps you would not usually think about and that was my reason for mentioning it. In terms of turning it round, as you are, and asking whether malaria usually presents with abdominal pain, I would say no, it is more likely to present with the other features.

Stones: One would probably highlight the enlarged spleen – bearing in mind that in many parts of the world malaria is endemic in pregnancy. It may be present but it may not be causal. In an area where malaria is endemic most women will have malaria parasites but that will not necessarily be relevant to their clinical presentation.

Whorwell: We see quite a lot of malaria in people coming back from abroad, and abdominal pain and diarrhoea are quite prominent. I wanted to mention airport malaria. Don't forget that if you live up to five miles from an airport you can get malaria without going out of the country.

MacLean: Professor Thornton, can I say how much I enjoyed your presentation? You prefaced it by saying that it was perhaps more relevant to people working outside the UK, but I don't think that is true. Following up the comments about the number of people who during pregnancy hop on planes and fly off, sometimes to see relatives in other countries or even, extraordinarily, go off on holiday because they think that is important. Certainly practising in London one comes across a number of people who have come from endemic areas, have had malaria, have lived here and have lost their innate resistance, then go back and spend some time abroad, and then come back here with exacerbations of malaria. There are enough immigrants coming into the UK so that tuberculosis is now a significant problem. Certainly you do not have to go very far from here to find TB sleeping out on the Embankment and elsewhere in London.

I also remember some years ago when I was working in Glasgow doing a clinic where I saw three patients in a row with porphyria and being amazed that this was happening, until I was informed that the Professor of Medicine in Glasgow, Sir Abraham Goldberg, was an international expert on porphyria and all these patients with porphyria seemed to end up in Glasgow, with the most incredible problems when it came to giving them hormones for contraception or to cope with their pregnancies. These are things that you see from time to time, and every trainee needs to take on the messages in your chapter.

Thornton: When I moved to Coventry I realised how common TB is. It is not infrequent for me to see TB in the antenatal clinic, and there are two patients with porphyria at the moment, so that is absolutely right. Thank you for emphasising that.

References

1.   Russell R, Groves P, Taub N, *et al.* Assessing long-term backache after childbirth. *BMJ* 1993; **306**:1299–1303.
2.   Snidvongs S, Holdcroft A, Berkley KJ. Pain from uterine contractions during breast feeding. *Dolor* 2000;**15**(suppl. 1):21.
3.   Potter H. Effect of an intense training programme for the deep antero-lateral muscles on rectus

abdominis diastasis: a single case study. In: *10th Biennial Conference Proceedings of the Manipulative Physiotherapists Association of Australia'Clinical Solutions'*. Victoria: Manipulative Physiotherapists Association of Australia; 1997.

4.   Sheppard, S. The role of transversus abdominis in post-partum correction of gross divarification recti. *Manual Therapy* 1996;**1**:214–6.

SECTION 8

PAIN RELIEF DURING LABOUR

Chapter 28

What does the woman want for her pain in labour?

Nancy Fletcher

Introduction

As a member of the Rugby Branch of the National Childbirth Trust (NCT) I have given postnatal support to several groups of new parents. I am also the Maternity Services Liaison Committee representative for the NCT in Rugby. I am in frequent contact with pregnant and recently delivered women. The discussion below is based on feedback from these women and a review of the literature of women's views on pain in labour.

The discussion takes the following structure:

- The role of pain in labour;

- Three perspectives on pain relief in labour: before, during and after labour;

- Conclusions and recommendations based on women's needs for pain relief.

The role of pain in labour

We have all read accounts of childbirth and barely a night's television goes by without a scene of intense labour accompanied by screams of anguish. Most first-time mothers have only seen labour and birth on television. Although I have not conducted extensive research in this field, it does seem that most dramatised deliveries do not give an accurate view of labour, in that usually the cervix dilates with spectacular speed and despite the 'high tech' delivery room there is only gas and air available for pain relief. This, along with the endless tales of childbirth from mothers, sisters and so-called friends, is not encouraging news for the mother-to-be.

Kirkman[1] supports this view: 'Women have been primed throughout life by stories from their mothers and others that childbirth involves the worst pain known to mankind'.

Women approach childbirth with the expectation of extreme pain. They start off anxious and afraid of the pain, of how they will behave in labour and concerned for the wellbeing of the baby and themselves. Given this starting point should we consider that all labour pain is 'bad' pain? Should we strive above all else to provide a pain free-experience? The evidence indicates that we should not be aiming to remove pain completely from the experience of childbirth. Women say time and time again that they consider that the pain engages them in the process, that it is in many ways a 'rite of passage'. A certain level of pain is to be anticipated and therefore tolerated. Rather than focusing on the drugs which can reduce pain we should be thinking more broadly about how we can make birth a positive experience.

While few women would say that they look forward to the pain of childbirth most women go into labour with the expectation that pain is inevitable. Indeed, many welcome the pain of early labour as a sign that something has started to happen. The onset of labour (provided it is not too rapid) is often associated with pleasurable feelings of excitement and anticipation. Moreover, the initial labour pains are a straightforward warning to find a place of safety in which to give birth.

Feelings about pain should also be considered in terms of the emotions aroused in those who support women in labour. In looking at this I have found Nicky Leap's work on pain to be a useful framework.[2] Leap reviews midwives' attitudes towards the pain women feel in terms of the 'pain relief' paradigm and the 'working with pain' paradigm. In summary her approach can be presented as:

- The 'pain relief' paradigm:

  - Personal discomfort experienced by practitioners who are around women in pain;

  - Reactions to the noise that women in labour make, particularly when they are frightened and alienated;

  - Paternalistic systems where practitioners want to be 'kind'.

- The 'working with pain' paradigm:

  - Pain marks the occasion,

  - Pain is a trigger of neuro-hormonal cascades,

  - Pain stops women and allows them to find a place of safety to give birth,

  - Pain summons support,

  - Pain develops altruistic behaviour in babies,

  - Pain heightens joy,

  - Pain as a transition to motherhood,

  - The triumph of going through pain,

  - The expression of pain gives clues to progress.

Mary Nolan also reflects on this as she states that: 'The medical profession also finds itself divided between practitioners who consider it an essential part of their vocation to relieve pain and those who make a distinction between pathological and physiological pain'.[3]

In the pain relief paradigm, pain is seen as a 'bad' thing and therefore should be reduced or removed completely. In the working with pain paradigm Leap suggests that pain should be seen as an integral part of childbirth and therefore it should be worked with. Underlying this analysis is the agreement that 'abnormal pain is associated with abnormal labour and that pain relief is usually appropriate in such cases'. Following Leap's argument, we should move away from a menu approach to pain relief and instead work on producing a culture around childbirth in which pain is seen as a positive part of the process of childbirth instead of wholly negative. I would like to emphasise here that Leap points out that midwives feel that it is important not to make generalisations in this area: 'midwives were quick to warn against an approach that engages in stereotyping around who will and who will not cope with pain in labour'.[2]

There is a great deal of literature available to suggest that women wish to minimise the pharmacological pain relief they use in labour. Conversely, we also see increasing rates of epidural analgesia. What does this say about women's wishes for pain relief? This is the crux of the matter. We are all different. Sample after sample has shown that pain relief choices do not correlate with age or social class, although some studies have indicated a positive correlation with ethnic origin. The key therefore is not that women want a particular type of pain relief but they want a means of meeting their needs.

Three perspectives on pain relief in labour

Planned pain relief: information, choice and control

Preparation for birth is critical to women's emotional response at this time. It is reassuring to know what will happen next, the signs to look out for and what to do in the early stages. Antenatal education varies considerably across the country in terms of availability and content. For this reason it has been extremely difficult to prove any kind of link between antenatal education and use of pain relief in labour. Mary Nolan's work supports this view and she quotes Shearer's conclusion that the validity of most studies into the effectiveness of classes is suspect because the classes themselves: 'vary widely in number of hours, instructor training and sponsorship (e.g. hospital-based versus independent) as well as by goals, focus and content'.[4]

However, women who have attended classes, read about labour, talked it through with family or a midwife, will feel more relaxed early in the labour than those who are unprepared for the onset of labour. There is plenty of evidence to suggest that increased anxiety in early labour may lead to the earlier use of pharmacological pain relief.

Pregnant women want information, choice and control when deciding what methods of pain relief to use. The reasons for choosing pain relief are many, varied and personal. Information should be available during pregnancy and in a variety of forms. While some women want to read, others prefer to discuss. Most of us like to do a bit of both. Information should give the pros and cons of each type of pain relief and the extent to which each one is available. For instance, if there is a pool for water birth, are there always enough staff for it to be used and if an epidural is requested how long might she have to wait for one.

The possible adverse effects of pain relief must be discussed. This should be in general terms as supported by research (e.g. drowsiness with pethidine and increased intervention with epidural) and in specific terms as related to the individual (e.g. blood pressure, previous reactions to drugs, back problems).

Once in possession of the facts, women can take decisions knowing the likely consequences. A poorly informed choice can result in long-lasting negative perceptions of birth. Nolan highlights the dilemma faced by many women as they prepare for labour: 'women have found themselves increasingly torn between a mistrust of pain which is part of their social consciousness and a new awareness of the possible adverse effects of intervention in labour'.[3]

On the one hand they have been brought up in a culture where pain is seen as a bad thing and is taken away wherever possible. On the other hand they are increasingly aware of the impact that intervention may have on their unborn child.

Control is vitally important when discussing what pain relief might be used. It must be considered in the planning stages as women should not feel that they are being railroaded into particular pain relief methods because they are the norm.

Most women seek pain relief that enables them to remain in control. They want to feel part of what is happening to them. I asked 15 women what the most important feature of pain relief was for them. Ten of those responses are listed in Table 28.1 and relate to staying in control during labour.

Kirkman has the following comments to make on the subject of control in labour:

'If one word could be extracted to express the main emotional concerns of labour to the women who are having the babies that word is control'.[1] Control is vital to women's perceptions of pain in labour and a woman who feels in control is likely to be able to invoke her own methods of pain relief. 'Such action is likely to involve certain coping strategies, such as relaxation, which the person has learned prior to the onset of pain'.[5]

Nonpharmacological methods of pain relief are generally viewed as first steps in pain relief. The list is lengthy and includes such things as mobility/changes of position, bathing/water birth, TENS, acupuncture, aromatherapy, reflexology and massage.

For consideration of these methods see Russell et al.[6] The nonpharmacological methods are often suggested by women themselves rather than medical professionals giving them care, although some hospitals now have midwives trained in acupuncture and reflexology. There is much debate as to the efficacy of these methods as little evidence-based research exists. However, the methods are increasingly popular. The women I talked to said they were encouraged to consider nonpharmacological methods of pain relief while they were pregnant. Some however expressed disappointment that once in labour they were not given more support in employing these methods.

Table 28.1.   Pain relief and control

What is most important to you about pain relief?
• Not to feel the pain but to be aware of the minute he came into the world
• To feel like I have some control
• Being in control
• I wouldn't want to be out of control or have anything to make me sick
• To understand the side effects and know that it is effective
• Possession of my brain (didn't like the idea of pethidine), that it is effective (i.e. reduces pain without detrimental effects)
• Quick and effective and helps you keep in control
• Still have my head but not the pain
• To be involved in the labour
• It enables me to stay in control, takes the edge off the pain, that the midwives/doctors support my decision regarding pain relief

Given that these kinds of pain relief are non-invasive it seems sensible to investigate their potential benefits further. In the first instance these therapies often provide considerable emotional support. If the woman is familiar with the routines of a certain therapy, that in itself can help her to feel in control. She is then bringing something of herself to the experience of childbirth rather than being subjected to processes. This in itself can contribute significantly to feelings of control.

One of the main requests made by women is that the chosen method of pain relief should not affect their involvement in the birth process. For instance they should be able to feel the urge to push and after the delivery they should be able to enjoy the newborn and, if they choose to, initiate breastfeeding.

As far as pharmacological pain relief is concerned, women are often presented with a list of options. Entonox is the most used form of pain relief and is generally offered first. However, many of the women I talked to reported feeling sick, being sick, extreme thirst and feeling unpleasantly drunk and this led to them feeling out of control and even more uncomfortable.

Pethidine and meperidine are often the next step up. Adverse effects here include sleepiness, feeling 'out of it' and possible problems with breastfeeding. Evidence suggests that mothers given pethidine are less likely to be breastfeeding at 6 weeks due to the newborn baby's reduced suckling instinct; 'breastfeeding was the nutrition method used at 6 weeks postpartum by 38% of women who received intrapartum meperidine and by 45% of women who did not'.[7]

Epidural anaesthesia is regarded as the most effective way of removing pain. Once a 'mobile' epidural is working, labouring women can talk, sleep and even move around, in fact behave 'as normal'. Most hospitals now offer epidurals on the 'pain relief menu' and most women are well aware of the positive outcomes. However, as Simkin[8] points out, not only does labour become more manageable for the mother, it becomes more manageable for those attending the mother. In the rush to see epidurals as the answer to all our problems the potential negative effects of epidurals have often been overlooked (increased use of forceps and ventouse and increased caesarean section rate). Several women I spoke to felt that once the epidural was in place the only thing left for them and their partner to do was to worry about what would happen next.

It is good to go into labour knowing that pain relief is there if you need it. It is not good to go into labour worrying that the pain relief you want is not or might not be available. It is also not good to fear that you may be offered a type of pain relief you really do not want and that you will not feel able to refuse.

Support and pain relief

In my view the most important aspect of managing pain in labour is provision of support. Pain relief of any kind should not be considered as a substitute for support. Women given relief and then left will have reduced physical pain but continue to feel anxiety and tension.

One of the main problems in discussing labour is that most of the time it is difficult to separate cause and effect. There are so many things that can affect the way a woman feels about her labour and delivery that it is hard for her to single out any individual actions that have brought about specific results. However, many of the women I spoke to did not refer to specific types of intervention but instead referred to the way their carers explained things and supported them through making a choice. Some women seemed more comfortable thinking back to a complex emergency procedure than those who felt they had been rushed into a relatively straightforward decision, such as taking pethidine or having an epidural. I would therefore suggest that we look at the work of Arulkumaran and Symonds[9] and avoid attributing positive outcomes to specific interventions in situations where a whole range of factors comes into play.

In recent years, the lack of correlation between increasing intervention in childbirth and the decrease of fetal morbidity and mortality has led to research into policies for the management of labour. In a review of several studies Arulkumaran and Symonds state that:

'Although there is some evidence to support the overall concept of active management of labour, the evidence that each of these steps are of benefit is less clear'.[9]

They go on to suggest that psychosocial support (support by an attendant throughout labour) could produce a better outcome. In their discussion, where there is psychosocial support particular reference is made to 'greater levels of satisfaction in the postpartum period' and the fact that 'Women's perception of control over their labour and delivery was better'. Continuous support was found to reduce the length of labour, the oxytocin augmentation rate and operative delivery rate.

Hodnett also concludes that continuous support: 'reduced the likelihood of medication for pain relief, operative vaginal delivery, caesarean delivery, and a 5-minute Apgar score less than 7'.[10] However, Arulkumaran and Symonds[9] suggest that although guidelines for psychosocial support exist, cost implications are such that continuous one-to-one care may not be available and therefore the rate of intervention continues to increase.

In discussing the role of caregivers in labour it is also important to consider the influence the companion has over a woman's choice of pain relief. To watch someone in pain is not a pleasant experience. The moment of birth is amazing, the onset and early stages of labour may be exciting but prolonged pain and exhaustion are definitely not pleasant. The natural response to pain is to attempt to relieve it. It is not therefore surprising that many caregivers guide labouring women towards pain relief.

Many women talk about how in established labour their mind can only work at a basic level. They mention 'instincts', 'urges' and 'feelings'. They find it virtually impossible to concentrate on things outside this immediate and overwhelming experience. The skill of an experienced supporter lies in following the woman's lead quietly, showing that she or he is at ease with the grunting, groaning and any other noises or behaviours of that woman's labour. She should do this without distracting her but enable her to disconnect from the outside world and concentrate on the world within.

Leap talks about the 'midwifery skill of being with women in pain'. 'Midwives with this approach feel that women can cope with the pain of 'normal' labour and that the experience and expression of pain gives women and midwives 'clues' to how labour is progressing'.[2]

Kirkman quotes Holldorsdottir and Karlsdottir,[11] stating that 'only the midwife who engaged fully with the client was seen to soothe and help reduce fear'.

Rajan suggests that midwives, doctors and anaesthetists are more likely to agree with each other over the effectiveness of pain relief than with the woman. She also suggests that different caregivers will advocate different methods of pain relief as a function of that caregiver's expertise: 'while these differing perceptions are perhaps inevitable they may give rise to limited responses to women's pain on the part of the professionals'.[12]

Rajan reflects on the differing perspectives of caregivers and women in labour.

Where the caregiver is a midwife, doctor or anaesthetist the woman's experience goes into a much wider frame of reference (all the women that the caregiver has previously attended). The woman in labour has however only her own experience to go by: 'For the woman in herself, labour will be one of the most painful and significant events she ever experiences'.[12]

The frame of reference argument may also explain why, in Rajan's study, doctors and anaesthetists rarely referred to nonpharmacological methods of pain relief. As they are rarely present when they are used it must be difficult for them to assess their effectiveness. I accept that there is not always evidence-based research to prove the individual contribution that a nonpharmacological method of pain relief can make. However, it does seem that there is a general reluctance to determine whether these methods help to provide a positive birth experience.

Mander makes the following statement about our understanding of pain relief: 'It is clear that while our knowledge of pharmacological pain control methods is more extensive than of their nonpharmacological counterparts, great gaps in our understanding of both interventions persist. These gaps apply particularly to the "softer" more woman-oriented effects'.[5]

Once in labour women often change their mind about the pain relief. It is critical that when this happens, the decision is that of the woman in labour, made for her own reasons and not that of those around her (be they friends, family or medical professionals). The problem with this is, of course, that once in labour it is not that easy to have a rational discussion. A woman in established labour is in no mood for an intellectual conversation on the relative merits of different forms of pain relief. Even if she feels up to the debate her input to the conversation will be necessarily less articulate as she will be interrupted by contractions. It is hard to take decisions at all and hard to argue against what seems like a foregone conclusion.

One woman I talked to said that she felt that the anaesthetist was not going to leave the antenatal ward until she had an epidural. She did have an epidural and accepted that it had provided good pain relief but she remained uncomfortable about the way the decision was taken. Another woman on arrival at hospital in the late evening was told 'You'll just be in pain all night, you might as well have an epidural'. There was no apparent consideration of whether the epidural would prolong labour or (as many studies have shown) increase the likelihood of intervention. In both cases it is hard to avoid the subtext that the night would be easier for all concerned if the epidural went in.

Although a birth plan will outline what a woman wanted before it all starts hurting, it cannot take account of the reality of labour. Women can prepare themselves by learning relaxation techniques and by planning their own strategies for managing the pain. It is only in established labour that they will know to what extent they are able to cope with the demands made on them. At this stage in labour women feel very vulnerable. On the one hand, will they feel that asking for pharmacological pain relief means they are weak and not real women? On the other hand, if they want to make a noise and move around will they be seen as an unco-operative crank? I should like to make it clear here that I do not think women only worry about what the medical profession will think. If anything, women can judge themselves and each other even more harshly in these matters. As a woman makes that pain decision she knows that at some point she will be asked about it. The more we can do to help women feel they have only themselves and the baby to answer to the better. No one else can feel their pain for them so ultimately no one should have more to say on the subject of relieving the pain than the woman herself.

Post-delivery perceptions of pain

In a medical situation pain relief is seen as normal. To deny someone pain relief when they are obviously suffering is by normal standards barbaric. When people are ill we do not have second thoughts about giving drugs to relieve pain. The problem with childbirth is that although it is painful there are some parts of it that we really want to participate in and not all pain-relieving drugs allow us to do that. Achieving the balance between those good emotions (the joy of giving birth) and bad emotions (trauma caused by pain) is the key to successful pain relief and it is difficult to achieve. This balance is critical in women's lasting perceptions of the birth as a positive experience.

Women in the the study by Arulkumaran and Symonds[9] were likely to describe the birth as both a distressing and a special experience. This flags up the particular skills required by the midwife in determining to what extent the pain the woman is feeling is damaging in terms of her perception of the birth as an experience. It seems to me that the great skill in supporting women in labour lies in interpreting their expression of the pain. The pain may be bad but bearable and forgotten quickly in the euphoria of birth. Alternatively it may be unbearable and a cause of serious and lasting trauma after the birth.

The National Childbirth Trust Access study[13] also found this contradiction in emotions. They found that women are likely to feel that while the birth was distressing it was also a special experience (Figure 28.1).

Similarly, Waldenström et al.[14] surveyed 278 women, 41% of whom said it was the worst imaginable pain but 28% experienced the pain in a positive way.

Oakley and Hood's earlier research also supports this finding of mixed emotions: 'Some women experience the pain of birth as violent and birth is remembered as a chaotic and destructive process. Others are given pain relief that relieves not only the pain but the possibility of ecstasy'.[15]

Level of distress

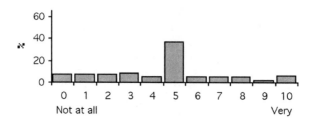

Level of specialness

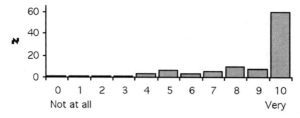

Figure 28.1. Women's rating levels of distress and of specialness during labour

We must return to the issue of control. McCrea and Wright[16] found that women were more likely to report satisfaction with pain relief if they felt they had been in control during labour. If women feel they have been in a position to influence the events around their labour they are more likely to feel positive about the experience. They may well have experienced pain but should recognise that this was part of the process. If they chose relief in the form, for example, of epidural they did this with an understanding of the possible consequences. This is closely linked to the fact that women who made choices about pain relief in labour made them with the support and guidance of a caregiver that they trusted.

Having accepted that pain is a normal part of giving birth it then becomes important not to create a system whereby requesting pain relief is seen as failure. All too often we hear 'I had to have an epidural', 'I couldn't manage on my own', as confessions. To have relief from pain is not a sign of weakness it is a choice. We need to take the judgements out of pain relief. A woman may be considered hippy/brave/insane by refusing pain relief. She may be left feeling a failure because she did have pain relief. She is none of those things; she is exercising a choice.

Having said this, it is too simplistic to say that all women are able to make a real choice about how their labour will be managed. This is not an ideal world. All too often the choices a woman makes are compromised by other external factors such as the culture of the unit where she delivers, the staffing levels of the unit at the time she delivers, the experience of the care givers and the availability of one-to-one care in labour.

Conclusions

Pain in childbirth is an expected part of the process. The overwhelming conclusion is that all women are different and therefore want different things for their pain in labour. There are however some common factors. The first is that women want to be able to choose what they have and when they have it. This choice is initially made while pregnant and then may be modified in labour. The process of the modification is critical to women's perceptions of the pain relief she had in labour. Too much, too little, too soon, or too late and pain is remembered not as pain but trauma. The second factor is that support is absolutely critical for women in labour. We need someone with us, next to us, helping, encouraging and explaining. Someone who is involved but not scared themselves. That may be a partner, a family member, a friend and almost certainly a midwife. This is someone who understands what the woman in labour needs as she focuses on her body and the pain.

Working with pain in labour would seem to be a more effective starting point for research into pain relief in labour. This enables us to move away from the assumption that all pain is bad. At present most of the models employed to consider the pain of childbirth are based around pharmacological relief. More attention should be directed towards ensuring continuous caregiver support through pregnancy and labour. Furthermore, we should be sure that nonpharmacological methods can be employed during labour. They should be considered in pregnancy and women should be given encouragement and help in using such techniques in labour.

The pain of childbirth will always exist and is an accepted fact. The important point is the response to that pain. Women should feel that they are in control of their pain management. Although no one can predict the path labour and childbirth will take it is vitally important that women feel they are part of the process and are able to influence what happens around them. Further research into the pain of labour should look at helping women to manage the pain rather than on removing the pain. It should focus on the way information on pain relief is given to women and how variations in planned pain relief are managed in labour.

References

1.   Kirkman S. The emotional pain of labour. *MIDIRS Midwifery Digest* 1998;September:328–31.
2.   Leap N. Pain in labour: towards a midwifery perspective. *MIDIRS Midwifery Digest* 2000;March: 49–53.
3.   Nolan M. *Antenatal Education: A Dynamic Approach*. London: Baillière Tindall Ltd; 1998.
4.   Shearer E. Commentary: randomized trials needed to settle question of impact of childbirth classes. *Birth* 1996;**23**:206–8.
5.   Mander R. *Pain in Childbearing and its Control*. Oxford: Blackwell Science Ltd; 1998.
6.   Russell R, Scrutton M, Porter J. In Reynolds F, editor. *Pain Relief in Labour*. London: BMJ Publishing Group; 1997.
7.   Rajan L. The impact of obstetric procedures and analgesia/anaesthesia during labour and delivery on breastfeeding. *Midwifery* 1994;**10**:87–103.
8.   Simkin P. What no one tells you about epidurals. *Mothering* 2000;December.
9.   Arulkumaran S, Symonds IM. Psychosocial support or active management of labour or both to improve the outcome of labour. *Br J Obstet Gynaecol* 1999;**106**:617–9.
10.   Hodnett ED. Caregiver support for women during childbirth. *Cochrane Database Syst Rev* 2000;CD000199
11.   Halldorsdottir S, Karlsdottir SI. Journeying through labour and delivery: perceptions of women who have given birth. *Midwifery* 1996;**12**:48–61.
12.   Rajan L. Perceptions of pain and pain relief in labour: the gulf between experience and observation. *Midwifery* 1993;**9**:136–45.
13.   Singh D, Newburn M. *Access to Maternity Information and Support*. London: National Childbirth Trust; 2000.
14.   Waldenström U, Bergman V, Vasell G. The complexity of labor pain: experiences of 278 women. *J Psychosom Obstet Gynaecol* 1996;**17**:215–28.
15.   Oakley A, Houd S. Helpers in childbirth. In: *Midwifery Today*. USA: Hemisphere Publishing Corporation; 1990.
16.   McCrea BH, Wright ME. Satisfaction in childbirth and perceptions of personal control in pain relief during labour. *J Advanced Nursing* 1999;**29**:877–84.

Chapter 29

Pain relief during labour: the role of the midwife

Edith M. Hillan

Introduction

Birth is a painful process and, although some women experience little or no pain, the majority will experience moderate to severe pain and use some form of analgesia to assist them. Pain relief may help a woman to remain in control of the process and to give birth the way she wants, or it may remove control and place her in the hands of others. Memories of labour and birth can remain with women for the rest of their lives and one of the most challenging aspects of midwifery care is to assist the woman to obtain the right form of pain relief at the right time.

In the 1990s, policy changes within the maternity services recommended that care should be woman-centred, offering more choice and control to women. With regard to the provision of pain relief in labour, a number of studies have shown that women are often faced with limited choices, controlled ultimately by those who provide them.[1-3] It is widely recognised that links exist between pain, anxiety and distress and how much control women have over their own pain relief. The major determinants of the use of pain relief in labour are the method planned by the woman and the duration of labour. These factors in turn are modulated by the mode of labour onset and the parity of the woman.[3]

Satisfaction in childbirth is not necessarily dependent on the complete absence of pain. Many women accept that some pain is inevitable, but they do not want it to overwhelm them. The ability to cope with the pain may be rated as more important than the actual level of pain experienced.[4] The need for a perceived sense of control during labour has been demonstrated in a number of studies.[5,6] Where loss of control during labour occurs this is associated with lower maternal satisfaction and postnatal wellbeing scores.[7]

In a prospective study of women's expectations and experiences of childbirth involving 825 women, the issues surrounding choice and control were explored.[7] A number of questions were asked about pain and pain relief before and after childbirth. Antenatally when women were asked 'are you worried about the thought of pain in labour?', 12% said they were 'very worried', 67% indicated they were 'a bit worried' and 22% stated that they were 'not at all worried'. Women were also asked about their general attitude towards drugs in labour and a number of options were given. Only 9% of the respondents wanted 'the most pain-free labour that drugs can give me'. The majority of women (67%) wanted 'the minimum quantity of drugs to keep the pain manageable' and the remaining 22% said they would prefer 'to put up with quite a lot of pain in order to have a completely drug-free labour'.[7]

Most women, regardless of educational level, planned to keep the drugs they used during labour to a minimum and wanted to be involved in decisions about pain relief. In practice, most women used gas and air and at least 10% of women felt under some pressure to use drugs. Women's own expectations and their support by staff affected drug use – women who ideally preferred to cope with only minimum drug use were more likely to do so than other women. In general, women were happier if they had not used a drug than if they had used it, over and above their antenatal wishes. Women who used pethidine or epidural analgesia were less fulfilled and satisfied than other women. The use of pethidine was also associated with low postnatal emotional wellbeing.[7]

Historical background

There were few serious attempts to relieve the pain of labour until the time of James Young Simpson. Thereafter, the usual anaesthetics were nitrous oxide, ether and chloroform.[8] These general anaesthetics were not really suitable for controlling the pain of labour, however, and no major advances in analgesia for labour occurred until the early 1900s. Carl Joseph Gauss developed a regimen of regular, repeated intramuscular doses of morphine and scopolamine which produced 'twilight sleep' – a state of clouded consciousness. This produced both pain relief and amnesia of many of the subjective events of labour. Although the combination of drugs was not without drawbacks for mother and baby, twilight sleep was a serious attempt to deal with a previously neglected problem of childbirth.[8]

A new approach to the issue of pain in labour came with the work of Grantly Dick-Read in 1933. He hypothesised that most of the pain of labour was due to fear, anxiety and apprehension. His basic premise was that ignorance of bodily functions and the process of labour leads to fear when contractions are experienced. Fear produces tension which in turn leads to pain and the experience of pain leads to fear of the next contraction. Dick-Read stated that removing ignorance was the key to removing fear. Teaching relaxation techniques would break the cycle and alter perception of the sensations as painful.[9] Grantly Dick-Read's methods were widely accepted in the USA but they encountered resistance in the UK.[10] It has been suggested that this might have been due to the societal, patriotic, medical and evangelical Christian influences on Dick-Read's approach to childbirth.[11,12] The National Childbirth Trust (NCT) was set up in 1956 (under the name of the Natural Childbirth Association) to promote Dick-Read's teachings and encourage women to approach labour free from ignorance and fear.[11] His approach was soon abandoned by the NCT in favour of a more active approach to prepared childbirth.

Nonpharmacological methods

Over the last 15 years there has been growing interest in the use of complementary therapies for the relief of labour pain. Complementary therapies offer a less invasive form of healthcare intervention than many types of nontraditional methods (Table 29.1).

This list of nonpharmacological pain control methods is by no means exhaustive. Forms of pain control are constantly developing and attitudes towards their use are ever changing. This can make it difficult for midwives to keep up to date with new methods.

The National Birthday Trust survey, conducted in 1990, found that only a small percentage of women used alternative methods of pain relief in labour. A number of comments were made on the use of transcutaneous electrical nerve stimulation (TENS). Although many women found it beneficial in the early stages of labour, it was less useful in the later stages. Practical and technical problems were also commonly encountered, such as leads becoming disconnected, batteries running out, incompatibility with electronic fetal monitoring and machines not being available when required. Such difficulties probably accounted for the fact that a higher proportion of women using it rated it negatively than those using any other method.[3]

In a comprehensive review of the literature in this area, Mander[10] concluded that many nonpharmacological pain control methods are inadequately researched or incompletely understood. However, since many women find them useful this should not preclude their use in clinical practice.

Table 29.1.   Nonpharmacological methods of pain relief (after Mander[10])

Intervention type	Method
Psychological	Relaxation Hypnotherapy Imagery Biofeedback Psychoprophylaxis Aromatherapy
Sensory modulation	Manual therapies • massage • therapeutic touch Quasi-manual therapies • acupressure • acupuncture
Non-manual interventions	TENS Music Hydrotherapy Homeopathy Aromatherapy Position, posture and ambulation The environment for labour

Inhalational analgesia

Nitrous oxide was used widely in anaesthesia during the 19th century but was not used in obstetrics until the 1930s. The development, in 1933, of the Minnitt machine for its administration allowed an adjustable concentration to be administered by midwives during labour. The concentrations used originally were 45% nitrous oxide to 55% air, although this was later altered to 50% of each.[3] Tunstall introduced premixed nitrous oxide (50%) in oxygen (50%) contained in a portable container.[3] This method combined the safety of a high concentration of oxygen with the efficacy of nitrous oxide. Premixed nitrous oxide and oxygen (Entonox®) was first produced in 1961 and is available in virtually all UK maternity units.[3]

Entonox is self-administered by the woman either via a mask or mouthpiece. It quickly reaches analgesic levels in the maternal circulation due to its low lipid solubility[13] and it is excreted quickly when inhalation ceases. Women normally begin self-administration at the onset of each uterine contraction so that its effect is maximal at the height of the contraction. According to Bonica and McDonald[14] this regimen provides 60% of women with good analgesia and a further 30% with partial analgesia.

The appropriateness of using nitrous oxide in the context of modern analgesia has been questioned. Nitrous oxide may contribute to increased nausea and vomiting.[15] Concerns have also been expressed related to safety issues from patient, occupational health and environmental perspectives.[15] Teratogenic and other effects on reproductive performance have been reported in groups of staff (including midwives) who frequently administer nitrous oxide.[16,17]

Although nitrous oxide is widely used in the UK as an analgesic in labour, few studies have examined its efficacy. In the 1990 National Birthday Trust survey,[3] inhalational analgesia was used by 60% of women, making it the most commonly used method of pain relief. Around 85% of women who used it found it helpful, although this was given not so much as a pain-relieving method but as a distraction and activity which assisted in relaxation and breathing exercises.[3,18] Some women in this study found it disorientating and felt that it had no effect on the pain. In the study by Green et al.,[7] 69% of the sample used Entonox, with 42% of these women finding it 'very effective' and 48% 'partly effective' in relieving pain.

Carstoniu et al.[19] conducted a randomised, double-blind, crossover placebo-controlled study of 26 women to assess the effect of intermittent nitrous oxide inhalation on labour pain and maternal haemoglobin oxygen saturation during the first stage of labour. They found no statistically significant differences in pain scores when nitrous oxide, as compared with compressed air, was administered. The authors concluded that nitrous oxide does not appear to predispose parturient women to haemoglobin oxygen desaturation but that its analgesic effect has yet to be clearly demonstrated. Therefore, although there has been a traditional acceptance of the place of nitrous oxide as an inhaled analgesic agent in labour, evidence surrounding its efficacy is unproven.

Opioids in labour

The National Birthday Trust survey, conducted in 1990, found that most women used some form of pain relief in labour, and of those, 38% used intramuscular opioids, mainly pethidine.[3] Pethidine was developed in Germany in 1939 and first used for the relief of pain in labour in the 1940s. Since 1950, midwives have been authorised to prescribe and administer the drug to women in labour. The effectiveness of pethidine in controlling labour pain has been questioned[13,20] and, although widely used, it has a number of adverse effects on both the mother and baby. It can cause confusion, drowsiness, nausea, vomiting and loss of control in the woman and respiratory depression and sedation in the baby after delivery.[13,20] The elimination half-life of pethidine in the baby is long, around 18–23 hours compared with five hours in the woman. This may account for the fact that its use is associated with a reduction in the proportion of babies who successfully establish breastfeeding.[3] In the study by Green et al.,[7] 53% of the sample used pethidine and of those who used it, 21% found it 'very effective'. However, 29% of women thought it was 'not at all effective' in relieving pain.

Diamorphine is beginning to overtake pethidine as the most popular opioid analgesia in labour, particularly in Scotland.[2] It is seen as producing maternal analgesia by raising the pain threshold and dampening pain perception without loss of consciousness.[21] It is also useful in relieving anxiety and enhancing relaxation. Adverse effects, such as nausea or vomiting and neonatal sedation, may occur, especially if it is given in large doses, however, it has been shown to have a very fast clearance time in women in labour, with low or undetectable concentrations in the newborn.[22] In the only randomised controlled trial which compared pethidine with diamorphine for pain relief in labour, intramuscular diamorphine was associated with less neonatal sedation and greater pain relief than intramuscular pethidine.[23] A more recent study, from Sweden, compared the analgesic and sedative effects of intravenous pethidine and morphine.[24] It concluded that labour pain is not sensitive to systemically administered morphine or pethidine and that the drugs only cause heavy sedation. However, the number of women studied ($n = 20$) was small and the data presented in the paper make it difficult to assess whether the authors' conclusions are justified. So, although only subjected to limited study, it appears that diamorphine has a number of advantages over other opioid analgesics in the control of labour pain.

In the conclusion of the *National Birthday Trust Report on Pain and its Relief in Childbirth*, diamorphine was dismissed as 'this addictive drug is still being used, mostly in Scotland. Its continued use in hospitals puts it at risk for theft for heroin has an active criminal market'.[3] No literature was found to support this statement.

Opioids in labour: mode of administration

Conventionally, opioids in labour are administered by the intramuscular route. In many maternity units protocols are used to determine the dosage and frequency of administration. This may mean that standardised dosages are given to women irrespective of maternal weight. Patient-controlled analgesia (PCA) refers to a relatively new approach to delivering analgesia that permits the recipient to self-administer small doses of intravenous opioids to achieve adequate levels of pain control. The technique was designed to overcome the highly variable analgesia requirements of individuals and the goal is for the recipient to titrate the drug dose to reach a level of tolerable pain rather than complete analgesia.[25] Compared with intramuscular delivery, more frequent and smaller doses provide a more even balance between pain and sedation[26] and prevent fluctuations in serum levels of opioids. The use of intravenous PCA also avoids the erratic and variable absorption observed with intramuscular administration.[21] It has been used successfully to control pain in other areas of health care; however, its use in the control of labour pain has been poorly evaluated. A meta-analysis of randomised controlled trials comparing PCA and intramuscular injections showed that patients significantly preferred PCA over conventional analgesia.[27]

With regard to the administration of opioid analgesia, a review of the literature suggests that there are a number of advantages of self-administration. The psychological influence of self-controlling analgesic administration appears to have a beneficial effect on the overall pain experience and may lead to a greater pain tolerance.[26] Perhaps even more importantly, it may enhance the woman's feeling of control in labour, leading to increased maternal satisfaction.

In Glasgow, we are currently conducting a randomised controlled trial comparing the efficacy of diamorphine administered by a patient-controlled pump with intramuscular administration. The specific objectives of the study are to compare the two modalities of administration with regard to the outcomes shown in Table 29.2. A pilot study was conducted to assess the feasibility of the study and the robustness of the data collection instruments. Twenty primigravidae were recruited and randomly allocated to the study and control groups. Preliminary results showed that the mean dose of diamorphine required in the PCA group was 4.8 mg (range 2.8–8.3 mg) compared with 9.0 mg in the control group. The proportion of women who required 7.5 mg of diamorphine or less was 90% in the study group (PCA) and 70% in the control group (intramuscular administration). Eight women required epidural analgesia (two in the PCA group and six controls). Adverse effects such as nausea, vomiting and sedation were more common in the control group, although this may be related to the higher dosage of diamorphine administered. The length of labour, need for augmentation and mode of delivery were similar between the groups. Women in the PCA group were more likely to be satisfied with their choice of pain relief. Four infants in the control group required Naloxone at delivery compared with none in the PCA group, otherwise there were no differences in the neonatal outcomes between the groups.

Assessment of pain in labour

The assessment of pain in labour is potentially problematic and a number of authors have preferred a method of pain recall post delivery in preference to interrupting the labour experience.[28,29] However, other authors have highlighted the problems women have in recalling their labour pain after the event,[30,31] which makes the use of retrospective pain measurement difficult and unreliable. Regular pain measurement has

Table 29.2. Outcome measures for patient administration and intramuscular diamorphine

Level	Outcome measure
Primary	• analgesia requirements during labour; • women's satisfaction with the method of pain relief.
Secondary	• women's perceptions of pain in labour; • presence of adverse effects e.g. nausea, vomiting, drowsiness, disorientation. • clinical outcomes for the mother and baby

been advocated to prevent missing subtle peaks and troughs of the pain experience.[6] In the Glasgow study, women are being asked to give a numerical rating (visual analogue scale)[32] as well as a verbal description (verbal descriptor scale)[33] of the pain intensity on an hourly basis throughout labour. The level of sedation and presence of adverse effects such as nausea, vomiting and dizziness are also recorded. In order to undertake a comprehensive evaluation of women's experiences of pain and its relief in labour, a follow-up study of the women will be undertaken six weeks postnatally. The questionnaire which will be utilised is an adaptation of that used for the National Birthday Trust Survey on pain in childbirth.[3] The questionnaire contains precoded questions covering information and choice about pain relief, the evaluation of pain relief, the general experience of childbirth and motherhood, physical and mental health since the birth and plans for a future confinement. Space is also included for any additional comments women care to make.

The role of the midwife in pain relief

The midwife is the main person in attendance at more than 75% of deliveries in the UK and is responsible for providing physical care and support to women during labour. Support encompasses both emotional and physical dimensions as well as assisting with instruction for breathing, relaxation and coping techniques. The constant presence of a support person in labour is one of the most effective forms of care introduced in the last 25 years and is associated with lower rates of analgesia and anaesthesia.[34]

Comparatively few studies have examined midwives' approaches to pain relief in labour; however, a number of more general studies have provided some information. In a study examining the factors which influence labour pain, Niven[35] found that midwives tended to emphasise pharmacological methods of pain relief and did not take any notice of women's personal coping strategies. Some midwives in this study considered themselves as the key decision maker in relation to pain relief, as opposed to the woman herself. Similar findings have been reported by other authors.[3,36-38]

In a small observational study, McCrea et al.[39] examined the influence of midwives' approaches to pain relief on women in labour. Three distinct types of midwife behaviour emerged, which were categorised as the 'cold professional', the 'disorganised carer' and the 'warm professional'. Midwives who displayed the cold professional approach tended to keep their distance, gave explanations in an objective and informed way but did not become involved in the decision-making process regarding pain relief. This approach was likely to be influenced by the woman's social class, with educated, informed women generally given information without having to ask for it. Cold professional midwives tended to spend a lot of time checking machines and monitors and did not work with women but rather 'did things' to them.

The midwife in the disorganised-carer category provided care in a haphazard way, giving bits of information in response to questions, although this was likely to be heavily influenced by her own opinions and personal experience rather than factual information on the benefits and risks associated with different courses of intervention. More time was spent on social chat than active listening and midwives in this category tended to spend considerable periods of time out of the room.

The third approach was categorised as the warm professional midwife. She provided adequate and appropriate information, taking time to give explanations and encouraging women to ask questions and seek clarification. Midwives in this category encouraged women and respected their choice of pain relief. The provision of emotional support and working in partnership with women was seen as important.

In McCrae's[39] study a number of other factors also influenced the midwife's approach to pain relief such as: the philosophy of care in the unit, staffing levels and continuity of care. The study was conducted in a unit which tended to adopt a medical approach to the management of labour. This meant that midwives tended to spend more time on technical aspects of care rather than on communicating effectively with women. Staffing levels in the labour ward affected the amount of time midwives had to spend with individual women, particularly during busy periods, which made it difficult to provide continuity of care.

Conclusion

Women's satisfaction with pain relief in labour is complex but appears to involve feelings of control over the pain experience. Control in labour is an important part of having a positive recollection of childbirth. Midwives have an important role to play in encouraging personal control in labour, however preparation should begin long before labour commences. Antenatal preparation is crucial to the concept of control as it can enhance the woman's confidence and ability to cope with the demands of labour. Women should be encouraged to use their personal coping resources and strategies during labour, but should also be given unbiased information about analgesia before the onset of labour so that they have realistic expectations about pain and pain relief. During labour, midwives should encourage women to be active and equal partners in the care process by involving them in decisions about pain relief and supporting them in the decisions they make about analgesia. There is good evidence to suggest that the constant presence of a support person results in lower rates of analgesia and anaesthesia use.

References

1.   Audit Commission. *First Class Delivery: Improving Maternity Services in England and Wales.* Oxford: Audit Commission Publications; 1997.
2.   CRAG Working Group on Maternity Services. *Report on Pain Relief in Labour (MSP 02/96).* Edinburgh: HMSO; 1996.
3.   Chamberlain G, Wraight A, Steer P. *Pain and its Relief in Childbirth.* Edinburgh: Churchill Livingstone; 1993.
4.   Ross A. Maternal satisfaction with labour analgesia. *Bailliere's Clin Obstet Gynaecol* 1998;**12**:499–512.
5.   Brewin C, Bradley C. Perceived control and the experience of childbirth. *Br J Clin Psychol* 1982;**21**:263–9.
6.   Green J. Expectations and experiences of pain in labour – findings from a large prospective study. *Birth* 1993;**20**:65–72.
7.   Green JM, Coupland VA, Kitzinger JV. Expectations, experiences and psychological outcomes of childbirth : a prospective study of 825 women. *Birth* 1990;**17**:15–24.
8.   Rhodes P. *A Short Textbook of Clinical Midwifery.* Hale: Books for Midwives Press; 1995.
9.   Bamfield T. Management of labour pain by midwives: a historical perspective. In: Moore S, editor. *Understanding Pain and its Relief in Labour.* Edinburgh: Churchill Livingstone; 1997.
10.   Mander R. *Pain in Childbearing and its Control.* Oxford: Blackwell Science; 1998.

11.   Kitzinger J. Strategies of the early childbirth movement: a case study of the National Childbirth Trust. In: Garcia J, Kilpatrick R, Richards MPM, editors. *The Politics of Maternity Care: Services for Childbearing Women in Twentieth Century Britain*. Oxford: Clarendon; 1989.

12.   Arney WR. *Power and the Profession of Obstetrics*. Chicago: University of Chigago Press; 1982.

13.   Dickersin K. Pharmacological control of pain during labour. In: Chalmers I, Enkin M, Keirse MJNC, editors. *Effective Care in Pregnancy and Childbirth*. Oxford: Oxford University Press; 1989, p. 913–50.

14.   Bonica JJ, McDonald JS. The pain of childbirth. In: Bonica JJ, Loeser CR, Chapman A, Fordyce WE, editors. *The Management of Pain,* 2nd edn. Philadelphia: FA Davis; 1990.

15.   Shaw ADS, Morgan M. Nitrous oxide : time to stop laughing. *Anaesthesia* 1998;**53**:213–15.

16.   Mills GH, Singh D, Longman M, O'Sullivan J, Caunt JA. Nitrous oxide exposure on the labour ward. *Int J Obstet Anaesth* 1996;**5**:160–4.

17.   Ahlborg G, Axelsson J, Bodin L. Shift work nitrous oxide exposure and subfertility among Swedish midwives. *Int J Epidemiol* 1996;**25**:783–90.

18.   Wraight A. Coping with pain. In: Chamberlain G, Wraight A, Steer P, editors. *Pain and its Relief in Childbirth*. Edinburgh: Churchill Livingstone; 1993.

19.   Carstoniu J, Levytam S, Norman P, Daley D, Katz J, Sandler AN. Nitrous oxide in early labor. Safety and analgesic efficacy assessed by a double-blind, placebo-controlled study. *Anesthesiology* 1994;**80**:30–35.

20.   Elbourne D, Wiseman RA. Types of intramuscular opioids for maternal pain relief in labour (Cochrane Review). *Cochrane Database Syst Rev* 2001;CD001237.

21.   Rayburn W, Zuspan FP. *Drug Therapy in Obstetrics and Gynecology*, 3rd edn. St Louis: Mosby; 1992.

22.   Gerdin E, Salmonson T, Rane A. Maternal kinetics of morphine during labour. *J Perinat Med* 1990;**18**:479–87.

23.   Fairlie FM, Marshall L, Walker JJ, Elbourne D. Intramuscular opioids for maternal pain relief in labour: a randomised controlled trial comparing pethidine with diamorphine. *Br J Obstet Gynaecol* 1999;**106**:1181–7.

24.   Olofsson C, Ekblom A, Ekman-Ordeberg G, Hjelm A, Irested L. Lack of analgesic effect of systemically administered morphine or pethidine on labour pain. *Br J Obstet Gynaecol* 1996;**103**:968–72.

25.   Welchew E. *Patient Controlled Analgesia*. London: BMJ Publishing Group; 1995.

26.   Ferrante FM, Orav E, Rocco AG, Galb J. A statistical model for pain in patient controlled analgesia and conventional intramuscular opiod regimes. *Anaesthesia* 1989;**67**:45.

27.   Ballantyne JC, Carr DB, Chalmers TC, Dear KB, Angelillo IF. Post-operative patient-controlled analgesia: meta-analyses of initial randomized controlled trials. *J Clin Anaesth* 1993;**5**:182–93.

28.   Melzack R, Kinch RA, Doblain P, Lebrun M, Taervier P. Severity of labour pain: influences of physical as well as psychological variables. *Canad Med Assoc J* 1984;**130**:579–84.

29.   Cogan R, Henneborn W, Klopfer F. Predictors of pain in prepared childbirth. *J Psychosom Res* 1990;**20**:523–33.

30.   Affonso DD, Stichler JF. Women's reactions following birth. *Am J Nursing* 1980; March:468–70.

31.   Niven C, Gijsbers K. A study of labour pain using the McGill Pain Questionnaire. *Soc Sci Med* 1984;**19**:1347–51.

32.   Price DD, Harkins SW. Psychophysical approaches to pain measurement and assessment. In: Turk D, Melzak R, editors. *Handbook of Pain Assessment*. New York: Guilford Press; 1992.

33.   Gaston-Johansson F. The measurement of pain. *J Pain Symptom Management* 1996;**12**:172–81.

34.   Hodnett, ED. Caregiver support for women during childbirth. In: *Cochrane Database Syst Rev* 2001;CD000199.

35.   Niven C. Factors affecting labour pain. Unpublished PhD Thesis; University of Stirling; 1996.

36.   Woolett A, Lyon L, White D. The reactions of East London women to medical intervention in childbirth. *J Reprod Infant Psychol* 1983;**1**:37–42.

37.   Williams S, Hepburn M, McIlwaine G. Consumer view of epidural analgesia. *Midwifery* 1985;**1**:32–6.

38.   McCrae BH, Wright ME. Satisfaction in childbirth and perceptions of personal control in pain relief during labour. *J Advanced Nursing* 1999;**29**:877–84.

39.   McCrae BH, Wright ME, Murphy-Black T. Differences in midwives' approaches to pain relief in labour. *Midwifery* 1998;**14**:174–80.

Chapter 30

Pain relief in labour and the anaesthetist

John A. Crowhurst and Felicity Plaat

Introduction

The International Association for the Study of Pain defines pain as: 'an unpleasant, subjective, sensory and emotional experience associated with real or potential tissue damage, or described in terms of such damage'.[1] From the patient's perspective: 'Pain is what hurts'; or 'What hurts is pain'. The neuropharmacology of pain; its psychological, physical, temporal effects and sequelae are presented elsewhere in this Study Group, and will not be discussed further in this chapter.

All pain is a subjective, emotional and personal perception, but in the public domain few pains are as well discussed as labour pain. Although normally not associated with disease or trauma, labour pain may be as severe as any other. In the mid-19th century, Sir James Young Simpson, an obstetrician and anaesthetist wrote: 'The distress and pain which women often endure while they are struggling through a difficult labour are beyond description, and seem to be more than human nature would be able to bear under any other circumstance.'[2]

Because Simpson had a new and effective method to eliminate such pain, he was among the first to focus the attention of the profession and the public on the pain of labour. Today, most societies agree that appropriate relief of all pain should be available to all as a basic right.[3]

Throughout history, obstetric pain has often been regarded as 'natural' and was not accorded the same degree of importance as pain due to surgery, injury, or disease until 1847, when Simpson developed chloroform anaesthesia. Despite this advance, opposition to the use of analgesia in labour persisted, and some still exists today. This debate over pain relief involves a wider controversy, namely: the involvement of doctors – both obstetricians and anaesthetists – in the care of the 'normal' parturient.

However, no pregnancy or labour, no matter how 'normal' it may seem, can be said to be low-risk or uneventful until it is over. Equally, pain in labour and its effects, which cannot be predicted, can only truly be assessed by the mother herself. Provision of efficacious and safe obstetric anaesthesia and analgesia is a prime example of one of the successes of modern obstetric care, but like most advances in quality of life, it is technologically complex, potentially hazardous and expensive, and still beyond reach of most women worldwide.

This chapter looks critically at present day techniques for providing relief of severe pain, their availability, safety and hazards, advantages and disadvantages, current research, and other issues concerning the roles of anaesthetists in providing these essential services.

Obstetric analgesia – current concepts and techniques

Pain relief strategies and methods:

Just as pain has emotional and subjective (mental and psychological) characteristics, so too do analgesic methods. Indeed, the patient, if conscious, must *believe* that her analgesia is effective. Without such belief, pain will not be relieved.

All successful analgesic regimens rely on one or both of two strategies:

- Those that reduce or eliminate pain *perception*

- Those that reduce or eliminate pain *transmission*.

Analgesic methods or techniques can be classified as psychological, physical, or pharmacological. Psychological methods include prenatal education and 'conditioning'; mental relaxation; 'breathing control'; hypnosis and others. In some subjects these methods may be augmented by drugs or other substances such as those used in aromatherapy. Physical techniques include massage; muscle relaxation; acupuncture and transcutaneous electrical nerve stimulation (TENS) and are frequently used in association with psychological methods. Indeed, to be effective, these techniques rely heavily on prenatal education, understanding and *belief* in the methods' efficacy. Psychological and physical methods have been discussed elsewhere and will not be considered further here.

Pharmacological techniques most reliably relieve and/or eliminate severe pain, and can be classified as:

- Systemic methods: these reduce the *perception* of pain by central neural mechanisms, most of which will reduce awareness and consciousness (chloroform and similar anaesthetics); or by inhibition of selective neural pain pathways (Entonox; opiates such as morphine; opioids such as pethidine or fentanyl; or other drugs such as ketamine).

- Regional techniques: neuraxial block (NAB)*, and also paravertebral, paracervical and pudendal block and perineal infiltration, block the neural *transmission* of pain at spinal cord level or more peripherally. Modern, low-dose, NAB has no significant effects on awareness and other central neural functions, and minimal

---

* The term *Neuraxial Block* (NAB) is used throughout this chapter to indicate all types of neuraxial block for labour *analgesia,* and for *anaesthesia* for spontaneous, assisted, or operative delivery, or other procedures. This term is preferred because since the early 1990s CSE has supplanted the use of both epidural and spinal (subarachnoid) block, for both *analgesia* and *anaesthesia*. NAB overcomes the difficulty of enumerating the plethora of terms such as: epidural, extradural, peridural, spinal, subarachnoid, intrathecal etc., all of which describe techniques of NAB.

effects on peripheral nervous system activity, such as co-ordination and motor function, permitting normal ambulation, voiding and bearing down.[4] Low-dose epidural or combined spinal–epidural (CSE) using mixtures of a local anaesthetic, usually bupivacaine, and a lipophilic opioid, usually fentanyl, are currently the most popular forms of NAB.

Although analgesic strategies and methods may be classified as above, there is much overlap in their use, with mothers and midwives choosing a method most suited for the circumstances, severity and type of pain.

It is perhaps unfortunate that the efficacy and popularity of NAB has impeded research and development of other simple analgesic methods. Existing psychological and physical methods remain popular for mild and moderately severe pain, but for *severe* first- and second-stage labour pain TENS and other methods have proved disappointing in many women. Existing systemic pharmacological analgesia too has many disadvantages, not the least of which are adverse effects on vital maternal central nervous system (CNS) functions such as awareness, co-operation and vital reflexes. There are also direct effects on the fetus, reduced uteroplacental bloodflow and gas exchange.

Nevertheless, current investigations of the ultra-short-acting opioid remifentanil and the volatile agent sevoflurane may offer promise for intermittent administration during labour.[5,6] These agents require drug administration to be co-ordinated with the tocograph (i.e. onset of uterine contractions), to provide analgesia only for the duration of the contractions, in the same way as self-administered Entonox®. Both drugs have better pharmacokinetics and potencies than Entonox. If such methods can be developed, they may provide simpler and cheaper alternatives to NAB in uncomplicated labours, when only pain relief is required.

Choice of analgesia, providing information and maternal consent

Prenatal education should enable expectant mothers to choose methods suitable for their own labour pain. In reality, the midwife, obstetrician and anaesthetist play a significant part in helping the mother make this choice, especially when factors such as interventions, disease, or pain severity increase the likelihood of an assisted delivery. Examples include induction and augmentation of labour, major systemic disease, multiple pregnancy and breech presentation (see also below). When severe pain is present, however, the informed mother herself will be more likely to choose the method of analgesia. If NAB is available, it is usually chosen, arguably because NAB is the most efficacious analgesic method available today.

Choice is influenced by many other factors, not the least of which are prenatal knowledge of pain, which analgesic methods are available and their safety and efficacy. Such knowledge may have been gleaned from either past experience, formal prenatal education classes or information gathered from friends, or the public media, including the Internet.

Since 1997, audit data from Queen Charlotte's & Chelsea Hospital indicate the parturient herself initiates 49% of requests for labour NAB.[7] These and other data suggest that public knowledge of pain and available techniques of analgesia may be a potent factor in determining demand.[8]

Who should provide information is a controversial topic, with many professional bodies competing, such as the Royal Colleges, the Obstetric Anaesthetists' Association, and commercial or other groups with various vested interests. A US survey in 2000 suggests that on the Internet, professional sites are greatly outnumbered by others, a matter which needs to be addressed.[9]

Obstetric anaesthetists, as experts in pain and its relief, have an ethical and professional responsibility to provide information on anaesthetic procedures and NAB for analgesia. This is needed not only to inform women, but also to satisfy the requirements necessary for informed consent.[10] Information should be provided in the antenatal period, in both antenatal classes and, when requested, in the consulting room on a one-to-one basis. Attempting to impart complex and lengthy information in labour is inappropriate, resulting in medico-legal consequences when complications or an unfavourable outcome occurs.

Information about pain, analgesia and anaesthesia can be classified as follows:

- Factual general information including pain causation, its severity and adverse effects on mother and fetus; descriptions of pain-relieving strategies and methods, along with their risks and disadvantages. If/when available, national statistical data on prevalence of analgesia use, efficacy, risks and complications should also be included. Such facts should be publicly available and kept updated, ideally on a website, which could be initiated by a representative committee of the Royal Colleges, the Obstetric Anaesthetists Association UK and other national bodies such as the Confidential Enquiry into Maternal Deaths (CEMD), the Confidential Enquiry into Stillbirths and Deaths in Infancy (CESDI) etc. A website with professional recognition and credibility would help to clarify the misinformation, and the anecdotal and incomplete information that is currently in the public domain, especially on the internet.

- Local NHS trust or individual obstetric unit services. Local information should include assistance and recommendations for those women who require more detailed information as their own individual circumstances dictate. For example, a woman who has had previous complications with NAB or anaesthesia should be informed how she may consult an anaesthetist. Department and clinic telephone numbers, etc. should be readily available. At a trust level, obstetric anaesthetists should provide a consultative service for individual patients, both ante- and postnatally.

Ideally, all women should be given these facts at booking and given the opportunity to attend formal antenatal education classes on pain, analgesia and anaesthesia. It is reasonable to suggest that better antenatal access to factual information, and at the local level, the opportunity of consultation with an experienced anaesthetist, are likely to reduce the frequency and cost of litigious actions. In obstetric anaesthetic practice, many such actions often result from a lack of communicating such types of information. (Examples will be cited in this chapter.)

Neuraxial methods of pain relief: current practices and research

Advantages and disadvantages of NAB

Today's low-dose NAB techniques have been developed and refined to provide complete analgesia with few adverse effects. These include incomplete analgesia, failure, pruritus, postdural puncture headache and motor block. More serious complications such as high block, collapse, local anaesthetic toxicity, neuropathy, spinal epidural haematoma and infection are infrequent nowadays with low-dose NAB. Clinically significant hypotension and fetal distress too are now uncommon.[11]

Nevertheless, despite the efficacy and relative safety of NAB analgesia, many controversies remain.

First, NAB is an invasive technique requiring skilled anaesthetists and support facilities. Second, NAB's effects on the mechanisms, progress and outcome of labour continue to be controversial, and although it is now widely accepted that there is an association between high-dose epidurals, and the incidence of increased labour duration and operative vaginal delivery, causation has not been proved.

To date, all randomised controlled trials, and their meta-analyses, have been flawed. The definitive scientific study to resolve this debate cannot be conducted because it is impossible to truly randomise women to receive NAB or not. Likewise, trials comparing NAB with other analgesic methods are flawed because no other analgesia is as efficacious as NAB, and crossovers to NAB are frequently so high as to be almost meaningless.[12,13] When NAB has been compared with other methods of analgesia, pain variations, exhaustion and other factors developing during labour bring into question results based on 'intention to treat'.[13] Results of such comparisons have provided useful data, but they do not answer the fundamental questions of whether and how low-dose NAB may affect labour mechanisms.

Local anaesthetics, opiates and other analgesic drugs may affect myometrial and neuroendocrine functions in labour,[14] although adverse effects are less likely to be significant with the low doses now beginning to be used for NAB, especially if pelvic floor tone is unaffected. Nevertheless, meaningful research in these areas is lacking.[15] As discussed below, if/when dystocia can be discounted these arguments may be resolved.

Another major problem with these types of studies is that dystocia is not easily defined and is a 'parameter' that cannot be measured objectively. Perhaps a clinical answer to the controversy is more likely to be found in impact studies in which only current low-dose NAB techniques are used.[16]

Third, the early use of NAB in many labours – perhaps as many as 10% – has reduced the urgent use of general anaesthesia, which is more hazardous, complex and expensive than topping-up an NAB for operative delivery or other surgical procedures. Undoubtedly, this feature of NAB in labour is a major factor in the reduction of maternal (and possibly of perinatal) anaesthetic-related morbidity and mortality.

Current NAB techniques and research

High-dose NAB does affect myometrial contractility and oxytocin release,[17] but the significance of these effects at the dose levels used in modern low-dose NAB is unknown. Clearly, more research is indicated.[15]

Over the past 30 years, the dose of local anaesthetic, usually bupivacaine, has been reduced by a factor of six, and low-dose NAB can be 'fine-tuned' to provide satisfactory relief of severe pain with minimal sympathetic, sensory and motor block of lumbar nerves. These low-dose regimens have been successful in minimising nerve block, especially of lumbar (leg) nerves, for two reasons.

- Lumbar nerve roots are much larger than thoracic or sacral roots, and local anaesthetics can now be administered in ways that result in local tissue concentrations below the minimal concentration necessary to block these large roots. Although these anatomical differences have been known for many years, their significance for NAB only became apparent in the 1970s when attempts were made to fine-tune tissue concentrations of local anaesthetics with lower doses, and the pharmacokinetics of local anaesthetics became clearer.[18,19]

- In the early 1970s it was discovered that opioids, which act on CNS receptors in pain pathways, were effective at the spinal cord level.[20,21] When administered intraspinally (epidurally or intrathecally), profound analgesia can be achieved with small doses that produced minimal systemic effects. When opioids and local anaesthetics are used together, they act synergistically, resulting in the need for much lower doses than if either is used alone.[22]

Both LAs and opioids with high lipid solubility are preferred for NAB, as neural elements have a high lipid content so such drugs are absorbed rapidly, which at low-dosage levels results in very low blood concentrations. Consequently, systemic effects in both mother and fetus are rare. However, local anaesthetics and opioids (in high doses) do cause marked sympathetic block, which reduces a mother's reflex ability to compensate for aorto-caval compression. This can largely be overcome by assuming an upright posture in labour with active low-dose CSE analgesia, but it remains a disadvantage of all NABs whenever some degree of sympathetic blockade is present.

Many researchers believe that local anaesthetics will need to be excluded to eliminate sympathetic blockade and retain normal function and tone of pelvic floor musculature. To date, attempts to use opioids alone have been unsuccessful, but such studies have not attempted to assess pelvic floor sensation or tone. Rather, they have concentrated on minimising lumbar and sympathetic blockade.[23]

Opioids and other cord-acting analgesics need to be delivered to the distal spinal cord in doses that achieve the tissue concentrations required to produce only analgesia. Many other cord-acting drugs, such as adenosine, benzodiazepines, verapamil and N-methyl-D-aspartate (NMDA) receptor antagonists, have yet to be studied in the context of labour NAB analgesia. Some, such as clonidine, have been researched, but like opioids, only as adjuvants to local anaesthetics.

The lowest effective doses of all can be realised only when the drugs are administered intrathecally, but some anaesthetists are reluctant to puncture the dura in parturients, for fear of headache and meningitis. Present data indicate that these complications are not significantly greater than an epidural if the procedure is carried out with due care and skill. CSE is increasing in popularity as efficacy and safety features become more widely appreciated. However, some studies to date suggest that low-dose epidural, without an initial spinal injection, has a profile similar to low-dose CSE, but epidural total doses are greater; onset time much longer, and failures and inadequate analgesia significantly more frequent.[24,25]

Long-acting analgesic drugs, especially cord-acting analgesics, or local anaesthetics in slow-release formulation (liposomes) are other possible avenues of NAB research.

Two techniques are currently available, in 2001, to achieve minimal drug concentrations at spinal cord level, but to date they have been researched only for surgical *anaesthesia*, with some success. These are epidural volume extension (EVE),[26] a recent CSE advance, and Continuous Spinal Anaesthesia (CSA).[27] Research of these mechanisms in the context of low-dose obstetric NAB is in its infancy, and they will be described in this chapter.

Arguably, the greatest advantage of continuous NAB in labour is the presence of a functioning catheter that can be used to induce full neuraxial anaesthesia in an emergency. In skilled hands, the need to convert to general anaesthesia in these circumstances is now less than 1%.[28] Although all techniques of NAB are relatively complicated and invasive, present and mooted refinements indicate that NAB, particularly low-dose CSE, will continue to increase in popularity and efficacy.

The concern that interventions, including NAB, may have on labour duration was highlighted in some articles in the public media in 2000, where it was claimed that a new induction drug would reduce pain and reduce the duration of nulliparous labours to two hours.[29,30] If true, then the need for NAB and similar analgesia may decrease, but to date, all induction techniques have failed in this regard.

In summary, there are many promising avenues of analgesia research being pursued. New systemic drugs, such as remifentanil and sevoflurane, and sophisticated patient-controlled delivery systems may result in a renaissance of effective, cheaper systemic analgesia techniques, especially for first-stage labour. For NAB, other analgesic drugs may displace local anaesthetics, at least for analgesia. A very-low-dose NAB, without effects on pelvic floor tone and without sympathetic blockade, will almost certainly be realised in the years ahead.

Ambulation

Ambulation during labour has been a topical subject for generations.[31] In recent times, studies comparing ambulation in women with low-dose NAB analgesia have failed to show that walking has any benefit concerning duration of labour and mode of delivery.[4,32]

Low-dose NABs have now been refined to provide near perfect analgesia with minimal motor block permitting normal ambulation, voiding and bearing down. To date, these low-dose, ambulatory NABs are used in only a few centres, but their use is increasing markedly. In 1998 in the UK, the use of low-dose CSE was estimated at 24% in 169 obstetric units, compared with 5% some five years earlier. While all of these centres used NAB for *anaesthesia*, 17% of the units used ambulatory, low-dose NAB for labour analgesia.[33] At Queen Charlotte's and Chelsea Hospital in London, low-dose CSE has been used for labour analgesia since 1992. Audits indicate that 95% of labour NABs are low-dose CSE, and the ability to walk is present in 93% of these, although some women choose not to do so.

Apart from improved maternal satisfaction, being upright or ambulant has been shown to have one major physiological advantage. Although low-dose NABs do invoke some sympathetic neural blockade, this is minimal. Indeed, and perhaps surprisingly, maternal systolic blood pressure is better maintained in labouring women who are upright, compared with those who remain recumbent, even in a lateral position. Moreover, uteroplacental bloodflow as assessed by blinded analysis of cardiotocograms (CTGs) is better maintained in the upright than the recumbent position in labour.[34] The mechanism believed to be responsible is that an upright posture offers better protection against aorto-caval compression, so optimising venous return, cardiac output and uteroplacental bloodflow.

Many clinicians remain sceptical about ambulation however, even though it does have positive benefits and does no harm. Most women who receive NAB in labour prefer not to have motor block, whether or not they ambulate. Low-dose NAB adds to the mothers' sense of being in control, and improves their overall satisfaction.[32]

NAB, altered coagulation, thromboembolism and thromboprophylaxis

Maternal mortality from most causes, especially anaesthesia, has declined, but thromboembolic complications and death appear to be increasing, both relatively and absolutely. In 1994–96, thromboembolism caused 2 deaths per 100 000 maternities, which equates to one-third of all direct maternal deaths (48/134), and 18% of all maternal deaths.[35] Undoubtedly, social factors such as obesity, an older parturient population, more sedentary life-style and higher operative delivery rates are contributing to this. However, the risk of thromboembolism is increased in almost all gravidae. In the parturient, all aspects of Virchow's triad are affected. Blood elements and clotting factors are increased, even though blood viscosity is reduced, at least up to about 34 weeks of gestation. Stasis in pelvic and leg veins is increased, by caval compression and reduced mobility in late pregnancy. (Greater mobility and ambulation in labour may be thromboprophylactic, but to date this has not been researched.) Vessel trauma also occurs during delivery.

At present, anticoagulants, usually heparins, are the main thrust of thromboprophylaxis. Aspirin and other anti-platelet drugs are less commonly used as primary agents for thromboprophylaxis, and although three cases of epidural-associated spinal epidural haematomas have been reported,[36] several large studies have demonstrated their relative safety in both surgical and obstetric patients receiving concurrent NAB.[37,38] In orthopaedic and other surgeries, low-dose aspirin prophylaxis is increasing in popularity, but its role in thromboprophylaxis in the pregnant population is not yet clear. Perhaps because of the risk of haemorrhagic complications?[39] While good evidence exists for the efficacy of prophylactic and therapeutic heparin regimens in surgical patients, their use has not been without hazard, especially in association with NAB. During the 1980s and 1990s, low-molecular-weight heparin (LMWH) gained popularity for prophylaxis, especially in patients undergoing hip or knee arthroplasty. In the USA, in 1993, over 40 cases of spinal epidural haematomas were reported when LMWH was used intra- or postoperatively with NAB. It was revealed that doses of LMWH used in the USA were 150% greater than those used in Europe, where the incidence of this complication had not increased. The incidence was estimated to be 1 in 3100 continuous epidural anaesthetics and 1 in 41 000 single-shot spinal anaesthetics. Timing of LMWH injection with respect to NAB administration and removal of an epidural catheter were also found to be of paramount importance.[40]

In the UK, Letsky reported that: 'Available evidence shows that the use of prophylactic heparin during the course of epidural or spinal anaesthesia does not increase the risk of local haematoma'.[41] De Swiet, Letsky and colleagues at Queen Charlotte's and Chelsea Hospital studied various regimens of LMWH and recommended a relatively simple regimen that to date has been used for some five years in more than 6000 (estimated) obstetric patients receiving concurrent NAB without any evidence of spinal epidural haematoma. It is now clear that heparin prophylaxis and concurrent NAB are safe, provided these guidelines are strictly adhered to.

Thromboembolism risk in pregnancy can be graded as follows:

1. High risk: (previous thrombosis +/– thrombophilia, recurrent fetal loss +/– anti-phospholipid syndrome, venous thromboembolism in current pregnancy)

2. Low risk: (only one previous episode of thromboembolism)

3. Third group: (caesarean delivery, age > 35 years, obesity, immobility).

Current QCCH Guidelines for thromboprophylaxis are as follows:

*   1. High risk group: antenatal and perinatal heparin;

*   2. Low risk group: antenatal low-dose aspirin;

*   3. Third group: perinatal heparin.

Heparin is administered as follows: unfractionated heparin 7500 subcutaneously every 12 hours; LMWH 40 mg subcutaneously, at 2200 hours. The dose may be adjusted according to maternal height.

NAB may be administered four hours after unfractionated heparin, or six to eight hours after LMWH. Similarly, epidural catheters may be removed safely after these intervals. Full heparinisation or abnormal coagulation is an absolute contraindication to NAB.

Clinical guidelines for the concurrent use of prophylactic heparins in patients will be presented and discussed in this chapter. It is now clear, that heparin prophylaxis and concurrent NAB are safe, provided these guidelines are strictly adhered to. Before leaving the question of thromboprophylaxis and NAB, it is important to realise that regional anaesthesia *per se* provides significant thromboprophylaxis.[42]

This was confirmed by a multinational group that reported the best evidence to date that when used for surgical *anaesthesia*, NAB is truly thromboprophylactic in surgical patients.[43] This Collaborative Overview of Randomised Trials of Regional Anaesthesia (CORTRA) study revealed most impressive improvements in thromboembolic morbidity and mortality rates in surgical patients. The authors concluded: 'These results support more widespread use of neuraxial blockade'.

It is therefore an enigma why such improvements are not obvious in obstetric patients, where NAB is by far the most commonly used mode of anaesthesia, prompting the question: 'If NAB is truly prophylactic in its own right, is additional systemic anti-coagulant prophylaxis necessary?'. To date, no attempt has been made to research this question, but because gravidae are more thrombogenic than many surgical patients, and because it is safe to use both NAB and heparins, it is understandable why both approaches are used in obstetrics.

Impact of current analgesic techniques on present-day obstetric practice

Quantifying the contribution that modern obstetric anaesthetic services have contributed to the low mortality and morbidity in developed countries is difficult, because in many countries where expert anaesthesia services are scanty, anaesthesia is rarely cited as a cause of death or injury.

The impact of modern NAB analgesia on morbidity is even less clear, but some university and teaching hospitals, such as Queen Charlotte's and Chelsea Hospital, now report NAB uptake rates of 70%, which figure was reported in Australia almost ten years ago.[44] In the developed world at least, Simpson's prophecy of 150 years ago has been realised.** But severe pain alone is not the only reason for the high utilisation of NAB.

** Simpson's prophecy was: 'Medical men may oppose for a time the superinduction of anaesthesia in parturition, but ... our patients will force the use of it upon the profession. The whole question is, even now, one merely of time.' Simpson JY: Notes on Chloroform (circa 1847).

Analysis of annual statistical returns to the Royal College of Obstetricians and Gynaecologists for 1997–98 demonstrated a NAB analgesia rate for labour of 23.6% (almost unchanged from 1996) and the rate for regional anaesthesia in caesarean sections, depending on urgency, was 70–86%.[45] These data indicate that anaesthetists were involved in more than 251 000 peripartum procedures, at least 63.8% of all maternities. In truth, the figure is nearer 70% if other procedures and surgery during pregnancy and the puerperium are included.

Thus, there is no doubt that the availability and provision of anaesthetic services in the UK are as essential to safe obstetric practice as blood transfusion, antibiotics and other essential support services.

Maternal expectations

As suggested above, informed mothers expect the best obstetric care, including access to satisfactory pain relief and anaesthesia when these are required. Arguably too, the popularity of NAB has been increased not only by improved safety and other developments, but by favourable media reports and published surveys such as the one in which a majority of obstetricians themselves opted for NAB for analgesia/anaesthesia for operative delivery.[46] Women, like all groups in society, will 'vote with their feet'. When they learn of something that will benefit them, they will demand it. When the best – low-dose, ambulatory NAB – is available, then that will be requested.

NAB analgesia in complicated labours

For some 30 years, the prophylactic value of an early NAB has been appreciated in women at risk for an instrumental or caesarean delivery – breech, multiple pregnancy, large fetus, cephalopelvic disproportion, vaginal birth after previous caesarean delivery, etc. Similarly, women with life-threatening diseases, especially cardio-respiratory and pre-eclampsia, benefit from early NAB to eliminate the stress responses to pain. Today, these circumstances constitute indications for the use of NAB, other than that of pain relief alone, and in some populations may account for 50% of the NABs administered in labour, if induction and augmentation of labour are included.[47]

Some of these indications continue to be debated. For example, should a NAB be used routinely for induction and augmentation of labour, which interventions themselves usually increase pain and the risk of an assisted delivery? Should an early NAB be requested for a vaginal birth after previous caesarean delivery trial of labour? Most anaesthetists (and perhaps obstetricians) would answer yes, because an elective NAB eliminates the 'panic' of urgent anaesthesia, which is more likely to be a general anaesthetic, and the increased risk of morbidity associated with emergency delivery and anaesthesia.

NAB analgesia in uncomplicated labours

The true prevalence of the use of NAB in 'normal', uncomplicated, spontaneous labours and spontaneous deliveries is not known accurately, but some QCCH data[47] indicate that in nulliparae it is 60%, and in multiparae, 35%. It is becoming clear that low-dose NAB does not significantly affect the rate of caesarean delivery, but it is less clear if the duration of labour or assisted delivery is affected.

Many studies have attempted to correlate duration of labour and mode of delivery with the degree of lumbar (legs and feet) motor block, but dystocia is believed to be related to pelvic floor tone rather than motor block in the legs. To date, it appears that small sacral nerve roots (S2–S5) are readily blocked by even very low doses of bupivacaine (1 mg intrathecal). Unfortunately, it is not yet clear if this sacral block of pelvic floor nerves is sensory alone, or both motor and sensory.[48]

If a block can be designed to spare sacral nerves and preserve pelvic floor tone, then the debate implicating dystocia may be resolved – see also section on Current techniques and research above.

The roles of the anaesthetist in obstetrics

Since 1998, the Royal College of Anaesthetists, the Obstetric Anaesthetists' Association and the Association of Anaesthetists of Great Britain & Ireland have issued clear guidelines on the roles and duties of anaesthetists in obstetrics.[49,50] These roles, compiled with the collaboration of obstetricians, midwives and others, are summarised below.

Physician (clinical and consultant) roles

Apart from providing and supervising anaesthetic and (pharmacological) analgesic administrations in the delivery suite, today's anaesthetists are trained as pre- and postnatal consultants. The safety of modern anaesthesia is based on optimisation of a patient's physiology. The CEMD has emphasised the need for early consultation, planning and optimisation for over 20 years. In this sense, safe anaesthesia care is the same as maternity care founded on sound antenatal monitoring and identification of risk factors. Testament to this is the fact that so-called 'emergency' anaesthesia has been a major cause of maternal death and anaesthetic morbidity.[51]

The demand for labour analgesia and anaesthesia is now such that 'ALL pregnant women are potential candidates for anaesthesia, (including epidurals) and 70% will receive it'.[44] Of this 70%, half are women who receive anaesthesia for caesarean and other operative or assisted deliveries, and other perinatal procedures, such as manual removal of placenta and repair of genital tract trauma. This fact indicates how imperative it is for anaesthetic risk factors to be identified early in all pregnancies, for anaesthetists to be consulted and for a mutually agreed plan for anaesthesia/analgesia to be documented that will minimise risk. Moreover, anaesthetists have a duty of care to see patients after anaesthesia.

Thus, as well as the familiar duties in the delivery suite and theatre, trusts and health authorities should make provision for obstetric anaesthetists to be able to see patients antenatally on request.

Resuscitation, intensive and high-dependency care

A skilled resuscitation service is mandatory in maternity units. Anaesthetists have such skills, and should lead the service and be active in the training and maintenance of these skills in other staff.

As already discussed, thromboembolism, haemorrhage and maternal disease are now the principal causes of maternal morbidity and anaesthetists play a key role in minimising and preventing these. In the UK, approximately 100 obstetric patients per month require intensive care,[45] but many more require high-dependency care, which is best provided by the perinatal management team, which includes a skilled anaesthetist. Ideally high-dependency care should be provided in the maternity unit, for transferring patients when afflicted by these complications is hazardous and likely to worsen outcome for both mothers and neonates. For modern obstetric anaesthesia, neonatal and other support services to be cost-effective, it is axiomatic that obstetric units have a 'critical mass' of at least 3000 deliveries per annum.[52]

Anaesthetists also contribute to neonatal resuscitation in many units, and while today's anaesthetists can and do contribute to the resuscitative care of neonates, such care is best provided by trained paediatricians.

Teaching, audit, research and development roles

Clearly, obstetric anaesthetists contribute to teaching all members of the perinatal team safe analgesic practices, pharmacology and physiology of pregnancy, resuscitation, acute care, patient monitoring, fluid management, equipment care and understanding, and other skills. In both the clinic and the classroom, today's anaesthetists teach how to identify anaesthesia risk factors relevant to both general anaesthesia and NAB, and how to safely prevent and treat adverse outcomes. Furthermore, the anaesthetist has a responsibility to contribute to public antenatal education at a national level, and locally, through audit, prenatal classes and individual consultation, as discussed.

Obstetrics is a fertile field of research in anaesthesia, pain and basic sciences such as physiology and pharmacology. Much useful clinical research in most specialties results from collaborative works with colleagues in relevant disciplines, which is certainly true in obstetrics, where the management-team concept is better developed than in most medical specialties. It is likely that only collaborative studies will settle many of the controversies cited and discussed in this paper and will be crucial to the future development of new analgesic systems and techniques. To achieve this development, we must realise better co-operation from midwives, obstetricians and expectant mothers during the antenatal period, when studies can be explained and subjects recruited.

Clinical audit, both at local and national levels, has a proud record in obstetrics. Anaesthetists and other support specialists have contributed to the success of the work of CEMD and CESDI, and to the subsequent impact such works have had on developing and implementing improved standards of care both at home and abroad.

Within anaesthesia, NAB techniques pioneered in obstetrics continue to lead the application of such techniques in surgical anaesthesia, and acute and chronic pain management.

Summary and conclusions

In this chapter we have attempted to identify the contribution the speciality of anaesthesiology makes to obstetrics and perinatal care. Obstetric anaesthesia is now a well-recognised sub-specialty, which continues to attract anaesthetists who gain much satisfaction from playing a team-management role, and who enjoy meeting the unique challenges of contributing to safe, pain-free, maternity care.

The future and improvement of today's safe obstetric anaesthesia, analgesia, critical care and related services rest squarely with collaboration within the perinatal management team, which has developed in obstetric practice over many decades. Team symposia and workshops such as this one are clearly the way ahead, as collaboration is the best approach for the many political, fiscal and economic challenges to obstetric and perinatal care.

References

1. Merskey H, Bogduk N. *Classification of Chronic Pain: Descriptions of Chronic Pain Syndromes and Definitions of Pain Terms*, 2nd edn. Seattle: IASP Press; 1994.
2. Moir DD, editor. *Obstetric Anaesthesia and Analgesia*, 2nd edn. London: Ballière Tindall; 1980, p. 2.
3. Cousins MJ. Pain relief – a basic human right. Joint Royal Colleges' Chloroform Sesquicentary meeting, Edinburgh; September 1997.
4. Collis RE, Baxandall ML, Srikantharajah ID, Edge G, Kadim MY, Morgan BM. Combined spinal epidural analgesia with ability to walk throughout labour. *Lancet* 1993;**341**:767–8.
5. Olufolabi AJ, Booth JV, Wakeling HG, Glass PS, Penning DH, Reynolds JD. A preliminary investigation of remifentanil as a labor analgesic. *Anesth Analg* 2000;**91**:606–8.
6. Yamakage M, Mori T, Tsujiguchi N, Kawana S, Namiki A. Inhibitory effects of halothane, isoflurane, and sevoflurane on contractility and intracellular calcium concentration of pregnant myometrium in rats. *Anesthesiology* 1998;**89**:3A.
7. Michail M, Razzaque M, Plaat F, Crowhurst JA. Neuraxial block, cervical dilatation and mode of delivery. European Society of Obstetric Anesthesiology meeting, Trinity College, Dublin, June 1999 (Poster).
8. Harding D. Making choices in childbirth. In: Page LA, editor. *The New Midwifery*. London: Churchill Livingstone; 2000. p. 71–85.
9. Weesner KA, Sutherland L, Madamangalam AS, Hess PE, Pratt SD, Soni AK *et al.* Labor epidural and the world-wide-web. *Anesthesiology (SOAP) Supplement*, April 2000;A88.
10. Association of Anaesthetists of Great Britain and Ireland. Information and Consent for Anaesthesia. London; 1999.
11. Rawal N, Van Zundert A, Holmström B, Crowhurst JA. Combined Spinal-Epidural Technique. *Reg Anesth* 1997;**22**:406–23.
12. Thorp JA, Hu DH, Albin RM, McNitt J, Meyer BA, Cohen GR, *et al.* The effect of intrapartum analgesia on nulliparous labour: A, randomised, controlled, prospective trial. *Am J Obstet Gynecol* 1993;**169**:851–8.
13. Loughman BA, Carli F, Romney M, Dore CJ, Gordon H. Randomized controlled comparison of epidural bupivacaine versus pethidine for analgesia in labour. *Br J Anaesth* 2000;**84**:715–19.
14. Bates RG, Helm CW, Duncan A, Edmonds DK. Uterine activity in the second stage of labour and the effect of epidural analgesia. *Br J Obstet Gynaecol* 1985;**92**:1246–50.
15. Eisenach JC. Obstetric anesthesia: what have you done for us lately? (Editorial). *Anesthesiology* 1999;**91**:907–8.
16. Impey L, McQuillan K, Robson F. Epidural analgesia need not increase operative delivery rates. *Am J Obstet Gynecol* 2000;**182**:358–63.
17. Goodfellow CF, Hull MG, Swaab DF, Dogterom J, Buijs RM., Hull MGR, *et al.* Oxytocin deficiency at delivery with epidural analgesia. *Br J Obstet Gynaecol* 1983;**90**:214–19.
18. Galindo A, Hernandez J, Benavides O, Ortegon de Munoz S, Bonica JJ. Quality of spinal extradural anaesthesia: the influence of spinal nerve root diameter. *Br J Anaesth* 1975;**47**:41–6.
19. Hogan Q, Toth J. Anatomy of soft tissues of the spinal canal. *Reg Anesth Pain Med* 1999;**24**:306–10.
20. Wang JK, Nauss LA, Thomas JE. Pain relief by intrathecally applied morphine in man. *Anesthesiology* 1979;**50**:149–51.
21. Behar M, Magora F, Olshwang D. Epidural morphine in treatment of pain. *Lancet* 1979;**1**:527–9.
22. Campbell DC, Camann WC, Datta S. The addition of bupivacaine to intrathecal sufentanil for labor analgesia. *Anesth Analg* 1995;**81**:305–9.

23. Shennan A, Cooke V, Lloyd-Jones F, Morgan B, deSwiet M. Blood pressure changes during labour and whilst ambulating with combined spinal-epidural analgesia. *Br J Anaesth* 1995;**102**:192.
24. Rawal N, Schollin J, Wesström G. Epidural versus combined spinal epidural block for caesarean section. *Acta Anaesthesiol Scand* 1988;**32**:61–6.
25. Rawal N, Holmström B, Crowhurst JA, VanZundert A. The combined spinal-epidural technique. *Anesthesiology Clin N Am* 2000;**18**:274.
26. Stienstra R, Dilrosun-Alhadi BZ, Dahan A, van Kleef JW, Veering BT, Burm AG, *et al.* The epidural 'top-up' in combined spinal-epidural anesthesia: the effect of volume versus dose. *Anesth Analg* 1999;**88**:810–14.
27. Rigler MI, Drasner K. Distribution of catheter-injected local anesthetic in a model of the subarachnoid space. *Anesthesiology* 1991;**75**:684.
28. Crowhurst JA, Plaat F. Labor analgesia for the 21st century. *Semin Anesth Periop Med Pain* 2000;**19**:3:164–70.
29. Thornton J. New drug could put an end to hard labour. Painless birth in 2 hours. *The Sun*, London; 5 December 2000.
30. Motluk A. First-time mums get a soft option. *New Scientist* 16 December 2000;24.
31. Williams JW. In: *Obstetrics: A Textbook for Students and Practitioners*, 1st edn, 1903; p. 282.
32. Collis RE, Harding SA, Morgan BM. Effect of maternal ambulation on labour with low-dose combined spinal-epidural analgesia. *Anaesthesia* 1999;**54**:535–9.
33. Burnstein R, Buckland R, Pickert J. A survey of epidural analgesia in the United Kingdom. *Anaesthesia* 1999;**54**:634–50.
34. Al-Mufti R, Morey R, Shennan A, Morgan B. Blood pressure and fetal heart rate changes with patient-controlled combined spinal epidural analgesia while ambulating in labour. *Br J Obstet Gynaecol* 1997;**104**:554–8.
35. Drife J, Lewis G. *Why Mothers Die: Report on Confidential Enquiries into Maternal Deaths in the United Kingdom 1994–1996*. London: HMSO; 1998.
36. Horlocker TT. Complications of spinal and epidural anesthesia. *Anesthesiology Clin N Am* 2000;**18**:461–85.
37. CLASP (Collaborative Low-dose Aspirin Study in Pregnancy): A randomised trial of low-dose aspirin for the prevention and treatment of pre-eclampsia among 9364 pregnant women. *Lancet* 1994;**343**:619–29.
38. Horlocker TT, Wedel DJ, Schroeder DR, Rose SH, Elliott BA, McGregor DG, *et al.* Preoperative antiplatelet therapy does not increase the risk of spinal epidural hematoma associated with regional anesthesia. *Anesth Analg* 1995;**80**:303–9.
39. Derry S, Yoon KL. Risk of gastrointestinal haemorrhage with long term use of aspirin: meta-analysis. (Editorial). *BMJ* 2000;**321**:1183–7.
40. Horlocker TT, Wedel DJ. Neuraxial block and low molecular weight heparin: Balancing perioperative analgesia and thromboprophylaxis. *Reg Anesth Pain Med* 1998;**23**:164–77.
41. Letsky EA. Peripartum prophylaxis of thrombo-embolism. *Ballière's Clin Obstet Gynaecol* 1997;**11**:523–43.
42. McKenzie PJ. Editorial. *Br J Anaesth* 1991;**66**:325.
43. Rodgers A, Walker N, Schug S, McKee A, Kehlet H, van Zundert A, *et al.* Reduction of postoperative mortality and morbidity with epidural or spinal anaesthesia: results from overview of randomised trials. *BMJ* 2000;**321**:1493.
44. Crowhurst JA: Anaesthesia in obstetrics – how safe? (Editorial). *Med J Australia* 1992;**157**:147.
45. Khor L, Jeskins G, Cooper GM, Paterson-Brown S. National obstetric anaesthetic practice in the UK 1997/1998. *Anaesthesia* 2000;**55**:1168–72.
46. Al-Mufti R, McCarthy A, Fisk NM. Survey of obstetricians' personal preference and discretionary practice. *Eur J Obstet Gynaecol Reprod Biol* 1997;**73**:1–4.
47. Queen Charlotte's and Chelsea Hospital Audit data, 2000. (Unpublished.)
48. Capogna G. Personal communication; 2000.
49. Royal College of Anaesthetists. *Guidelines for Anaesthetic Services*. London; 1999.
50. Obstetric Anaesthetists' Association and the Association of Anaesthetists of Great Britain and Ireland. *Guidelines for Obstetric Anaesthesia Services*. London; 1998.
51. Dept. of Health Welsh Office, Scottish Office Dept. of Health, Dept. of Health and Social Services, Northern Ireland. *Report on Confidential Enquiries into Maternal Deaths in the United Kingdom 1991–1993*. London: HMSO; 1994.
52. Bromage P. Epidural analgesia: demand and supply. In: Doughty A, editor. *Epidural Analgesia in Obstetrics – A Second Symposium*. London: Lloyd-Luke; 1980. p. 7.

Chapter 31

Pain relief during labour

Discussion

Discussion following papers of Mrs Fletcher, Professor Hillan and Dr Crowhurst

Berkley: Both speakers were talking about the dynamic of the delivery situation, and one of the things that happens in this dynamic is the interaction between the different professionals and the woman herself. There are no female obstetricians here at this meeting and I was just wondering about the dynamics of the sex difference issues. Can anyone speak to that? Have there been studies or thoughts?

Stones: We know in gynaecology that pain outcomes are not related to the gender of the gynaecologist; some data on that was presented yesterday. But that does not relate to labour pain.

MacLean: Can I ask Professor Hillan? One of the interesting things that is happening among our trainee midwives is the appearance of male midwives. One always had some concern whether they were able to play a full role. Do they need chaperoning, for instance, during assessment? And is there any difference in the rapport that a woman has with her female midwife and with the male midwife? That perhaps is greater interaction than happens between a male or female obstetrician.

Hillan: I do not think there is any research evidence. The numbers of male midwives are still comparatively small and you tend to have just one or two working in any given unit. Anecdotally I don't think there have been any major problems. I can only speak in the context of Glasgow, but sometimes some ethnic women prefer not to have a male midwife look after them in labour. However, that is for other reasons. I believe they are accepted now as part of the team in many labour wards where they work.

Thornton: That has been our experience in Coventry where we have had a male midwife.

Stones: What are people's feelings about nalbuphine? Does anyone have any experience of that agent? I gather it is used quite a lot in France for obstetric anaesthesia. As we heard yesterday, it is one of the more κ-active opioids. I gather it is not licensed for obstetric use in the UK but it is in a number of other countries and is widely used.

Fernando: I have not used it personally. Is nalbuphine a partial agonist?

Crowhurst: It is both an agonist and an antagonist.

Stones: But it has activity at κ, which you emphasise is not the case with the ones that we use.

Fernando: From most of the data that I have seen on these partial agonists, they are not very efficacious used in an obstetric setting anyway.

Crowhurst: One of the big problems with partial agonist–antagonist opioids in obstetrics – and I am old enough to go back to the days of pentazocine and phenazocine – is that if you get a baby, or even a mother, that becomes grossly depressed with those sorts of drugs, they are very difficult to reverse. That is why we prefer to use pure agonists of the morphine, diamorphine, fentanyl–remifentanil type. They can be completely reversed immediately with Naloxone®, but partial agonist–antagonist drugs cannot.

Stones: We feel that κ-active agents may be more relevant to visceral pain and, as I understand it, the idea is that the pain of labour is not necessarily morphine sensitive or opioid sensitive.

Crowhurst: I take your point. If we can look at some of these drugs perhaps even in animal models with some of the new techniques of getting them on to the cord in appropriate doses – not much bigger doses than have been used in the past but using the sort of things I have shown you today – we may get some answers about that and about visceral pain. It is a pity Beverly is not here to comment on that. At the moment I do not think we have the data.

Grace: I am a little perplexed by the juxtaposition of the papers presented by Mrs Fletcher and Dr Crowhurst. Mrs Fletcher, you had an analysis and you presented some ideas based on your own work on the idea that women are not so much demanding a totally pain-free labour and are not demanding to be both awake and pain-free in the way that Dr Crowhurst was suggesting. Yet, Dr Crowhurst, you were saying that women are demanding this. I am rather confused by these two quite different perspectives on this issue and would be interested to hear what either of you have to say about that juxtaposition.

I should add that I was disturbed by your suggestion, Dr Crowhurst, that women demand this, therefore we provide it. As a university lecturer, I could say that the students demand to pass their courses and they demand to have high grades. You use the analogy of televisions and microwaves. Those consumerist analogies are not necessarily the kinds of things to which we should be responding as professionals surely, so there is another curious juxtaposition in there, too, which has to do with women's choice, where that choice comes from, what it represents and how we respond to it.

I should appreciate your comments on those issues.

Fletcher: One thing that might throw some light on it goes back to the idea of the frame of reference in that by the time you are seeing people for epidural they may already have decided that they want an epidural: it is already part of their care pattern. I very often see people right at the very beginning, I see the whole range of women, and certainly I believe it would be unlikely for a woman to say 'I want an epidural'. I have not heard anyone say to me 'I want an epidural' in the sense of 'I want an epidural, come what may.' I have heard lots of women say 'I was in labour for ten hours and I had an epidural', and they have been perfectly happy with that. It is important that that is not seen as a criticism.

It could perhaps be a regional variation. The women that I deal with used to use a local hospital where they could not have an epidural. It is only within the last four years that they have moved to hospitals where epidural analgesia was more widely available. That in itself may be a factor, because people who are having their second and third children locally would not have one if they had not had one before – they would not think about it necessarily. Even so, generally I do not believe that people go out with a shopping list for an epidural.

To come briefly to the microwave comments, that also concerns me. I have a microwave in my kitchen and I am constantly worried that it is going to microwave my kidneys. It is there and it is usable, but there is that element of discomfort. I have the same level of discomfort when I think about epidurals. They are there and I accept that they provide very good pain relief, but I would like to qualify that: they provide very good pain relief for the women who are in the circumstances that require it.

Crowhurst: There are great differences depending on which pocket of the population you look at. In West London where I am, the mean age of primiparity in our area, Chiswick, Hammersmith, Richmond and so on, is just over 30 years. The national figure is 27 point something years for women to have their first baby. When I did my obstetrics in the 1970s, before I did anaesthesia, in Australia it was 21.3 years. Age is a big factor. As we get older a lot of things happen. Mrs Coldron did not mention too much about the change with age, but the musculoskeletal system is less supple and so on, and because they are older women are more knowledgeable, at least in the population with which I work day to day. That is also a big factor.

Just about all the women I deal with – if they wanted to go to America or Australia they would not go down to Southampton and catch the ship any more. They would go to Heathrow and catch the Boeing, because it is there. They know it is there and they know it is safe. That is what I mean about consumerism. You say we should not be driven by consumerism, but we are in medicine. Once something is there and it has been shown to be safe and effective, people will want it. They do want it. I was reading a story coming in on the train today about fetal cell transplants in the USA for people with Parkinson's disease. They are hardly safe, but they are there. If people have something and they know it is there, they will want it. Consumerism is an active thing in the world today. The population I work with are out there on the Web. I see them in the clinic antenatally, not just those with problems but in the antenatal classes as well – and it is the same in California and Florida and everywhere else. Women come in and say, 'I want my epidural', sometimes before the contractions start. Surveys of obstetricians in this country, and recently in North America, have shown a large number of obstetricians and/or their partners, asked if they were having a baby this year or next year, how would they like to have the baby, electing to have a caesarean section with one of these low-dose blocks. Large numbers of obstetricians are selecting that. People know about these things out there.

I am not selling it. The less I have to get up in the middle of the night to do these things, the better, but it is a fact that consumerism is out there and it is very active – but quantitatively different in different parts of the country, in different communities.

Hillan: I want to make two points. There is evidence to suggest that not all women would want to go straight for an epidural from the outset of labour. Dr Whorwell reflected this when talking in a different context. Quite often people will want an incremental approach and know that it is available if they get to the point where they feel that they need it.

The other issue that we have to take note of is that many women in the UK do not give birth in centres that have access to such facilities. The issue of small maternity units is a bit of a political 'hot potato' right now, but in Scotland there are many small maternity units where these facilities will never be available, where epidural services are not available at all. We should not lose sight of that either.

MacLean: One of the differences that Dr Grace has identified is that in some facilities the availability of a midwife to give one-to-one service can be almost guaranteed. Rather sadly, the challenge in London increasingly is that you cannot have a midwife per patient. There is a chronic shortage, and the midwives that you are working with today may not be people who have worked in the unit with you before. This causes anxieties not only for the medical staff working there but also for the patients. Many patients come in in labour with perceptions that quickly disappear because they do not have the support. I don't know what the Royal College of Midwives can do to reverse this, but it is going to be one of the critical things that influences obstetric care over the next decade.

Hillan: I am on the Council of the Royal College of Midwives and this issue is hotly debated. They despair at the lack of influence that they appear to have over this issue. However, I would also say that unless you have appropriate clear structures for midwives it is unlikely that we will be able to recruit and retain people in the profession.

SECTION 9

RECOMMENDATIONS

Chapter 32

Recommendations arising from the 41st Study Group: Pain in Obstetrics and Gynaecology

Recommendations fall into three categories:

1. Recommendations for **clinical practice** (principally aimed at Fellows and Members of the Royal College of Obstetricians and Gynaecologists) based upon research evidence (where available) and the consensus view of the Group. The clinical practice recommendations have been graded from 'A' to 'C' according to the strength of evidence on which each is based (Table 32.1). The scheme for the grading of recommendations is based on the system adopted by both the NHS Executive and the Scottish Intercollegiate Guidelines Network.

2. Recommendations for **future research** in those clinical areas where the Group identified a need for further evidence on which to base practice.

3. Recommendations relating to **health education** and **health policy**.

Recommendations for clinical practice

1. There should be support for specialist obstetrics and gynaecology pain clinics and for a transdisciplinary approach with a true diversity of specialists involved (Grade C).

Table 32.1. Grading of recommendations

Grade	Recommendation
A	Requires at least one randomised controlled trial as part of the body of literature of overall good quality and consistency addressing the specific recommendation.
B	Requires availability of well-conducted clinical studies but no randomised clinical trials on the topic of recommendation.
C	Requires evidence from expert committee reports or opinions and/or clinical experience of respected authorities. Indicates absence of directly applicable studies of good quality.

2.   The setting in which consultations for pelvic pain take place need adequately to reflect the referral pattern: patients with long-standing or disabling symptoms require extended consultation time and access to other advice and treatment resources, as in a multidisciplinary model (Grade B).

3.   Clinicians need to be aware of the importance of the initial medical consultation with women with chronic pelvic pain as a factor influencing the outcome from investigation and treatment. While consulting styles reflect the individual personality of the doctor, clinicians need to be aware of their own underlying attitudes and how these might enter into the dynamics of the consultation (Grade B).

4.   Women presenting with pelvic pain in whom no clear diagnosis is present, or where diagnoses overlap, need to be given clear explanations which do not undermine the legitimacy of their experience of pain or convey a message of dismissal (Grade B).

5.   Treatments need to be individualised and regularly reviewed on the basis of each patient's needs and aspirations. This takes place in some centres, which need to be identified to gynaecologists and to those in primary care. As well as offering the best available treatment for patients whose symptoms are proving difficult to manage, these would develop greater expertise in treatment and provide advanced training for the range of healthcare professionals involved in endometriosis care (Grade C).

6.   Patients with severe endometriosis should be referred to specialist treatment centres with experience in advanced laparoscopic surgery (Grade B).

7.   Laparoscopic treatment of stage I–III endometriosis is a safe procedure and has been shown in a double blind randomised controlled trial to be effective in a large proportion of patients. It requires the complete removal of disease not only from the peritoneum but also from the utero-sacral ligaments (Grade B).

8.   There appears to be no evidence at present that denervation procedures confer any additional benefit to the excellent results of laparoscopic ablation of ectopic endometriotic implants and deeply infiltrating disease (Grade A).

9.   Optimum selection of drug therapy can make a difference to treatment outcome despite the complexity of pain management and the need to take account of various other factors (Grade C).

10.   Collaborative working will lead to improved palliative care for cancer patients (Grade C).

11.   The anaesthetist should ensure individual preoperative assessment of postoperative analgesic requirements (Grade C).

12.   Anaesthetists (as well as other clinicians) should increase the use of simple analgesics and multimodal analgesia (Grade A).

13.   There should be increased involvement of acute pain teams in managing post-operative pain (Grade C).

14.   Education in back care and instruction in stability exercises by a physiotherapist should be available to all pregnant women (Grade B).

15. Women presenting with peripartum spinopelvic pain should be referred to a specialist physiotherapist for individual examination, assessment and clinical practice treatment (Grade B).

16. Consider imaging to investigate abdominal pain during pregnancy and surgical intervention as soon as appropriate (Grade C).

17. Continuous caregiver support from a single individual should be available to women in labour (Grade A).

18. Midwives must involve women in decisions about analgesia in labour and recognise the value of promoting personal control (Grade C).

Recommendations for future research

1. It is known that physiology involves co-coordinative interactions between various internal organs, muscles and skin. However, less is understood about how pathophysiology in one structure influences those interactions and influences both the nervous system's control of bodily functions and its mechanism of pain. Recent studies show that these influences may be profound, evidencing themselves in ways that impair proper diagnosis and treatment. Therefore, dialogue between neuroscientists and researchers who study the physiology and pathophysiology of different organs is recommended. This will improve our understanding of viscero-visceral and viscero-somatic interactions in health and illness, and their influence of the nervous system.

2. There should be support for research on the role of sociocultural meanings, processes and constructs involving chronic pain in obstetrics and gynaecology, with initial emphasis on sound methodology.

3. Chronic pelvic pain (CPP) is common in the general population but the reasons why some women and not others seek health care need to be determined.

4. Further studies are required on the relationship between consulting style and patient outcomes, perhaps using observational techniques such as video recording of consultations. Research is needed to clarify the importance of elements in the patient's experience such as continuity of care and the contribution of different members of a multidisciplinary team.

5. Consensus diagnostic criteria for common painful gynaecological disorders should be established.

6. Research aimed at standardising examination techniques for painful disorders, e.g. using pressure transducers to standardise palpation of the abdominal muscles, levators, should be encouraged.

7. Prospective research is needed into the endocrine mechanisms of pelvic congestion as a functional disorder of the menstrual cycle.

8. The development of mechanism-based classification of vulval pain is required.

9. Tools for reliable and valid measures of treatment outcome in vulval and pelvic pain, including psychometric measures and measures of quantitative sensory threshold (QST) should be developed.

10. Additional studies on the prevalence of various vulval pain disorders are required. Only one study is known to be under way that is population-based.

11. Establish multicentre, multidisciplinary groups to run randomised clinical trials in the treatment of vulval pain.

12. Collect evidence about the efficiency of existing and new treatment modalities to prevent peritoneal formation.

13. Epidemiological studies are needed on the incidence and morbidity of chronic gynaecological diseases and cost/benefit analysis.

14. The precise healthcare, and the indirect costs (e.g. effect on quality of life, ability to work) of CPP need to be estimated.

15. Collaborative multidisciplinary research projects into the causes and management of peri-partum spino-pelvic pain should be undertaken with the obstetric team.

16. Maternity services should be encouraged to research the 'working with pain' framework suggested by Leap.[1]

17. Further research is required into the most appropriate drug for labour use and most appropriate method of administration.

18. More collaborative research (and audit) into pain and analgesia is needed among all members of the perinatal management team.

Recommendations for health education and policy

1. There should be greater awareness of the necessity to provide pain relief in acute and chronic situations in obstetrics and gynaecology.

2. The role of establishing whether pain is 'real' or not should be rejected, as chronic pain may be a diagnosis as well as a symptom.

3. Health professionals should discard dualistic notions of pain being either physical or psychological, and adopt a biopsychosocial model of pain instead. The biopsychosocial model of pain is especially important with regard to chronic pain in women, where there is been a greater tendency to label unexplained pains as manifestations of psychiatric illness.

4. Referral patterns from primary to secondary care must be understood better to plan resource allocation and develop evidence-based protocols.

5. Tertiary referral clinics in which gynaecologists and psychologists work together are necessary to treat effectively some of the more complex cases of pelvic pain in women. These clinics should be supported by the NHS regionally.

6. Gynaecology departments with interests in pain management need to employ a psychologist as part of the treatment team. Ideally, the psychologist should be also a member of the clinical psychology department. The International Association for the Study of Pain recommends that medically and psychologically trained professionals should treat chronic pain.

7. There is an apparent disparity between the existence of physiological and symptom 'cross talk' between organs (viscero-visceral or viscero-somatic interactions). To understand this disparity we need to convene multi-specialist discussion groups, i.e. obstetricians-gynaecologists, urologists, gastro-enterologists, cardiologists, neurologists, rheumatologists, anaesthetists, pain nurses, physiotherapists, psychologists, psychotherapists and psychiatrists.

8. The variety, the intensity and the destructive effects of chronic pelvic pain need to be recognised. Treatment strategies that directly address this problem are urgently needed. These should be disseminated to clinicians and patients alike. Patients must participate in the control of symptoms and not be regarded as unfeeling recipients of prescription.

9. All prescribers, especially for pain relief, should understand the pharmacological basis of the drugs they prescribe.

10. The final selection of drugs should take account of the fact that drug therapy is only one option in pain management.

11. The continuing pain that endometriosis can produce is a strong indication of the need for radical review of the current understanding and treatment of this disease. In order to develop treatments that are not exclusively based on the clinical model of medicine, psychologists need to be involved (at every level) in the design and implementation of research projects as well as the design and delivery of patient care and clinical training.

12. Effective teamwork should be taught as a keystone for pain control in palliative care.

13. There is a need to increase awareness of the breadth of conditions during pregnancy that require surgery.

14. Maternity services should make sure that women have access to written and verbal information on pain relief and should support women in their choices of pain relief.

15. Maternity services should respect women's wishes to remain in control in labour and to have some control over their pain relief.

16. Improve public information and data on pain and analgesia with professional, collaborative websites.

17. NHS Trusts should review and improve the integration of obstetric anaesthesia and support services into women's health.

Training

18. Gynaecologists should be taught psychological pain management theory and skills as part of their training and should take more time for in-depth assessment.

19. There should be dissemination of existing information from psychology sources to both clinicians and patients.

20. The RCOG and the British Psychological Society should set up a joint education committee to develop the content of a training programme in psychogynaecology, for trainees and staff, in obstetrics, gynaecology and psychology.

21. Study guides need to emphasise the importance of attention to the patient's needs for treatment objectives and explanation, rather than an exclusive pursuit of a pathological diagnosis. Consulting styles that address these needs can be taught in role-play and evaluated in OSCE formats, as can the communication skills required to convey diagnostic uncertainty or negative findings without undermining the patient's confidence.

22. The RCOG should create a subspecialty of benign gynaecological surgery and funding should be available to ensure an adequate number of such centres throughout the UK.

23. Educational programmes in vulval disorders, vulval pain and chronic pelvic pain should be promoted.

24. Gynaecologists need to be educated to take a full history including a full gastroenterological history.

25. There should be an awareness of the ethical issues in the management of pain.

Reference

1.   Leap N. Pain in labour: towards a midwifery perspective. *MIDIRS Midwifery Digest* 2000; March:49–53.

Index